Hot Topics in Small Animal Medicine

Editor

LISA L. POWELL

VETERINARY CLINICS OF NORTH AMERICA: SMALL ANIMAL PRACTICE

www.vetsmall.theclinics.com

May 2022 • Volume 52 • Number 3

ELSEVIER

1600 John F. Kennedy Boulevard • Suite 1800 • Philadelphia, Pennsylvania, 19103-2899
http://www.vetsmall.theclinics.com

**VETERINARY CLINICS OF NORTH AMERICA: SMALL ANIMAL PRACTICE Volume 52, Number 3
May 2022 ISSN 0195-5616, ISBN-13: 978-0-323-96185-1**

Editor: Stacy Eastman
Developmental Editor: Axell Ivan Jade Purificacion

Veterinary Clinics of North America: Small Animal Practice (ISSN 0195-5616) is published bimonthly by Elsevier Inc., 360 Park Avenue South, New York, NY 10010-1710. Months of issue are January, March, May, July, September, and November. Business and Editorial Offices: 1600 John F. Kennedy Blvd., Ste. 1800, Philadelphia, PA 19103-2899. Customer Service Office: 3251 Riverport Lane, Maryland Heights, MO 63043. Periodicals postage paid at New York, NY and additional mailing offices. Subscription prices are $369.00 per year (domestic individuals), $980.00 per year (domestic institutions), $100.00 per year (domestic students/residents), $465.00 per year (Canadian individuals), $1029.00 per year (Canadian institutions), $503.00 per year (international individuals), $1029.00 per year (international institutions), $100.00 per year (Canadian students/residents), and $220.00 per year (international students/residents). To receive student/resident rate, orders must be accompanied by name of affiliated institution, date of term, and the *signature* of program/residency coordinator on institution letterhead. Orders will be billed at individual rate until proof of status is received. Foreign air speed delivery is included in all *Clinics* subscription prices. All prices are subject to change without notice. **POSTMASTER:** Send address changes to *Veterinary Clinics of North America: Small Animal Practice*, Elsevier Health Sciences Division, Subscription Customer Service, 3251 Riverport Lane, Maryland Heights, MO 63043. Customer Service (orders, claims, online, change of address): Elsevier Periodicals Customer Service, Elsevier Health Sciences Division Subscription **Customer Service 3251 Riverport Lane Maryland Heights, MO 63043. Tel: 1-800-654-2452 (U.S. and Canada); 314-447-8871 (outside U.S. and Canada). Fax: 314-447-8029. E-mail: journalscustomerservice-usa@elsevier.com (for print support); journalsonlinesupport-usa@elsevier.com (for online support).**

Reprints. For copies of 100 or more of articles in this publication, please contact the Commercial Reprints Department, Elsevier Inc., 360 Park Avenue South, New York, NY 10010-1710. Tel.: 212-633-3874; Fax: 212-633-3820; E-mail: reprints@elsevier.com.

Veterinary Clinics of North America: Small Animal Practice is also published in Japanese by Inter Zoo Publishing Co., Ltd., Aoyama Crystal-Bldg 5F, 3-5-12 Kitaaoyama, Minato-ku, Tokyo 107-0061, Japan.

Veterinary Clinics of North America: Small Animal Practice is covered in *Current Contents/Agriculture, Biology and Environmental Sciences, Science Citation Index, ASCA, MEDLINE/PubMed (Index Medicus), Excerpta Medica,* and *BIOSIS.*

Contributors

EDITOR

LISA L. POWELL, DVM
Diplomate, American College of Veterinary Emergency and Critical Care; Associate Emergency and Critical Care Clinician, BluePearl Veterinary Partners, Senior Consultant, Critical Consults, LLC, Eden Prairie, Minnesota, USA

AUTHORS

JOSEPH W. BARTGES, DVM, PHD
Professor of Internal Medicine, Interventional Radiology, and Nutrition, Department of Small Animal Medicine and Surgery, College of Veterinary Medicine, University of Georgia, Athens, Georgia, USA

CELESTE CLEMENTS, DVM
Diplomate, American College of Internal Medicine - Small Animal Internal Medicine; IDEXX Laboratories, Inc, Westbrook, Maine, USA

LEAH A. COHN, DVM, PhD
Diplomate, American College of Internal Medicine - Small Animal Internal Medicine; Professor at University of Missouri College of Veterinary Medicine, Columbia, Missouri, USA

GILLES DUPRÉ DVM, Dr Med Vet, Dr Hc
Professor, Diplomate, European College of Veterinary Surgery; Department for Small Animal and Equine, Vetmeduni Vienna, Veterinary Medicine University, Vienna, Austria

DAVID L. DYCUS, DVM, MS, CCRP
Diplomate, American College of Veterinary Surgeons – Small Animal; Department of Orthopedic Surgery, Nexus Veterinary Bone & Joint Center, Baltimore, Maryland, USA

SONYA G. GORDON, DVM, DVSc
Diplomate, American College of Veterinary Internal Medicine (Cardiology); Professor Cardiology, Eugene Ch'en Chair in Cardiology, Department of Small Animal Clinical Science, College of Veterinary Medicine and Biomedical Sciences, Texas A&M University, College Station, Texas, USA

RAGNVI HAGMAN, DVM, PhD
Associate Professor in Small Animal Surgery, Department of Clinical Sciences, Swedish University of Agricultural Sciences, Uppsala, Sweden

KATE HOPPER, BVSC, PhD
Diplomate, American College of Veterinary Emergency; Critical Care Professor of Small Animal Emergency and Critical Care, Department of Veterinary Surgical and Radiologic Sciences, University of California, Davis, Davis, California, USA

AMY J. KAPLAN-ZATTLER, DVM, CVMA, MRCVS
Diplomate, American College of Veterinary Emergency and Critical Care; VETgirl, Tampa, Florida, USA

DOROTHEE KRAINER, Dr Med Vet, MBA(hons)
Diplomate, European College of Veterinary Surgery; Head of Small Animal Surgery; AniCura Tierklinik Hollabrunn, Researcher Department for Small Animal and Equine, Vetmeduni Vienna, Veterinary Medicine University, Vienna, Austria

JUSTINE A. LEE, DVM, DABT
Diplomate, American College of Veterinary Emergency and Critical Care; VETgirl, Tampa, Florida, USA

DAVID LEVINE, PT, PhD, DPT, CCRP, FAPTA
Department of Physical Therapy, University of Tennessee at Chattanooga, Chattanooga, Tennessee, USA

REBEKAH MACK, DVM
Diplomate, American College of Internal Medicine - Small Animal Internal Medicine; IDEXX Laboratories, Inc, Westbrook, Maine, USA

DENIS J. MARCELLIN-LITTLE, DEDV
Diplomate, American College of Veterinary Surgeons; Diplomate, American College of Veterinary Sports Medicine and Rehabilitation; Department of Clinical Sciences, College of Veterinary Medicine, University of California, Davis, Davis, California, USA

ELISA MAZZAFERRO, DVM, MS, PhD
Cornell University Veterinary Specialists, Stamford, Connecticut, USA

HELEN MICHAEL, DVM, PhD
Diplomate, American College Clinical Pathology; IDEXX Laboratories, Inc, Westbrook, Maine, USA

SHELLY J. OLIN, DVM
Associate Professor of Internal Medicine, Department of Small Animal Clinical Sciences, College of Veterinary Medicine, University of Tennessee, Knoxville, Tennessee, USA

MARIANA A. PARDO, BVSc, MV
Diplomate, American College of Veterinary Emergency and Critical Care; White Plains Hospital, Veterinary Emergency Group, White Plains, New York, USA

LISA L. POWELL, DVM
Diplomate, American College of Veterinary Emergency and Critical Care; Associate Emergency and Critical Care Clinician, BluePearl Veterinary Partners, Senior Consultant, Critical Consults, LLC, Eden Prairie, Minnesota, USA

BARBARA ESTEVE RATSCH, DVM, PhD, CCRP
Evidensia Sørlandet Animal Hospital, Hamresanden, Norway

LINDA ROSS, DVM, MS
Diplomate, American College of Veterinary Internal Medicine (SAIM); Associate Professor Emerita, Department of Clinical Sciences, Cummings School of Veterinary Medicine, Tufts University, North Grafton, Massachusetts, USA

ASHLEY B. SAUNDERS, DVM
Diplomate, American College of Veterinary Internal Medicine (Cardiology); Professor Cardiology, Department of Small Animal Clinical Science, College of Veterinary Medicine and Biomedical Sciences, Texas A&M University, College Station, Texas, USA

DONALD SZLOSEK, MPH
IDEXX Laboratories, Inc, Westbrook, Maine, USA

LUIS H. TELLO, MV, MS, DVM
Tigard Animal Hospital, National Veterinary Associates, Tigard, Oregon, USA

KATRINA R. VIVIANO, DVM, PhD
Diplomate, American College of Veterinary Internal Medicine; Diplomate, American College of Veterinary Clinical Pharmacology; Department of Medical Sciences, University of Wisconsin-Madison, School of Veterinary Medicine, Madison, Wisconsin, USA

SONYA R. WESSELOWSKI, DVM, MS
Diplomate, American College of Veterinary Internal Medicine (Cardiology); Assistant Professor Cardiology, Department of Small Animal Clinical Science, College of Veterinary Medicine and Biomedical Sciences, Texas A&M University, College Station, Texas, USA

Contents

> Urinary tract infection (UTI) is commonly encountered in small animal general practice. Within the past 5 years, there have been changes to terminology, such as the renaming of asymptomatic bacteriuria to subclinical bacteriuria, as well as paradigm shifts in the management of UTI. In general, there is an emphasis for responsible antimicrobial stewardship and selecting treatment based on urine culture and sensitivity and treating symptomatic bacterial UTI with a shorter duration of antimicrobials. In addition, for most cases, treatment of subclinical bacteriuria is not indicated.

> Symmetric dimethylarginine (SDMA) is a valuable surrogate marker for decreased glomerular filtration rate (GFR) and is incorporated into the International Renal Interest Society (IRIS) guidelines for diagnosing, staging, and treating chronic kidney disease (CKD). SDMA increases above the reference interval with smaller reductions in GFR rate than does creatinine and persistent mild increases in SDMA can be used to diagnose early-stage CKD. Evaluation of both SDMA and creatinine is recommended for diagnosis and monitoring of animals with CKD.

 Video content accompanies this article at http://www.vetsmall. theclinics.com.

> Pyometra is a common disease in intact bitches and queens and occurs, although less frequently, in most other female pets. The illness is generally diagnosed within 4 months after estrus, in middle-aged to older bitches and queens. Hormonal and bacterial factors are important for the disease development, and progesterone plays a key role. The diagnosis is based on case history, clinical signs, and findings on physical examination, laboratory analyses and diagnostic imaging. Pyometra is potentially life-threatening and considered a medical emergency. Surgical

lead to an abnormal development or to progressive degeneration of the femoral head and dorsal acetabular rim. Osteoarthritis and its clinical impact progress over time. Changes to the femoral head and neck and the acetabulum and the impact on joint motion and pain vary widely among dogs. The rehabilitation of dogs with hip dysplasia includes rehabilitation therapy in dogs managed conservatively and the rehabilitation of dogs managed with surgery.

Dorothee Krainer and Gilles Dupré

 Video content accompanies this article at http://www.vetsmall. theclinics.com.

Dogs presenting with brachycephalic obstructive airway syndrome suffer from multilevel obstruction of the airway as well as secondary structural collapse. Stenotic nares, aberrant turbinates, nasopharyngeal collapse, soft palate hyperplasia, macroglossia, tonsillar hypertrophy, laryngeal collapse, and left bronchial collapse are described as the most common associated anomalies. Rhinoplasty and palatoplasty as well as newer surgical techniques and prudent preoperative and postoperative care strategies have resulted in significant improvement even in middle-aged dogs.

Elisa Mazzaferro and Lisa L. Powell

Water is essential for life. Without adequate fluid intake, normal body functioning becomes impaired and ultimately can lead to death. A fluid therapy plan should be considered for any small animal patient that has either inadequate fluid intake, excessive fluid loss, or both. A simplified approach to fluid therapy begins with an understanding of the composition of fluid and its distribution within the body. Next, consideration of electrolyte loss, acid-base disturbances, perfusion impairment, and loss of protein also becomes important when replenishing deficits by using various fluids that are commercially available to small animal practitioners.

Katrina R. Viviano

The treatment of immune-mediated diseases in dogs and cats continues to evolve as new therapies are adapted from human medicine. Glucocorticoids remain the first-line treatment followed by second-line therapies including cyclosporine, azathioprine (dogs), chlorambucil, or mycophenolate. Second-line therapies are introduced due to the patient's lack of response or intolerable effects to glucocorticoids or may be introduced early in the disease treatment due to the patient's severe life-threatening clinical presentation. The goals of immunosuppressive treatment are to achieve disease remission while minimizing drug side effects. Ultimately, gradual drug tapering to the lowest dose to maintain disease remission or successful drug withdrawal.

Degenerative valve disease (DVD) is the leading cause of heart disease and heart failure in the dog. The first consensus statement published in 2009 by the American College of Veterinary Internal Medicine was updated in 2019 and provides guidelines for the diagnosis and treatment of DVD. These updated guidelines recommend treatment with pimobendan in stage B2 DVD characterized by sufficient left heart enlargement. Asymptomatic dogs with DVD that do not meet or exceed the definition of stage B2 are considered stage B1. No treatment is recommended in stage B1 DVD. This article discusses the relevant scientific background and practical application of the updated DVD guidelines related to stage B. In addition, management of common sequelae of DVD that can result in clinical signs unrelated to congestive heart failure will be reviewed. The impact of new evidence on current recommendations and a glimpse into novel diagnostic approaches and possible future therapies will also be addressed.

VETERINARY CLINICS OF NORTH AMERICA: SMALL ANIMAL PRACTICE

SERIES OF RELATED INTEREST

Veterinary Clinics: Exotic Animal Practice
https://www.vetexotic.theclinics.com/

THE CLINICS ARE NOW AVAILABLE ONLINE!
Access your subscription at:
www.theclinics.com

Erratum

In the article, "Focused Ultrasound Examination of Canine and Feline Emergency Urinary Tract Disorders," by Laura Cole, Karen Humm, and Helen Dirrig, published in the November 2021 issue (Volume 51, number 6, pages 1233-1248), the running head should be "Focused Ultrasound Examination of Canine and Feline Emergency Urinary Tract Disorders."

Vet Clin Small Anim 52 (2022) xiii
https://doi.org/10.1016/j.cvsm.2022.03.003
0195-5616/22/© 2022 Elsevier Inc. All rights reserved.

Preface

Hot Topics in Small Animal Veterinary Medicine: 2010–2018

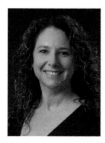

Lisa L. Powell, DVM
Editor

This issue of *Veterinary Clinics of North America: Small Animal Practice* contains the most read articles from 2010 to 2018. It is notable that 3 of the 12 articles are on the topic of fluid therapy, illustrating the importance of this treatment modality in our small animal patients. All topics have been updated, including a discussion about novel high-flow oxygen therapy, new therapies for the treatment of asymptomatic canine degenerative valve disease, and updated recommendations for the treatment of urinary infections.

As we continue to navigate the ever-changing veterinary world, especially as impacted by the COVID-19 pandemic, it is refreshing to have new and updated content to help us continue to provide exceptional care to emergent and ill dogs and cats. Increasing and overwhelming veterinary caseloads during the pandemic have caused daily emergency clinic pauses and closures, and appointments, in both general practice and specialty medicine, are booked out for many weeks. At this time in veterinary medicine, I feel it is important to remember why we chose to be involved in this great profession and give ourselves grace as we continue to do our best to provide high-quality medical and surgical care to our small animal patients.

I want to thank Elsevier for inviting me to be guest editor of this issue and also, thanks to the amazing authors that took the time to share their knowledge and update the information contained in their articles.

Lisa L. Powell, DVM
BluePearl Veterinary Partners, Critical Consults, LLC
7717 Flying Cloud Drive, Eden Prairie, MN 55344, USA

E-mail address:
ervet1@gmail.com

https://doi.org/10.1016/j.cvsm.2022.02.001
0195-5616/22/© 2022 Published by Elsevier Inc.

vetsmall.theclinics.com

Urinary Tract Infections Treatment/Comparative Therapeutics

Shelly J. Olin, DVM[a],*, Joseph W. Bartges, DVM, PhD[b]

KEYWORDS

- Canine • Feline • Pyelonephritis • Prostatitis • Urinary tract infection

KEY POINTS

- Preferred terminology for urinary bacterial infection is sporadic or recurrent bacterial cystitis. Recurrent infections are further defined as relapsing, refractory/persistent, reinfection, or superinfection.
- Asymptomatic bacteriuria was renamed subclinical bacteriuria, and treatment is not recommended.
- Antimicrobials are the cornerstone of treatment of symptomatic bacterial urinary tract infection (UTI) and, ideally, are selected based on culture and sensitivity; shorter duration of antimicrobial treatment is recommended.
- Analgesics, such as a nonsteroidal anti-inflammatory drug, should be used pending culture results to alleviate clinical signs.
- Urine culture is no longer recommended following treatment for sporadic UTI if clinical signs resolve.
- There is limited literature to support preventative therapies; identification and resolution of underlying causes are essential.

INTRODUCTION

Urinary tract infection (UTI) occurs when there is a compromise of host defense mechanisms and a virulent microbe adheres, multiplies, and persists in a portion of the urinary tract. Host defenses include normal micturition, anatomic structures, the mucosal barrier, properties of urine, and systemic immunocompetence. Most commonly UTI are caused by bacteria, but fungi and viruses also may infect the urinary tract. UTI may involve more than one anatomic location, and the infection should be categorized as upper urinary tract (kidneys and ureters) versus lower urinary tract (bladder, urethra,

[a] Department of Small Animal Clinical Sciences, College of Veterinary Medicine, University of Tennessee, 2407 River Drive, Knoxville, TN 37996, USA; [b] Department of Small Animal Medicine and Surgery, College of Veterinary Medicine, University of Georgia, 501 DW Brooks Drive, Athens, GA 30602, USA
* Corresponding author.
E-mail address: solin@utk.edu

Vet Clin Small Anim 52 (2022) 581–608
https://doi.org/10.1016/j.cvsm.2022.01.002
0195-5616/22/© 2022 Elsevier Inc. All rights reserved.

and vagina or prostate). Most bacterial UTI occur as a consequence of ascending migration of pathogens through the genital tract and urethra to the bladder, ureters, and one or both kidneys. Rectal, perineal, and genital bacteria serve as the principal reservoirs for infection.[1,2]

Bacterial Isolates

A single bacterial pathogen is isolated from approximately 75% infections; 20% of UTI are caused by 2 coinfecting species, and approximately 5% are caused by 3 species.[3–5]

The bacteria that most commonly cause UTI are similar in dogs and cats (**Fig. 1**).[3,6–8] *Escherichia coli* is most common, followed by gram-positive cocci, and then various others, including *Proteus, Klebsiella, Pasteurella, Pseudomonas, Corynebacterium,* and several other rarely reported genera.[3,6] *Enterococcus* spp are the fourth to fifth most common bacterial isolate in dogs and commonly associated with anatomic abnormalities, urolithiasis, or neoplasia.[9] Only 50% of dogs will display clinical signs.[9] *Mycoplasma* spp are isolated from urine of dogs with clinical signs of lower urinary tract in less than 5% of samples; whether *Mycoplasma* spp are associated with urinary tract disease in cats is controversial.[3,10–12]

Cats may be infected with a unique strain of *Staphylococcus, Staphylococcus felis,* and commercial phenotypic identification systems may not differentiate between *S felis* and other coagulase-negative *Staphylococcus* spp.[7,8] One study found that *S felis* was the third most common isolate based on 16S rDNA sequencing (n = 25/106, 19.8% of bacterial isolates cultured), suggesting *S felis* is the most common Staphylococcal species causing UTI in cats.[7]

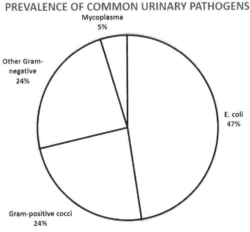

PREVALENCE OF COMMON URINARY PATHOGENS

Fig. 1. Prevalence of common urinary pathogens: 33% to 50% *E coli*, 25% to 33% gram-positive cocci (*Staphylococcus* sp, *Streptococcus* sp, *Enterococcus* sp), 25% to 33% other gram-negative (*Proteus* sp, *Klebsiella* sp, *Pasteurella* sp, *Pseudomonas* sp, *Corynebacterium* sp), less than 5% *Mycoplasma* sp. (*Data from* Ling GV, Norris CR, Franti CE, et al. Interrelations of organism prevalence, specimen collection method, and host age, sex, and breed among 8354 canine urinary tract infections (1969–1995). J Vet Intern Med 2001;15:341-7; and Barsanti J. Genitourinary infections. In: Greene CE, editor. Infectious diseases of the dog and cat. 4th edition. St Louis (MO): Elsevier Saunders; 2012. p. 1013-31.)

Pyelonephritis

Pyelonephritis, or infection of the renal pelvis and parenchyma, is most commonly due to ascending infections from the lower urinary tract in dogs and cats, but hematogenous spread is possible (**Fig. 2**).[13] E coli is the most commonly isolated bacteria.[13] In addition to the components of immunity that protect urinary tract in general, the kidneys are protected from bacterial infection by vesicoureteral flap valves, relatively long ureters that usually allow only one-way flow of urine via peristalsis, and generally hypoxic environment of the renal medulla.

Prostatitis

Inherent prostatic defense mechanisms against infection include local immune factors, such as immunoglobulin A and antibacterial proteins, retrograde flow of prostatic fluid and urine, and urethral peristalsis, and the urethral high pressure zone.[14,15] Dogs with bacterial prostatitis often have alteration of normal defenses, such as underlying benign prostatic hyperplasia, prostatic cysts, or neoplasia.[16] Most commonly prostatitis develops from ascending bacterial infection and may result in prostatic abscessation in addition to prostatic parenchymal infection (**Fig. 3**). Hematogenous spread and prostatitis secondary to cystitis are also possible. Bacterial pathogens are similar to those causing bacterial cystitis with E coli being the most common (see **Fig. 1**). Brucella canis should also be considered, especially for intact male dogs, as a cause for both acute and chronic prostatitis.[16]

Catheter-Associated Urinary Tract Infection

Normal host defense mechanisms are effective in preventing bacterial UTI; however, they are not impenetrable. Normal host defenses may be overwhelmed if large quantities of a virulent uropathogen are introduced into the urinary tract during diagnostic and therapeutic procedures. Catheter-associated bacterial UTI is a common complication of indwelling urinary catheters, especially if an open-ended system is used. In a clinical study, infection developed in 30% to 52% of dogs and cats with indwelling urinary catheters; risk of infection increased with duration of catheterization.[17,18] The risk of infection is further compounded if the patient has preexisting urinary tract disease. Use of indwelling urinary catheters during diuresis or corticosteroid administration is particularly dangerous.

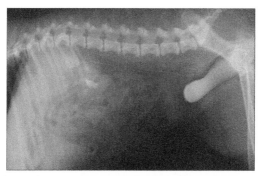

Fig. 2. Lateral abdominal excretory urography showing a pelvically displaced urinary bladder and renal pelvic dilation (pyelonephritis) owing to ascending E coli urinary tract in a 4-year-old spayed female mixed breed dog.

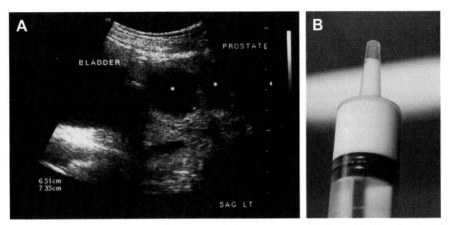

Fig. 3. (*A*) Sagittal ultrasonographic image of the prostate and urinary bladder showing 2 cystic lesions that were abscesses (asterisk) and (*B*) purulent prostatic wash fluid owing to *E coli* in a 6-year-old intact male Rhodesian ridgeback.

Fungal Urinary Tract Infection

Fungal UTI is uncommon. As with bacterial UTI, fungal UTI occurs because of temporary or permanent breaches in local or systemic immunity of the lower urinary tract. Funguria may be due to primary infections of the lower urinary tract or secondary to shedding of fungal elements into the urine in animals with systemic infections. Primary fungal UTI is most commonly due to *Candida* spp, a commensal inhabitant of the genital mucosa, upper respiratory tract, and gastrointestinal tract.[19,20] *Candida albicans* is the most commonly identified species, followed by *Candida glabrata* and *Candida tropicalis*; other ubiquitous fungi may also occasionally cause primary fungal UTI, including *Aspergillus* spp, *Blastomycosis* spp (**Fig. 4**), and *Cryptococcus* spp.[21] Risk factors for *Candida* UTI include antimicrobial administration within the past month and immunosuppression.[22]

Viral Urinary Tract Infection

Viral-induced disease in humans is increasingly recognized, especially of the upper urinary tract. However, it can be difficult to determine cause-and-effect relationships

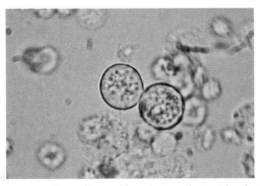

Fig. 4. *Blastomyces* spp organisms observed by microscopic examination of urine sediment from a 2-year-old castrated male Doberman pinscher (Unstained, original magnification ×100).

because viral-induced disease may occur in the absence of detectable replicating virus. Several viruses have been implicated in canine and feline disease (**Box 1**).[23]

PATIENT EVALUATION OVERVIEW
Clinical Signs

Lower urinary tract infection: bacterial, fungal, viral
Lower bacterial colonization may be symptomatic (UTI) or asymptomatic/subclinical, and clinical signs are indistinguishable from other causes of lower urinary tract disease. Nonspecific clinical signs of lower urinary tract disease include, but are not limited to, pollakiuria, dysuria, stranguria, hematuria, and inappropriate urination.[24]

Prostatitis. Acute prostatitis is usually associated with systemic illness, including fever, anorexia, vomiting, and lethargy. Dogs with acute disease may also have caudal abdominal pain, stiff gait, and preputial discharge and be unwilling to breed.[14–16] In contrast, dogs with chronic prostatitis are usually not systemically ill or febrile.[15]

Commonly, recurrent UTI or preputial bloody discharge is the only clinical sign of chronic prostatitis.[16] Other presentations include stiff gait, discomfort with rising, infertility, or orchiepididymitis, or dogs may be asymptomatic.[15]

Upper urinary tract infection
Pyelonephritis. Pyelonephritis may have an acute or chronic presentation. Acute pyelonephritis is usually associated with signs of severe systemic illness (eg, uremia, fever, painful kidneys, possible nephromegaly, or sepsis). In contrast, chronic pyelonephritis usually has a more insidious presentation: slowly progressive azotemia that may not be associated with uremia, progressive kidney damage, and ultimately, renal failure if untreated. Bacterial pyelonephritis may be associated with hematuria only.

Diagnosis

Bacterial urinary tract infection
In addition to clinical signs, results of a complete urinalysis may provide evidence of a bacterial UTI. Hematuria, pyuria, and bacteriuria are often present unless there is suppression of immune response because of underlying disease or drugs (**Fig. 5**).

Microscopic examination of unstained urine sediment is less sensitive and specific than examining urine sediment stained with a modified Wright stain.[25]

A positive urine culture is the "gold standard" for diagnosing bacterial UTI, and a sample collected by cystocentesis is preferred. Immediate sample submission is recommended.[26] If immediate submission is not possible, then refrigerating the sample is

---

Box 1
Viruses associated with urinary tract disease in dogs and cats

Species	Upper Urinary Tract Disease	Lower Urinary Tract Disease
Canine, feline	Canine adenovirus type I	Feline calicivirus
	Canine herpesvirus	Bovine herpesvirus-4
Feline, foamy (syncytium-forming) virus	Feline coronavirus	Feline foamy (syncytium-forming) virus
	Feline immunodeficiency virus	
	Feline leukemia virus	

Adapted from Kruger JM, Osborne CA, Wise AG, et al. Viruses and urinary tract disease. In: Polzin D, Bartges JW, editors. Nephrology and urology of small animals. Chichester (United Kingdom): Blackwell Publishing Ltd; 2011. p. 725-33.

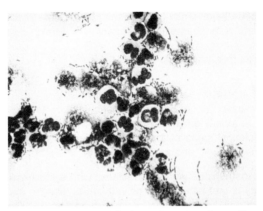

Fig. 5. Microscopic examination of a modified Wright stain urine sediment from a dog with *E coli* bacterial cystitis showing white blood cells and bacteria (Wright's stain, original magnification ×100).

recommended, but it is important to recognize that storage time and temperature can influence quantitative bacterial culture.[26] A quantitative urine culture includes isolation and identification of the organism and determination of the number of bacteria (colony-forming units per unit volume). Quantitation of bacteria enables interpretation as to the significance of bacteria present in a urine sample. Caution should be exercised when interpreting quantitative urine cultures obtained by midstream voiding or manual expression of urine.[24] Furthermore, a positive quantifiable urine culture may be present with subclinical bacteriuria (SB); therefore, culture results must be interpreted in conjunction with the patient's clinical status and results of diagnostic testing.

Several novel and bedside tests have been developed to diagnose UTI. A rapid diagnostic test to confirm UTI is attractive because of improved choice in empirical therapy, and more rapid resolution of the patient's clinical signs; therefore, the practitioner should be cautious. Some of the available tests have similar turnaround times to the gold-standard culture, such as a urine dipstick paddle (Uricult Veterinary System; LifeSign, Skillman, NJ, USA) and compartmented bacteriologic culture and susceptibility plate (Flexicult VET; Atlantic Diagnostics, Miami, FL, USA).[27,28] Others, such as a rapid catalase-based test (Accutest Uriscreen; Jant Pharmaceuticals, Mundelein, IL, USA), require culture to confirm infection and are neither sensitive nor specific.[29] However, a rapid immunoassay test kit (RapidBac Vet; Silver Lake Research Corp, Monrovia, CA, USA) accurately detected UTI, compared with the reference bacterial culture, and could be considered during a routine office visit.[30] Molecular-based diagnostic testing is also becoming available using polymerase chain reaction (PCR) either in-house (SeptiFastH; Roche Diagnostics GmbH, Penzberg, Germany) or as a send out to a laboratory, which increases speed of turnaround of sample analysis. PCR may be combined with routine antimicrobial techniques or with PCR-based detection of antimicrobial resistant genes with an identified bacterial organism.[31,32] Of note, susceptibility testing is still recommended for positive tests to optimize the antimicrobial treatment plan.

Terminology updates
Previously, the terminology used to describe bacterial cystitis was adopted from human medicine, and infections were named as uncomplicated or complicated. A simple uncomplicated UTI was thought to occur sporadically in an otherwise healthy animal with a normal structural and functional urinary tract.[33] In contrast, infection was

complicated if there is (1) involvement of the upper urinary tract and/or prostate, (2) an underlying comorbidity that alters the structure or function of the urinary tract, such as an endocrinopathy or chronic kidney disease (CKD), or (3) recurrent infection.[33,34] However, in the recent International Society for Companion Animal Infectious Disease (ISCAID) consensus statement, the use of this terminology can be confusing because it is unknown if truly "uncomplicated" disease occurs in dogs or if there is an underlying risk factor for most cases.[35]

Sporadic bacterial cystitis. Sporadic bacterial cystitis (previously simple, uncomplicated UTI) describes the occasional *symptomatic* UTI in an otherwise healthy animal (nongravid or neutered male) without any known anatomic or functional abnormalities to the urinary tract or predisposing comorbidities (ie, endocrinopathy or intervertebral disk disease). If the animal has greater than 3 sporadic infections within 12 months, these should be considered recurrent.[35]

Recurrent bacterial cystitis. Recurrent bacterial cystitis is defined as greater than 3 sporadic infections within the preceding 12 months; usually, there is an underlying or predisposing condition.[35] However, the underlying cause can only be found in approximately 25% of animals.[9] Recurrent infections are further categorized as relapsing, refractory/persistent, reinfection, or superinfection (**Table 1**).[33–35] Additional laboratory testing and imaging studies are often required for recurrent infections (**Box 2**).[24]

Feline urinary tract infection. Feline UTI historically were considered to be complicated infections because of the frequent comorbidities and increased incidence in geriatric cats.[24] However, there is no evidence to suggest that sporadic UTI in cats are necessarily more complicated to manage than in dogs. Therefore, management of feline UTI is similar to that of dogs. The practitioner should note that most young cats with lower urinary tract signs will have feline idiopathic cystitis or urolithiasis rather than bacterial cystitis.[35]

Pyelonephritis. Diagnosis of pyelonephritis is usually presumptive based on positive urine culture, concurrent consistent renal diagnostic imaging abnormalities (eg, pyelectasia, distortion of the collection system, increased echogenicity of the renal medulla and pelvis),[36] and improvement in degree of azotemia following antimicrobial therapy. Although a positive culture is helpful for the diagnosis, a negative urine culture does not rule out pyelonephritis, and pyelonephritis can have a subtle presentation.[13] In a recent retrospective study, fever was more common in dogs with histologically subacute pyelonephritis compared with chronic disease. However, the presence or absence of azotemia or leukocytosis did not distinguish the severity or duration of pyelonephritis.[13] Predisposing factors for pyelonephritis include conditions altering the uroepithelium, obstructive uropathies, immunosuppressive therapy, neurogenic disorders of micturition, incontinence, and altered urine composition.[33] Leptospirosis should be considered in endemic regions.[35]

Prostatitis. All intact dogs with a bacteriuria or bacterial cystitis should be evaluated for bacterial prostatitis. Recommended diagnostics include a complete physical examination, including rectal examination, and a minimum database with complete blood count, chemistry panel, urine analysis, and urine culture.[35] Abdominal radiographs and ultrasound are useful to determine the size, shape, location, and architecture of the prostate as well as if any cysts or abscesses are present (see **Fig. 3**A).[16] Prostatic fluid should be evaluated for cytology and bacterial culture and sensitivity

Table 1
Definitions for sporadic and recurrent urinary tract infections

	Definition	Underlying Cause
Sporadic UTI	• Healthy individual, normal urinary tract anatomy and function • <3 per year	• Spontaneous

Comorbidity	• Disease that alters the structure or function of the urinary tract
	 • Relevant comorbidity predisposes to persistent infection, recurrent infection, or treatment failure
		• Endocrinopathies
		  ○ Diabetes mellitus
		  ○ Hyperadrenocorticism
		  ○ Hyperthyroidism
		 • CKD
		 • Urinary or reproductive tract anatomic abnormality
		 • Immunocompromised
		 • Neurogenic bladder
		 • Pregnancy

Recurrent infection	• ≥3 infections per year	

Relapsing	• Recurrence within weeks to months of a successfully treated infection
	 • Sterile bladder during treatment
	 •Same organism
		Failure to eradicate pathogen
		 • Deep-seated niche
		  ○ Pyelonephritis
		  ○ Prostatitis
		  ○ Bladder submucosa
		  ○ Stone
		  ○ Neoplasia

Refractory/persistent	• Persistently positive culture with original pathogen despite in vitro antimicrobial susceptibility • No elimination of bacteriuria during or after treatment	Rare • Failure of host defenses • Structural abnormality • Patient/client incompliance • Abnormal metabolism/excretion of antimicrobial

Reinfection	• Recurrence with different organism
	 • Variable time course after previous infection
		• Poor systemic immune function
		  ○ Endocrinopathy
		  ○ Immunosuppressed
		 • Loss of urine antimicrobial properties
		  ○ Glucosuria
		  ○ Dilute urine
		 • Anatomic abnormality
		 • Physiologic predisposition
		  ○ Neurogenic bladder
		  ○ Urinary incontinence

Superinfection	• Infection with different pathogen during treatment of the original infection	• Cystotomy tube • Indwelling urinary catheter • Neoplasia

Adapted from Weese JS, Blondeau J, Booth D, et al. International society for companion animal infectious disease (ISCAID) guidelines for the diagnosis and management of bacterial urinary tract infections in dogs and cats. Vet J 2019;247:8-25; and Barsanti J. Multidrug-resistant urinary tract infection. In: Bonagura JD, Twedt DC, editors. Current veterinary therapy XIV. St Louis (MO): WB Saunders; 2009. p. 921-5.

(see **Fig. 3**B). Options for prostatic fluid sampling are discussed elsewhere, but include semen evaluation of the third fraction, prostatic wash, fine-needle aspiration, and prostatic biopsy.[16] There can be discordance between culture results from urine and prostatic fluid.[35] Intact males should be screened for *Brucella* spp with rapid slide

---

Box 2
Diagnostic testing for recurrent urinary tract infections

Extended diagnostic testing may be required for complicated infections

- Urine analysis

- Urine culture (ideally, cystocentesis sample)

- Complete blood count

- Chemistry profile with electrolytes

- Digital rectal examination

- Feline leukemia virus/feline immunodeficiency virus (cats)

- Thyroid testing
  - Cats: total T4

- Adrenal testing
  - Low-dose dexamethasone suppression test
  - Adrenocorticotropic hormone stimulation test

- Abdominal radiographs

- Abdominal ultrasound

- Contrast radiology
  - Excretory urography
  - Contrast cystourethrography
  - Double-contrast cystography
  - Contrast vaginourethrography

- Prostatic wash

- Cystoscopy with bladder wall culture

Adapted from Bartges JW. Diagnosis of urinary tract infections. Vet Clin North Am Small Anim Pract 2004;34:927-29; and Weese JS, Blondeau JM, Boothe D, etal. Antimicrobial use guidelines for treatment of urinary tract disease in dogs and cats: antimicrobial guidelines working group of the international society for companion animal infectious diseases. Vet Med Int 2011;2011:2,4.

---

agglutination test (RSAT), tube agglutination test, or immunofluorescent antibody test. Confirmatory tests include 2-mercaptoethanol RSAT or agar gel immunodiffusion assay using an internal cytoplasmic antigen.[37]

Catheter-associated urinary tract infection. There is no evidence to support routine urine culture or culture of the urinary catheter tip following removal in asymptomatic patients; such cultures do not predict the development of catheter-associated infection.[33,35] In contrast, urine culture is always indicated for a patient with clinical signs of UTI, fever of undetermined origin, or abnormal urine cytology (ie, hematuria, pyuria). If the patient develops new clinical signs or fever after a urinary catheter has been placed, then, ideally, the urine catheter is removed and a cystocentesis is performed to provide a sample for culture once the bladder fills. Alternatively, the original urinary catheter is replaced, and a urine sample is collected through the second catheter. It is less ideal to sample the urine through the original catheter, and a sample from the collection bag should never be used.[33,35]

Subclinical bacteriuria. Subclinical bacteriuria, previously called asymptomatic bacteriuria or occult bacteriuria, refers to the presence of bacteria in the urine, based on positive urine culture, but the absence of lower urinary tract clinical signs.[35] SB in healthy dogs and cats is not uncommon with prevalence up to 13% in reportedly healthy animals.[35,38–42] Animals with underlying comorbidities, such as diabetes mellitus, or CKD, or recurrent infection, have increased prevalence of SB, up to 30%[41,43–46] to 50%.[47] Hyperthyroidism is not a risk factor for SB.[48]

In humans, there are extensive studies to support not treating SB with antimicrobials in almost all groups of patients; an exception is patients undergoing transurethral surgery.[35] Human meta-analysis has shown that treatment of SB does not benefit this patient population, but is associated with increased adverse reactions and promotes antimicrobial resistance.[49] Similar recommendations exist for veterinary patients, and treatment for SB is not recommended except in a few situations (**Box 3**). There is no evidence that SB progresses to clinical cystitis and/or predisposes to ascending infections.[33] Likewise, there is no evidence that treatment of a multidrug-resistant bacteria is beneficial if the animal is subclinical.[50] In one prospective study of dogs with SB, 50% had transient colonization, and 50% had persistent bacteriuria over a 3-month time period; no dog developed clinical signs at any time point.[39]

In some dogs and cats, such as the paralyzed patient or those with unobservant owners, it might be challenging for the practitioner to confidently assess if the dog or cat has lower urinary tract signs. In such scenarios, the practitioner must use their best clinical judgment to determine if antimicrobial treatment is warranted. It is noteworthy that change in urine odor and pyuria are not indications for treatment in people.[51]

Cats with CKD and SB are another population in which the decision whether to treat can be challenging. It is reasonable to try appropriate antibiotic therapy based on culture and susceptibility for 2 weeks to rule out pyelonephritis. However, if there is stable renal function but persistent SB, the practitioner might elect not to treat further and instead monitor.[52]

Fungal urinary tract infection
Diagnosis of fungal UTI most commonly occurs by identification of fungal elements during routine or concentrated urine sediment examination. Fungal culture and sensitivity are ideal before treatment, especially in cases other than *C albicans*, which tend to be more resistant.[21]

Viral urinary tract infection
Routine diagnostic tests, including urine analysis and light microscopy, cannot identify viruses or viral-induced disease. Virus isolation is the gold standard for diagnosis, but

---

Box 3
When to treat subclinical bacteriuria[35,52]

- Suspected pyelonephritis
- Undergoing surgical procedure of urinary tract
- Undergoing endoscopic procedure if bleeding is expected
- If the bladder is suspected to be site of extraurinary infection
- If diabetic animal and subclinical bacteriuria are thought to be the cause of insulin resistance or ketosis
- If *C urealyticum* because this has been associated with encrusting cystitis
- If urease-producing organism (ie, *Staphylococci* spp) because of association with struvite urolithiasis

this technique is expensive and time-consuming and requires live replicating virus. Diagnostic PCR assays are rapid and sensitive, but methods to optimize nucleic acid preparation are essential because the nucleic acids are easily degraded in urine.[23]

PHARMACOLOGIC TREATMENT OPTIONS
Antimicrobials

Antimicrobial drugs are the cornerstone of treatment of UTI. In most cases, the antimicrobial agent chosen should be based on susceptibility testing of the uropathogen, and urine culture is recommended for all patients with clinical signs. Overuse and misuse of antimicrobial drugs may result in the emergence of resistant organisms, a situation that has implications for successful treatment of infections in the patient as well as overall veterinary and human health.

A paradigm shift in the management of UTI is to start analgesics, such as a nonsteroidal anti-inflammatory drug (NSAID), initially while waiting for the results of culture and susceptibility. As clinical signs are the results of urinary tract inflammation, analgesics alone can be equally as effective as antimicrobials for uncomplicated cases in humans.[35] Patients with clinical signs severe enough to merit therapy before results of urine culture and sensitivity testing should receive a broad-spectrum antimicrobial that has excellent urine penetration. Suggested "first-line" antimicrobials for uncomplicated UTI include amoxicillin, cephalexin, or trimethoprim-sulfamethoxazole (**Table 2**). The use of fluoroquinolones, nitrofurantoin, or extended-release cephalexin (ie, cefovecin) is inappropriate for most sporadic UTI and should be reserved for resistant infections (**Table 3**).

Combination Therapies

If multiple bacteria are isolated, then the relative importance of each must be assessed based on quantification and suspected pathogenicity. Ideally, an antimicrobial effective against all pathogens is selected. If this is not possible, then combination therapy with multiple antimicrobials may be considered.[33] Assuming there is no evidence of pyelonephritis or increased risk of ascending infection, then targeting antimicrobial

Table 2	
Summary of first-line antimicrobial options for urinary tract infections in the dog and cat	
Infection	**First-Line Drug Options**
Sporadic or recurrent UTI	Start analgesics, such as NSAID, while waiting for culture results. Consider as sole therapy, especially in cats and in dogs, if mild clinical signs, pending culture Antimicrobial choice guided by culture and susceptibility testing. Consider amoxicillin or trimethoprim-sulfonamide initially while results are pending. Amoxicillin with clavulanic acid can be considered if amoxicillin is not available
Subclinical bacteriuria	Antimicrobial therapy not recommended. If treatment needed, treat as per sporadic UTI
Pyelonephritis	Start with a fluoroquinolone, with reassessment based on culture and susceptibility testing
Prostatitis	Trimethoprim-sulfonamide, enrofloxacin, chloramphenicol

Adapted from Weese JS, Blondeau J, Booth D, et al. International society for companion animal infectious disease (ISCAID) guidelines for the diagnosis and management of bacterial urinary tract infections in dogs and cats. Vet J 2019;247:8-25.

Table 3
Antimicrobial treatment options for urinary tract infection in dogs and cats

Drug	Dose	Comments
Amoxicillin	11–15 mg/kg q8h, po	Good first-line option for UTI. Excreted in urine predominantly in active form if normal renal function is present. Ineffective against β-lactamase–producing bacteria. Not recommended for pyelonephritis or prostatitis
Amikacin	Dogs: 15–30 mg/kg q24h, IV/IM/SC Cats: 10–14 mg/kg q24h, IV/IM/SC	Not recommended for routine use but may be useful for treatment of multidrug-resistant organisms. Potentially nephrotoxic. Avoid in animals with renal insufficiency
Amoxicillin/clavulanate	12.5–25 mg/kg q8h, po (dose based on combination of amoxicillin + clavulanate)	Not established whether there is any advantage over amoxicillin alone. Not good for *E coli* in tissue (ie, bladder wall)
Ampicillin		Not recommended because of poor oral bioavailability. Amoxicillin is preferred
Cephalexin, cefadroxil	12–25 mg/kg q12h, po	Enterococci are resistant. Resistance may be common in *Enterobacteriaceae* in some regions
Cefovecin	8 mg/kg single SC injection. Can be repeated once after 7–14 d	Should only be used in situations where oral treatment is problematic. Enterococci are resistant. Pharmacokinetic data support the use in dogs and cats, with a duration of 14 d (dogs) and 21 d (cats)
Cefpodoxime proxetil	5–10 mg/kg q24h, po	Enterococci are resistant
Ceftiofur	2 mg/kg q12–24h, SC	Approved for treatment of UTI in dogs in some regions. Enterococci are resistant
Chloramphenicol	Dogs: 40–50 mg/kg q8h, po Cats: 12.5–20 mg/kg q12h, po	Reserved for multidrug-resistant infections with few other options. Myelosuppression can occur, particularly in cats and with long-term therapy. Avoid contact by humans because of rare idiosyncratic aplastic anemia. Not a first line for pyelonephritis or prostatitis

(continued on next page)

Table 3
(continued)

Drug	Dose	Comments
Ciprofloxacin	25–30 mg/kg q24h, po	Sometimes used because of lower cost than enrofloxacin. Lower and more variable oral bioavailability than enrofloxacin, marbofloxacin, and orbifloxacin. Difficult to justify over approved fluoroquinolones. Dosing recommendations are empirical
Doxycycline	5 mg/kg q12h, po	Highly metabolized and excreted through intestinal tract, so urine levels may be low. Not recommended for routine uses. Can cause esophageal stricture
Enrofloxacin	Dogs: 10–20 mg/kg q24h, po Cats: 5 mg/kg q24h, po	Excreted in urine predominantly in active form. Reserve for documented resistant UTI. Good first-line choice for pyelonephritis (dogs 20 mg/kg po q24h). Limited efficacy against enterococci. Associated with risk of retinopathy in cats. Do not exceed 5 mg/kg/d of enrofloxacin in cats
Imipenem-cilastatin	5 mg/kg q6–8h, IV/IM	Reserve for treatment of multidrug-resistant infections, particularly those caused by *Enterobacteriaceae* or *Pseudomonas aeruginosa*. Recommend consultation with a urinary or infectious disease veterinary specialist or veterinary pharmacologist before use
Marbofloxacin	2.7–5.5 mg/kg q24h, po	Excreted in urine predominantly in active form. Reserve for documented resistant UTI. Good first-line choice for pyelonephritis. Limited efficacy against *Enterococcus* spp

(continued on next page)

Table 3
(continued)

Drug	Dose	Comments
Meropenem	Dogs: 8.5 mg/kg q12h, SC or q8h, IV Cats: 10 mg/kg q12h SQ, IV, IM	Reserve for treatment of multidrug-resistant infections, particularly those caused by *Enterobacteriaceae* or *P aeruginosa*. Recommend consultation with a urinary or infectious disease veterinary specialist or veterinary pharmacologist before use
Nitrofurantoin	4.4–5 mg/kg q8h, po	Good second-line option for sporadic UTI, particularly when multidrug-resistant pathogens are involved. Do not use for pyelonephritis where tissue drug concentrations (vs urine) are needed
Orbifloxacin	Tablets: 2.5–7.5 mg/kg q24h, po; oral suspension: 7.5 mg/kg q24h, po (cats) or 2.5–7.5 mg/kg q24h, po (dogs)	Excreted in urine predominantly in active form. Reserve for documented resistant UTI. Good first-line choice for pyelonephritis. Limited efficacy against *Enterococcus* spp
Pradofloxacin	Dogs: 3 mg/kg q24h, po[a] Cats: 5 mg/kg q24h, po[a]	Good first-line option for pyelonephritis in cats. Not associated with feline blindness like the other fluoroquinolones. May cause bone marrow suppression resulting in severe thrombocytopenia and neutropenia in dogs. Not recommended for *Enterococcus* spp

(continued on next page)

	Table 3 (continued)	
Drug	**Dose**	**Comments**
Trimethoprim-sulfadiazine	15 mg/kg q12h, po Note: dosing is based on total trimethoprim + sulfadiazine concentration	Good first-line option. Concerns regarding idiosyncratic and immune-mediated adverse effects in some patients, especially with prolonged therapy. If prolonged (>7 d) therapy is anticipated, baseline Schirmer tear testing is recommended (dogs), with periodic reevaluation and owner monitoring for ocular discharge. Avoid in dogs that may be sensitive to potential adverse effects, such as keratoconjunctivitis sicca, hepatopathy, hypersensitivity, and skin eruptions. An option for prostatitis

Abbreviations: IM, intramuscularly; IV, intravenously; PO, orally, SC, subcutaneously.
   [a] Dose extrapolated from previous studies.[53]
   Adapted from Weese JS, Blondeau J, Booth D, et al. International society for companion animal infectious disease (ISCAID) guidelines for the diagnosis and management of bacterial urinary tract infections in dogs and cats. Vet J 2019;247:8-25.

therapy against the pathogen with the most clinical relevance is reasonable. For example, anecdotally, resolution of *Enterococcus* sp infection is often possible after treatment of concurrent infection.[33]

Pyelonephritis

Antimicrobial therapy should be initiated while waiting for the culture and sensitivity results. Empirical antimicrobials should have efficacy against gram-negative bacteria, the most common pathogens; fluoroquinolones or cefpodoxime are good first choices (see **Table 2**). Acute pyelonephritis requires hospitalization for parenteral antimicrobial therapy and intravenous fluids. Parenteral therapy should be continued until patients will eat and drink normally and azotemia is no longer improving with intensive therapy. If the animal is systemically well and eating and drinking, then oral antimicrobial therapy can be used, and the patient does not require hospitalization.[35] Patients with chronic pyelonephritis often do not require hospitalization at the time of diagnosis. When interpreting the culture and susceptibility results, *serum* breakpoints rather than urine breakpoints should be used.[35]

Prostatitis

The blood-prostate barrier is compromised with acute prostatitis, and an appropriate antimicrobial should be selected based on culture and sensitivity. Antimicrobials must be selected more carefully in cases of chronic prostatitis because the blood-prostate barrier is generally intact (see **Table 2**). Nonionized, basic, lipid-soluble antimicrobials have the best penetration into the prostatic tissue.[14–16] Drugs such as trimethoprim-sulfadiazine, chloramphenicol, and enrofloxacin (but not ciprofloxacin) are excellent choices. Examples of drugs with low-lipid solubility and poor diffusion across the blood-prostate barrier include penicillin and cephalothin.[14–16] *Serum* rather than urine breakpoints should be used when interpreting the culture and susceptibility.[35] Culture of prostatic fluid should be performed before and after discontinuation of antimicrobials.[14–16]

Castration is recommended as an adjunctive treatment to medical management to help reduce the prostatic size, speed recovery, and decrease recurrence.[14–16] Finasteride, a 5a-reductase inhibitor, may be considered in valuable breeding animals or for owners that refuse surgery.[54]

Catheter-Associated Urinary Tract Infection

Although it seems logical to administer antimicrobial agents while an indwelling urinary catheter is inserted in an effort to decrease iatrogenic infection, the practice is strongly discouraged. Concomitant oral or parenteral administration of antimicrobial agents during indwelling urethral catheterization does not prevent development of bacterial UTI and promotes infection caused by multidrug-resistant bacteria.[17]

Antifungals

Fluconazole is recommended as initial treatment in most patients because of the high margin of safety, sensitivity of most strains of *Candida* spp, and excretion of active drug into urine in high concentrations (**Table 4**).[21] *Candida* spp other than *C albicans* are more likely to be resistant to fluconazole, and antifungal sensitivity testing is recommended to determine if a higher dose of fluconazole is appropriate or if another drug should be used. Although amphotericin B is renally excreted and achieves

Table 4
Treatment of fungal cystitis

For all cases	Identify and correct underlying predisposing factors	• Breaches in local or systemic immunity
If *C albicans*	Fluconazole 5–10 mg/kg po q12h for 4–6 wk	• Urine sediment and culture at 2- to 3-wk intervals to confirm resolution •Urine sediment and culture 1 and 2 mo after therapy discontinuation
If non–*C albicans*	Therapy based on culture and sensitivity	•Monitor as above •Consider drug penetration into urine when selecting therapy
If initial treatment fails	Repeat culture and sensitivity	Consider: •Intravesicular infusion 1% clotrimazole or amphotericin B •IV or SQ amphotericin B •Combination fluconazole at maximum dose plus terbinafine •Benign neglect, regular monitoring for disease progression

Adapted from Pressler BM. Urinary tract infections–fungal. In: Polzin D, Bartges JW, editors. Nephrology and urology of small animals. Ames (IA): Blackwell Publishing; 2011. p. 719-21.

high concentration in urine, it is not often used because it is parenterally administered and nephrotoxic. Other commonly used antifungal drugs, including itraconazole and ketoconazole, are not renally excreted in active form.[21]

Secondary fungal UTI occurs because of shedding of organisms into urine in patients with systemic infections. Organisms most commonly associated with urine shedding are *Aspergillus* spp in dogs (particularly German shepherd dogs) and *Cryptococcus* spp in cats.[55–58] These patients should be treated with antifungal agents standardly recommended for systemic infections.

Antivirals

Antiviral drugs have not been evaluated for animals with viral-induced urinary tract disease, and management of these patients is limited to supportive care.[23]

EVALUATION OF OUTCOME AND LONG-TERM RECOMMENDATIONS
Treatment Duration and Monitoring

It is important for the practitioner to recognize that the primary goal of treating a UTI is to resolve clinical signs. Achieving microbiological cure (elimination of the organism) is desirable but might not be achieved and is not necessarily required in order to have clinical resolution. These therapeutic goals provide prospective for the movement toward shorter "courses" of antimicrobial therapy and withholding treatment for cases with SB.

Sporadic bacterial urinary tract infection

The previous treatment recommendation for dogs with uncomplicated UTI was 7 to 14 days of an appropriate antimicrobial agent.[33] In human medicine, short-duration antimicrobial therapy, commonly, trimethoprim-sulfamethoxazole or fluoroquinolone, has become the standard treatment of acute uncomplicated bacterial cystitis in women.[59] The recommendations are antimicrobial-specific because not all antimicrobials have comparable efficacy when given as only a 3-day treatment. Benefits of shorter therapy include better compliance, lower cost, and decreased adverse effects.[56] The goal of treatment is to decrease the bacterial load enough to control clinical signs with the immune system eliminating remaining organisms. There are some studies in dogs to support the effectiveness of shorter dosing regimens.[60,61]

Updates. As reflected in the 2019 ISCAID consensus statement, the current recommendation is to treat sporadic UTI for 3 to 5 days (**Table 5**).[35] If the proper antimicrobial is chosen and administered at the appropriate dosage and frequency, clinical signs are expected to resolve within 48 to 72 hours. If there is not clinical improvement, then investigation is warranted to confirm that cystitis is indeed present and to identify any confounding factors. Empirically changing to a different antimicrobial is not recommended. Urine culture following cessation of antimicrobial therapy is no longer recommended if there is resolution of clinical signs.[35]

Recurrent bacterial urinary tract infection, pyelonephritis, prostatitis

Previous recommendations for recurrent or complicated infections, including pyelonephritis and prostatitis, were to treat with antimicrobials for a minimum of 3 to 6 weeks[33,34] and periodically reculture urine during and after therapy to document efficacy and resolution.

Updates. Categorizing recurrent infections as reinfections or relapsing infections is important to determine the optimal management strategy. Reinfections can be treated as for sporadic UTI with a short duration, 3 to 5 days, of antimicrobials (see **Table 5**). In

Table 5
Treatment duration and monitoring

	Treatment Duration	Monitoring Urine Culture
Sporadic bacterial UTI	3–5 d	Not recommended if resolution of clinical signs
Reinfection	3–5 d	Not recommended if resolution of clinical signs
Reinfection or refractory/ persistent infection	7–14 d	Reculture urine 5–7 d following cessation of treatment
Pyelonephritis	10–14 d	Physical examination, serum creatinine, urinalysis, urine culture 1–2 wk following treatment
Prostatitis	4–6 wk	Castration. Drain abscess, if present. Reassess prostate size and architecture after 8–12 wk
Catheter-associated UTI	3–5 d, if symptomatic	Not recommended if resolution of clinical signs

Data from Refs.[21,24,35]

such cases, urine culture after completion of treatment is not recommended. If there is relapsing or persistent UTI, then longer duration, 7 to 14 days, of treatment is indicated. Urine culture 5 to 7 days following longer duration of treatment can be considered; if positive, then further investigation into why the bacteria has not been eliminated is warranted (ie, compliance issue, appropriate antimicrobial choice in light of culture and susceptibility and tissue penetration, pyelonephritis). If clinical signs are resolved and there is SB, additional treatment might not be indicated.[35]

The recommended treatment duration for pyelonephritis is 10 to 14 days (see **Table 5**). Recheck physical examination, serum creatinine, urinalysis, and urine culture is recommended 1 to 2 weeks after discontinuing antimicrobials. If there is resolution of clinical signs and azotemia, the finding of SB might not necessitate continued antimicrobial treatment.[35]

The duration of treatment for prostatitis is a minimum of 4 weeks for acute prostatitis and 4 to 6 weeks for chronic prostatitis, potentially longer if there is abscessation present (see **Table 5**).[35] Prostatic abscesses should be drained either percutaneously with ultrasound guidance or with surgical debridement, omentalization, and marsupialization.[62] Castration is recommended, if possible. If castration is not an option, then medical therapies to reduce hormonal influence, such as finasteride, androgen receptor antagonists, or GnRH agonists, can be considered. Reassessment of prostatic size and architecture with ultrasound is recommended 8 to 12 weeks after starting treatment.[35]

Catheter-associated urinary tract infection
It is not necessary to treat bacteriuria associated with an indwelling catheter if there is no clinical or cytologic evidence of infection. For patients that develop a catheter-associated UTI, treatment is more likely to be successful if the catheter can be removed. Urine culture should be performed on a sample collected by cystocentesis, or after placing a new indwelling urinary catheter with care to discard the first 3 to 5 mL of urine. Urine culture *should not* be performed on urine collected from the collection system or bag. Likewise, culture of the catheter tip is not recommended. If the patient is clinical for UTI, then treat as a sporadic infection.[35]

Fungal urinary tract infection
Primary fungal UTI should always be treated with a minimum of 6 to 8 weeks of anti-fungal therapy and regular monitoring during and after cessation of therapy.[21]

PREVENTION
Catheter-Associated Urinary Tract Infection

There are several strategies to decrease the risk of catheter-associated UTI (**Box 4**).

Recurrent Urinary Tract Infection

Several strategies have been evaluated to prevent recurrent UTI, but unfortunately, there are no effective and recommended therapies for prevention (**Table 6**). If possible, identify and correct any underlying structural (ie, ectopic ureters, recessed vulva) or functional abnormalities (ie, urinary incontinence).

Local Therapy

Local infusions with antimicrobials, antiseptics, and dimethyl sulfoxide can be irritating and are not retained within the urinary bladder.[33] Anecdotally, instillation of dilute chlorhexidine (1:100, 0.02%) and/or EDTA-tromethamine (EDTA-Tris)[69] via cystotomy tube may decrease the incidence of bacterial UTI (JW Bartges, 2014, personal communication,). In a small human study, bladder irrigation with dilute 0.02% chlorhexidine significantly decreased postoperative bacteriuria, although it did not elimi-nate preexisting infection and did not appear to damage the bladder mucosa.[70] It has been postulated that EDTA-Tris has synergistic effects with systemic antimicro-bials[71] as well as local chlorhexidine irrigation.[70] Proposed mechanisms included divalent ion binding causing alteration of bacterial DNA synthesis, cell wall perme-ability, and ribosomal stability. In additional, in vitro studies suggest that the presence of EDTA-Tris reduces the minimum inhibitory concentration for various antimicrobial drugs.[71] In a small study (n = 17 dogs, n = 4 with chronic cystitis), daily local infusion via sterile urinary catheter (25 mL EDTA at 37°C) for 7 days was well tolerated, and dogs had negative urine cultures up to 180 days after treatment.[71] Additional studies are needed to determine the short- and long-term effects of EDTA-Tris therapy. Currently, the ISCAID guidelines do not recommend infusion of antimicrobials, anti-

---

Box 4
Strategies to prevent catheter-associated urinary tract infection

- Avoid indiscriminate use of urinary catheters. Carefully assess the need for placing and retaining catheter

- Always use hand hygiene

- Use a closed collection system for indwelling catheters

- Sterile catheter placement

- Minimize duration of catheterization

- Avoid indiscriminate antimicrobial use

- Try to avoid an indwelling urinary catheter in immunocompromised patients

- Be cautious with indwelling catheter use in patients undergoing diuresis

Adapted from Siddiq DM, Darouiche RO. New strategies to prevent catheter-associated urinary tract infections. Nat Rev Urol 2012;9:305 to -14; with permission.

Table 6
Prevention strategies for recurrent urinary tract infection

Therapy	Proposed Mechanism of Action	Evidence	Recommendation[33]
Low-dose or pulse antibiotic therapy		Promotes antimicrobial resistance	Not recommended
D-mannose	D-mannose sugar competitively binds to mannose-fimbriae on certain E coli strains, thereby inhibiting adhesion to the uroepithelium[63]	No veterinary studies of efficacy	Not recommended
Methenamine	Urinary antiseptic. Converted to bacteriostatic formaldehyde in an acidic environment	Veterinary studies of safety, efficacy, and appropriate dosing are lacking	Not recommended
Cranberry	Proanthocyanidin, the "active ingredient" in cranberry, alters the genotypic or phenotypic expression of fimbriae, which subsequently inhibits E coli adherence to human bladder and vaginal epithelial cells[64]	In vivo studies are not as promising as in vitro. Limited veterinary studies.[65–67] Concerns for variable quality and potency in available formulations Most recently, a randomized, placebo-controlled, blinded clinical trial in dogs with acute disk herniation did not show any benefit[68]	Not recommended, although no contraindication and supplements appear safe

inflammatories, or biocides into the bladder because there is lack of evidence for efficacy and the potential to cause iatrogenic trauma, infection, and irritation.[35]

TREATMENT RESISTANCE/COMPLICATIONS
Treatment Resistance

Several factors can result in treatment failure, including inappropriate antimicrobial selection, pharmacokinetic issues (ie, biofilm formation, deep-seated infection), a complicated infection, or multidrug resistant bacteria.[72]

Bacterial resistance

The emergence of multidrug-resistant bacteria is concerning and has important implications for both the patient and the public health. There are trends toward increasing resistance in both fecal and environmental reservoirs.[73] In addition, there is growing concern of shared bacterial isolates between animals and humans, and several studies have shown that dogs and cats can share uropathogenic bacteria with other members of the household.[74] Examples of clinically and epidemiologically important

resistance mechanisms include extended spectrum beta-lactamase, cephalospori-
nases, peptidoglycan transpeptidase (PBP2a), and high-level gentamicin resistance
biofunctional enzyme.[74] In addition to acquiring resistance genes via plasmids, there
are other bacterial strategies for persistence within the urinary tract. For example, uropathogenic *E coli* can invade and persist within the superficial bladder wall epithelial
cells.[73] These bacteria may remain dormant for a period of time followed by
recrudescence.

Biofilms. Some bacteria have the capacity for biofilm formation, which facilitates colonization.[75–77] *E coli* isolates are frequently capable of biofilm formation, and the potential for biofilm formation should always be considered.[78,79] A biofilm is composed of
organisms adhered together by a self-produced polysaccharide matrix.[75] It has
been suggested that the bacteria within the biofilm become sessile; they are protected
from the immune system, are antimicrobial, and inherently are resistant to shear forces
of removal.[75] In humans, bacteria with the capacity to produce biofilms have been
associated with SB.[73,75] Biofilms are also implemented in the development of
catheter-associated UTI[78] and with the development of resistant bacterial isolates.[80]

Strategies to prevent catheter-associated biofilms include using (1) materials that
are less amendable to biofilm formation and (2) coatings or surface modifications
that decrease biofilm formation. For example, silicone catheters are preferred over latex because scanning electron microscope imaging reveals that latex surfaces are
more irregular and promote microbial adherence.[81,82] An example of an agent used
for catheter coating is the antiseptic chlorhexidine. In a veterinary prospective study
(n = 26 dogs) evaluating biofilm formation on indwelling urinary catheters,
sustained-release varnish of chlorhexidine-coated urinary catheters statistically
decreased biofilm formation.[80] There are an array of other catheter coatings and modifications to decrease bacterial adherence and biofilm formation that have primarily
been studied in a research setting, including silver coating, nanoparticles, iontopho-
resis, antimicrobials, urease and other enzyme inhibitors, liposomes, and bacterio-
phages. Other novel strategies include quorum sensing inhibitors and vibroacoustic
stimulation. A detailed discussion of comparison is beyond the scope of this article,
and the reader is referred elsewhere.[81]

Fungal resistance

Infections that fail to respond completely to fluconazole should be recultured and antifungal sensitivity testing performed (see **Table 3**). Some susceptible isolates may
respond to intravesicular administration of 1% clotrimazole or amphotericin
B.[21,83,84] Urinary alkalinization has also been historically proposed as adjunctive therapy in patients with fungal UTI, because increased urine pH may inhibit fungal growth.
However, this is not currently favored for treatment of fungal UTI in humans and is of
questionable efficacy in veterinary patients.[21]

Complications

Magnesium ammonium phosphate (struvite) urolithiasis

Staphylococcus spp and *Proteus* spp, and more rarely *Corynebacterium* spp, *Klebsiella* spp, and *Ureaplasma* spp, may produce urease (**Box 5**). This enzyme hydrolyzes
urea to ammonia, which buffers urine hydrogen ions, forming ammonium ions,
increasing urine pH, and increasing dissolved ionic phosphate. In the presence of
magnesium, magnesium ammonium phosphate (struvite) may precipitate around a
nidus to form uroliths (**Fig. 6**). Bacteria are incorporated into the urolith matrix, and
thus, should be considered complicated UTI because of poor antimicrobial penetration. Greater than 90% of struvite uroliths in dogs are induced by urease-producing

---

Box 5
Complications of urinary tract infection

Potential complications of UTI
- Resistant infection
- Polypoid cystitis
- Emphysematous cystitis
- Magnesium ammonium phosphate (struvite) urolithiasis
- Pyelonephritis
- Prostatitis
- Prostatic abscess

---

bacteria, whereas struvite uroliths in cats are commonly sterile (ie, not associated with bacterial UTI). Struvite uroliths can be dissolved through a combination of dietary therapy and appropriate antimicrobial therapy; following dissolution or removal, preventing urolith recurrence requires preventing reinfection. For dogs that are uncomfortably symptomatic from urocystolithiasis and/or fail medical management, minimally invasive procedures, such as laser lithotripsy, laparoscopic-assisted cystotomy, or cystotomy, may be considered. The reader is referred to the open-access 2016 American College of Veterinary Internal Medicine Small Animal Consensus recommendations on the treatment and prevention of uroliths in dogs and cats.[85]

Polypoid cystitis

Chronic bacterial infections may induce microscopic or macroscopic bladder mucosal proliferation and intramural accumulation of inflammatory cells. Polypoid cystitis occurs when epithelial proliferation is severe, resulting in masslike lesions or diffuse thickening of the bladder wall (**Fig. 7**).[86,87] Gross differentiation of polypoid cystitis from bladder wall neoplasms is not reliable; however, polypoid cystitis is more likely to develop in the bladder apex (vs transitional cell carcinomas, which are more commonly found in the bladder trigone), is more commonly botryoid in appearance rather than fimbriated, and is not as grossly vascular as transitional cell carcinomas. Proteus spp may be more commonly associated with development of these lesions.[86,87] Polypoid cystitis lesions are niduses of deep-seated bacterial infection. In some cases, long-term antimicrobial therapy may result in successful resolution of lesions. However, partial cystectomy results in more rapid resolution of clinical signs, is likely associated with improved rates for long-term resolution of infection, and allows shorter antimicrobial treatment courses.[87] There is a recent case report

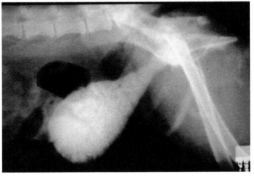

Fig. 6. Lateral survey abdominal radiograph of infection-induced struvite urocystourethroliths in a 3-year-old spayed female Irish setter.

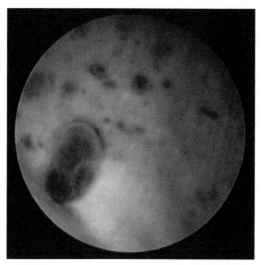

Fig. 7. Cystoscopic image of a urinary bladder polyp with cystitis due to *E coli* in a 6-year-old spayed female Irish setter.

of a young dog with presumptive malignant transformation of polypoid cystitis into transitional cell carcinoma.[88]

Emphysematous cystitis

Emphysematous cystitis refers to an accumulation of air within the bladder wall and lumen secondary to infection with glucose-fermenting bacteria. Most cases are due to *E coli* infection, but *Proteus* spp, *Klebsiella* spp, *Clostridium* spp, and *Aerobacter aerogenes* have also been reported.[89–91] Emphysematous cystitis most commonly develops in dogs and cats with diabetes mellitus because of the high concentration of fermentable substrate.[90] The ideal duration of treatment is unknown, but a minimum of 4 weeks is generally considered; if glucosuria is present, then appropriate treatment should be initiated for the underlying cause. A good prognosis can be achieved with early diagnosis and appropriate medical management.[91]

Pyelonephritis

Although no systematic reviews of pyelonephritis in dogs or cats have been performed, animals with systemically compromised immunity (ie, hyperadrenocorticism, diabetes mellitus), dogs or cats with CKD, and patients with any cause of vesicoureteral reflux are likely predisposed to development of pyelonephritis. Chronic pyelonephritis is likely underdiagnosed as a cause of renal failure in dogs and cats and should be especially considered in patients with previously stable CKD that have unexpected worsening of azotemia (ie, "acute-on-chronic" renal failure).

Prostatic abscessation

Prostatic abscessation is a sequela to prostatitis and is characterized by purulent fluid accumulations within the prostatic tissue. Clinical signs are variable and dependent on the size and extent of the abscess as well as systemic involvement. Prostatic abscesses are generally easily identified with ultrasonography, and the goal of therapy is to provide drainage through either ultrasound-guided percutaneous drainage or surgery. Surgical options include partial prostatectomy and prostate omentalization.[16]

SUMMARY

- Urinary tract infections can be sporadic or recurrent. Recurrent infections are further characterized as relapsing or refractory/persistent.
- Treatment of subclinical bacteriuria is not recommended.
- Antimicrobials are the cornerstone of treatment of bacterial UTI and, ideally, selected based on culture and sensitivity; shorter duration of antimicrobial treatment is recommended.
- There is limited literature to support preventative therapies; identification and resolution of underlying causes are essential.

DISCLOSURE

Dr Bartges current funding includes the following – these are not in conflict with the topic of this article: UGA Small Animal Medicine and Surgery Research Grant, UGA CVM Georgia Veterinary Scholars Program, Companion Animal Wellness Institute, Every Cat Foundation, Integrity Laboratories, IDEXX Laboratories, NHV Pet Products, Nutramax.

REFERENCES

1. Johnson JR, Kaster N, Kuskowski MA, et al. Identification of urovirulence traits in Escherichia coli by comparison of urinary and rectal E. coli isolates from dogs with urinary tract infection. J Clin Microbiol 2003;41:337–45.
2. Osborne C, Caywood D, Johnston G, et al. Perineal urethrostomy versus dietary management in prevention of recurrent lower urinary tract disease. J Small Anim Pract 1991;32:296–305.
3. Ling GV, Norris CR, Franti CE, et al. Interrelations of organism prevalence, specimen collection method, and host age, sex, and breed among 8,354 canine urinary tract infections (1969-1995). J Vet Intern Med 2001;15:341–7.
4. Bartges D, Blanco L. Bacterial urinary tract infections in cats. Compend Std Care 2001;3:1.
5. Davidson A, Ling G, Stevens F, et al. Urinary tract infection in cats: a retrospective study 1977-1989. Calif Vet 1992;46:32–4.
6. Barsanti J. Genitourinary infections. In: Greene CE, editor. Infectious diseases of the dog and cat. 4th edition. St Louis (MO): Elsevier Saunders; 2012. p. 1013–31.
7. Litster A, Moss SM, Honnery M, et al. Prevalence of bacterial species in cats with clinical signs of lower urinary tract disease: recognition of Staphylococcus felis as a possible feline urinary tract pathogen. Vet Microbiol 2007;121:182–8.
8. Litster A, Thompson M, Moss S, et al. Feline bacterial urinary tract infections: an update on an evolving clinical problem. Vet J 2011;187:18–22.
9. Wood M, Lepold A, Tesfamichael D, et al. Risk factors for enterococcal bacteriuria in dogs: a retrospective study. J Vet Intern Med 2020;34:2447–53.
10. Jang S, Ling G, Yamamoto R, et al. Mycoplasma as a cause of canine urinary tract infection. J Am Vet Med Assoc 1984;185:45–7.
11. Ulgen M, Cetin C, Senturk S, et al. Urinary tract infections due to Mycoplasma canis in dogs. J Vet Med A Physiol Pathol Clin Med 2006;53:379–82.
12. Abou N, van Dongen A, Houwers D. PCR-based detection reveals no causative role for mycoplasma and ureaplasma in feline lower urinary tract disease. Vet Microbiol 2006;116:246–7.
13. Bouillon J, Snead E, Caswell J, et al. Pyelonephritis in dogs: retrospective study of 47 histologically diagnosed cases (2005-2015). J Vet Intern Med 2018;32:249–59.

14. Prostatic disease Kustritz MR. In: Polzin D, Bartges JW, editors. Nephrology and urology of small animals. 1st edition. Ames (IA): Blackwell Publishing; 2011. p. 787–96.

15. Feldman EC, Nelson RW. Prostatitis. In: Kersey R, LeMelledo D, editors. Canine and feline endocrinology and reproduction. St Louis (MO): Elsevier Publishing; 2004. p. 977–86.

16. Smith J. Canine prostatic disease: a review of anatomy, pathology, diagnosis, and treatment. Theriogenology 2008;70:375–83.

17. Barsanti J, Blue J, Edmunds J. Urinary tract infection due to indwelling bladder catheters in dogs and cats. J Am Vet Med Assoc 1985;187:384–8.

18. Hugonnard M, Chalvet-Monfray K, Dernis J, et al. Occurrence of bacteriuria in 18 catheterised cats with obstructive lower urinary tract disease: a pilot study. J Feline Med Surg 2013;10:843–8.

19. Jin Y, Lin D. Fungal urinary tract infections in the dog and cat: a retrospective study (2001-2004). J Am Anim Hosp Assoc 2005;41:373–81.

20. Pressler BM, Vaden SL, Lane IF, et al. Candida spp. urinary tract infections in 13 dogs and seven cats: predisposing factors, treatment, and outcome. J Am Anim Hosp Assoc 2003;39:263–70.

21. Pressler BM. Urinary tract infections—fungal. In: Polzin D, Bartges JW, editors. Nephrology and urology of small animals. Ames (IA): Blackwell Publishing; 2011. p. 717–24.

22. Reagan K, Dear J, Kass P, et al. Risk factors for *Candida* urinary tract infection in dogs and cats. J Vet Intern Med 2019;33:648–53.

23. Kruger JM, Osborne CA, Wise AG, et al. Viruses and urinary tract disease. In: Polzin D, Bartges JW, editors. Nephrology and urology of small animals. Chichester (United Kingdom): Blackwell Publishing Ltd; 2011. p. 725–33.

24. Bartges JW. Diagnosis of urinary tract infections. Vet Clin North Am Small Anim Pract 2004;34:923–33.

25. Swenson CL, Boisvert AM, Kruger JM, et al. Evaluation of modified Wright-staining of urine sediment as a method for accurate detection of bacteriuria in dogs. J Am Vet Med Assoc 2004;224:1282–9.

26. Acierno M, Partyka M, Waite K, et al. Effect of refrigeration of clinical canine urine samples on quantitative bacterial culture. J Am Vet Med Assoc 2018;253(2):177–80.

27. Olin S, Bartges J, Jones R, et al. Diagnostic accuracy of a point-of-care bacteriologic culture test in dogs. J Am Vet Med Assoc 2013;243:1719–25.

28. Ybarra W, Sykes J, Wang Y, et al. Performance of a veterinary urine dipstick paddle system for diagnosis and identification of urinary tract infections in dogs and cats. J Am Vet Med Assoc 2014;244:814–9.

29. Kvitko-White H, Cook A, Nabity M, et al. Evaluation of a catalase-based urine test for the detection of urinary tract infections in dogs and cats. J Vet Intern Med 2013;27:1379–84.

30. Jacobs M, Crowell M, Fauls M, et al. Diagnostic accuracy of a rapid immunoassay for point-of-care detection of urinary tract infection in dogs. Am J Vet Res 2016;77(2):162–6.

31. Lehmann LE, Houser S, Marlinka T, et al. Rapid qualitative urinary tract infection pathogen identification by SeptiFast real-time PCR. PlosONE 2011;6(2).

32. DiBasio ED, Steward D, Wang Z, et al. MiQLAB bacterial and AMR test for rapid detection of UTI pathogens at the veterinary clinic (abstract). J Vet Emerg Crit Care 2021;31:S212.

33. Weese JS, Blondeau JM, Boothe D, et al. Antimicrobial use guidelines for treatment of urinary tract disease in dogs and cats: antimicrobial guidelines working

group of the International Society for Companion Animal Infectious Diseases. Vet Med Int 2011;2011:263768. Available at: http://www.hindawi.com/journals/vmi/% 202011/263768/.

34. Barsanti J. Multidrug-resistant urinary tract infection. In: Bonagura JD, Twedt DC, editors. Current veterinary therapy XIV. St Louis (MO): WB Saunders; 2009. p. 921–5.

35. Weese JS, Blondeau J, Booth D, et al. International Society for Companion Animal Infectious Disease (ISCAID) guidelines for the diagnosis and management of bacterial urinary tract infections in dogs and cats. Vet J 2019;247:8–25.

36. Kearly J, McAllister H, Graham P. Ch 2 the abdomen. In: Diagnostic radiology and ultrasonography of the dog and cat. 5th edition. Elsevier; 2011. p. 23–198.

37. Crosford K. Brucella canis: an update on research and clinical management. Can Vet J 2018;59:74–81.

38. McGhie J, Stayt J, Hosgood G. Prevalence of bacteriuria in dogs without clinical signs of urinary tract infection presenting for elective surgical procedures. Aust Vet J 2014;92:33–7.

39. Wan SY, Hartmann FA, Jooss MK, et al. Prevalence and clinical outcome of subclinical bacteriuria in female dogs. J Am Vet Med Assoc 2014;245:106–12.

40. Eggertsdottir AV, Ssvik BK, Halvorsen I, et al. Occurrence of occult bacteriuria in healthy cats. J Feline Med Surg 2011;13:800–3.

41. Litster A, Moss S, Platell J, et al. Occult bacterial lower urinary tract infections in cats—urinalysis and culture findings. Vet Microbiol 2009;136:130–4.

42. Moberg F, Langhorn R, Bertelsen P, et al. Subclinical bacteriuria in a mixed population of 179 middle-aged and elderly cats: a prospective cross-sectional study. J Feline Med Surg 2020;22(8):678–84.

43. Mayer-Roenne B, Goldstein RE, Erb HN. Urinary tract infections in cats with hyperthyroidism, diabetes mellitus and chronic kidney disease. J Feline Med Surg 2007;9:124–32.

44. White JD, Stevenson M, Malik R, et al. Urinary tract infections in cats with chronic kidney disease. J Feline Med Surg 2013;15(6):459–65.

45. McGuire NC, Schulman R, Ridgway MD, et al. Detection of occult urinary tract infections in dogs with diabetes mellitus. J Am Anim Hosp Assoc 2002;38:541–4.

46. Koutinas A, Heliadis N, Saridomichelakis M, et al. Asymptomatic bacteriuria in puppies with canine parvovirus infection: a cohort study. Vet Microbiol 1998;63: 109–16.

47. Seguin MA, Vaden SL, Altier C, et al. Persistent urinary tract infections and reinfections in 100 dogs (1989-1999). J Vet Intern Med 2003;17:622–31.

48. Peterson M, Li A, Soboroff P, et al. Hyperthyroidism is not a risk factor for subclinical bacteriuria in cats: a prospective cohort study. J Vet Intern Med 2020;34:1157–65.

49. Kőves B, Cati T, Veeratterapillay R. Benefits and harms of treatment of asymptomatic bacteriuria: a systematic review and meta-analysis by the European Association of Urology Urological Infection Guidelines Panel. Euro Urol 2017;72:865–8.

50. Johnstone T. A clinical approach to multidrug-resistant urinary tract infection and subclinical bacteriuria in dogs and cats. New Zeal Vet J 2020;68(2):69–83.

51. Hill T, Baverstock R, Carlson K, et al. Best practices for the treatment and prevention of urinary tract infection in the spinal cord injured population: the Alberta context. Can Urol Assoc 2013;7:122–30.

52. Dorsch R, Teichmann-Knorrn S, Lund H. Urinary tract infection and subclinical bacteriuria in cats. J Fel Med Surg 2019;21:1023–38.

53. Lees P. Pharmacokinetics, pharmacodynamics and therapeutics of pradofloxacin in the dog and cat. J Vet Pharmacol Ther 2013;36:209–21.

54. NiZanski W, Levy X, Ochota M, et al. Pharmacological treatment for common prostatic conditions in dogs-benign prostatic hyperplasia and prostatitis: an update. Reprod Domest Anim 2014;49:8–15.

55. Gerds-Grogan S, Dayrell-Hart B. Feline cryptococcosis: a retrospective evaluation. J Am Anim Hosp Assoc 1997;33:118–22.

56. Kabay M, Robinson W, Huxtable C, et al. The pathology of disseminated Aspergillus terreus infection in dogs. Vet Pathol 1985;22:540–7.

57. Kahler J, Leach M, Jang S, et al. Disseminated aspergillosis attributable to Aspergillus deflectus in a springer spaniel. J Am Vet Med Assoc 1990;197:871–4.

58. Jang S, Dorr T, Biberstein E, et al. Aspergillus deflectus infection in four dogs. Med Mycol 1986;24:95–104.

59. Nicolle LE. Short-term therapy for urinary tract infection: success and failure. Int J Antimicrob Agents 2008;31:40–5.

60. Westropp J, Sykes J, Irom S, et al. Evaluation of the efficacy and safety of high dose short duration enrofloxacin treatment regimen for uncomplicated urinary tract infections in dogs. J Vet Intern Med 2012;26:506–12.

61. Clare S, Hartmann F, Jooss M, et al. Short- and long-term cure rates of short-duration trimethoprim-sulfamethoxazole treatment in female dogs with uncomplicated bacterial cystitis. J Vet Intern Med 2014;28:818–26.

62. Boland L, Hardie R, Gregory S, et al. Ultrasound-guided percutaneous drainage as the primary treatment for prostatic abscesses and cysts in dogs. J Am Anim Hosp Assoc 2003;39:151–9.

63. Kranjcec B, Papes D, Altarac S. D-mannose powder for prophylaxis of recurrent urinary tract infections in women: a randomized clinical trial. World J Urol 2014; 32:79–84.

64. Gupta K, Chou M, Howell A, et al. Cranberry products inhibit adherence of p-fimbriated Escherichia coli to primary cultured bladder and vaginal epithelial cells. J Urol 2007;177:2357–60.

65. Howell AB, Griffin DW, Whalen MO. Inhibition of p-fimbriated Escherichia coli adhesion in an innovational ex-vivo model in dogs receiving a bioactive cranberry tablet (Crananidin TM). In: Programs and abstracts of the Am College Vet Intern Med. Anaheim (CA): 2010. p. 660.

66. Smee N, Grauer GF, Schermerhorn T. Investigations into the effect of cranberry extract on bacterial adhesion to canine uroepithelial cells. In: Programs and abstracts of the Am College Vet Intern Med. Denver (CO): 2011. p. 722-723.

67. Chou H, Chen K, Wang H, et al. Effects of cranberry extract on prevention of urinary tract infection in dogs and on adhesion of Escherichia coli to Madin-Darby canine kidney cells. Am J Vet Res 2016;77(4):421–7.

68. Olby N, Vaden S, Williams K, et al. Effect of cranberry extract on the frequency of bacteriuria in dogs with acute thoracolumbar disk herniation: a randomized controlled clinical trial. J Vet Intern Med 2017;31:60–8.

69. King J, Stickler D. The effect of repeated instillations of antiseptics on catheter-associated urinary tract infections: a study in a physical model of the catheterized bladder. Urol Res 1992;20:403–7.

70. Ball A, Carr T, Gillespie W, et al. Bladder irrigation with chlorhexidine for the prevention of urinary infection after transurethral operations: a prospective controlled study. J Urol 1987;138:491–4.

71. Farca A, Piromalli G, Maffei F, et al. Potentiating effect of EDTA-Tris on the activity of antibiotics against resistant bacteria associated with otitis, dermatitis and cystitis. J Small Anim Pract 1997;38:243–5.

72. McGovern D, Gaschen F, Habil D, et al. Antimicrobial susceptibility patterns and clinical parameters in 208 dogs with positive urine cultures (2012-2014). J Am Anim Assoc 2019;55:306–13.

73. Thompson MF, Litster AL, Platell JL, et al. Canine bacterial urinary tract infections: new developments in old pathogens. Vet J 2011;190:22–7.

74. Marques C, Belas A, Franco A, et al. Increase in antimicrobial resistance and emergence of major international high-risk clonal lineages in dogs and cats with urinary tract infection: 16 year retrospective study. J Antimicrob Chemother 2018;73:377–84.

75. DiCicco M, Neethirajan S, Singh A, et al. Efficacy of clarithromycin on biofilm formation of methicillin-resistant Staphylococcus pseudintermedius. BMC Vet Res 2012;8:225.

76. Nam EH, Chae JS. Characterization and zoonotic potential of uropathogenic Escherichia coli isolated from dogs. J Microbiol Biotechnol 2013;23:422–9.

77. Hancock V, Ferrieres L, Klemm P. Biofilm formation by asymptomatic and virulent urinary tract infectious Escherichia coli strains. FEMS Microbiol Lett 2007;267:30–7.

78. Kern Z, Jacob M, Gilbertie J, et al. Characteristics of dogs with biofilm-forming *Escherichia coli* urinary tract infections. J Vet Intern Med 2018;32:1645–51.

79. Oliveira M, Dias F, Pomba C. Biofilm and fluoroquinolone resistance of canine *Escherichia coli* uropathogenic isolates. BMC Res Notes 2014;7(499):1–5.

80. Segev G, Bankirer T, Steinberg D, et al. Evaluation of urinary catheters coated with sustained-release varnish of chlorhexidine in mitigating biofilm formation on urinary catheters in dogs. J Vet Intern Med 2013;27:39–46.

81. Siddiq DM, Darouiche RO. New strategies to prevent catheter-associated urinary tract infections. Nat Rev Urol 2012;9:305–14.

82. Flores-Mireles A, Hreha T, Hunstad D. Pathophysiology, treatment, and prevention of catheter-associated urinary tract infection. Top Spinal Cord Inj Rehabil 2019;25(3):228–40.

83. Forward ZA, Legendre AM, Khalsa HD. Use of intermittent bladder infusion with clotrimazole for treatment of candiduria in a dog. J Am Vet Med Assoc 2002;220:1496–8.

84. Toll J, Ashe CM, Trepanier LA. Intravesicular administration of clotrimazole for treatment of candiduria in a cat with diabetes mellitus. J Am Vet Med Assoc 2003;223:1156–8.

85. Lulich J, Berent A, Adams L, et al. ACVIM small animal consensus recommendations on the treatment and prevention of uroliths in dogs and cats. J Vet Intern Med 2016;30(5):1564–74.

86. Johnston S, Osborne C, Stevens J. Canine polypoid cystitis. J Am Vet Med Assoc 1975;166:1155–60.

87. Martinez I, Mattoon JS, Eaton KA, et al. Polypoid cystitis in 17 dogs (1978-2001). J Vet Intern Med 2003;17:499–509.

88. Butty E, Hahn S, Labato M. Presumptive malignant transformation of chronic polypoid cystitis into apical transitional cell carcinoma without BRAF mutation in a young female dog. J Vet Intern Med 2021;35:1551–7.

89. Petite A, Busoni V, Heinen MP, et al. Radiographic and ultrasonographic findings of emphysematous cystitis in four nondiabetic female dogs. Vet Radiol Ultrasound 2006;47:90–3.

90. Root C, Scott R. Emphysematous cystitis and other radiographic manifestations of diabetes mellitus in dogs and cats. J Am Vet Med Assoc 1971;158:721.

91. Fumeo M, Manfredi S, Volta A. Emphysematous cystitis: review of current literature, diagnosis, and management challenges. Vet Med Res Rep 2019;10:77–83.

Symmetrical Dimethylarginine: Evaluating Chronic Kidney Disease in the Era of Multiple Kidney Biomarkers

Helen Michael, DVM, PhD, DACVP[a], Donald Szlosek, MPH[a],
Celeste Clements, DVM, DACVIM[a], Rebekah Mack, DVM, DACVIM[a],*

KEYWORDS

- Nephrology • Veterinary • Creatinine • SDMA • Glomerular filtration rate

KEY POINTS

- Symmetric dimethylarginine (SDMA) is incorporated into the International Renal Interest Society guidelines for diagnosing, staging, and treating chronic kidney disease (CKD).
- Persistent mild increases in SDMA can be used to diagnose CKD.
- SDMA and creatinine correlate well with each other and with GFR.
- SDMA is affected by fewer nonrenal influences than creatinine.

INTRODUCTION

The diagnosis and management of chronic kidney disease (CKD) is a routine part of the clinical small animal practice. CKD is a common cause of morbidity and mortality in older cats and dogs.[1–3] The prevalence of CKD in cats rises sharply with age, with an estimated prevalence of less than 1% in young cats, 30% to 40% in cats more than 9%, and 60% in geriatric cats.[2,4–6] In dogs, the prevalence of CKD is lower and believed to be less than 1.5% and, similar to cats, is more common in older dogs.[7,8] Diagnosis of CKD is multifactorial involving clinical signs, physical examination, kidney biomarkers, urinalysis, and kidney imaging. The International Renal Interest Society (IRIS) is a globally recognized group of experts that provide education to practitioners around CKD and guidelines to standardize staging and management of cats and dogs with CKD.[9–11] CKD monitoring and management goes beyond renal biomarkers alone to include serum calcium and phosphorus, electrolytes, urine and serum protein, and blood pressure.[10,11]

---

[a] IDEXX Laboratories, Inc, 1 IDEXX Dr, Westbrook, ME 04092, USA
* Corresponding author.
E-mail address: rebekah-mack-gertig@idexx.com

Vet Clin Small Anim 52 (2022) 609–629
https://doi.org/10.1016/j.cvsm.2022.01.003
0195-5616/22/© 2022 Elsevier Inc. All rights reserved.
vetsmall.theclinics.com

CKD stage at diagnosis impacts survival and prognosis for cats and dogs and patients with earlier stages of CKD have longer survival following diagnosis[8,12–14] and recognition at early stages may slow the progression of CKD.[8,15,16] Although recognition of CKD in early stages has the potential to improve the prognosis, it can be difficult due to subtle changes in patients' clinical presentation and kidney biomarkers concentrations. In cats and dogs with IRIS stage 1 and 2 CKD, serum or plasma creatinine (sCr) is often within laboratory reference intervals (RI) and proteinuria, clinical signs, and changes to urine concentrating ability and urine specific gravity (USG) are variable and often absent.[9,17] Symmetric dimethylarginine (SDMA) is often the only kidney biomarker increased above the RI in animals with these early stages of CKD.[9] Single SDMA concentrations can detect smaller declines in glomerular filtration rate (GFR) than traditional kidney biomarkers sCr and blood urea nitrogen (BUN) concentrations.[18–20] Since becoming commercially available SDMA has been explored extensively in acute, chronic, and active kidney disease in cats and dogs, resulting in a large body of literature describing the use of SDMA in diagnosis, treatment, and monitoring of kidney disease in companion animals. Additionally, a recent systematic review and consensus statement of feline CKD treatment trials recommended that SDMA be included in the Core Outcome Set for minimum data collected in those research studies.[21]

Historically, CKD has been thought of as an irreversible, continuously progressive disease process characterized by a linear progression of indirect biomarkers recognizing the regression of GFR. While recent studies still describe CKD as irreversible and progressive, it is often proposed that a series of subtle and clinically impactful active injuries advance the decline in GFR and lead to CKD and CKD-linked sequelae.[22,23] These injuries can lead to nonlinear progression and there can be periods of partial recovery of kidney function between injuries.[24,25] Over the past decade, this changing paradigm and advancements in kidney biomarker availability and improvements in technology have enhanced practitioners' ability to detect more subtle CKD. The addition of SDMA and more frequent inclusion of urine protein to creatinine ratios (UPC) into CKD diagnosis and staging have improved detection and staging of early CKD in the general practice setting. Wide availability of high-quality ultrasound equipment, widespread imaging training, and more robust practice management and medical records software have contributed to improved assessment of patients.[2,26] Electronic medical records software often includes chronologic analyte concentrations and easier visualization of patient trends. There is strong evidence that serial assessment or trending of kidney biomarkers (including SDMA, sCr, USG, and UPC) shortens time to diagnosis and can lead to early intervention and potentially improved outcomes for cats and dogs with CKD.[7,27] Overall, the addition of SDMA, improvements in technology, and updated educational materials and IRIS guidelines have provided clarity around the diagnosis of CKD in early stages and, therefore, provided opportunities to improve outcomes for cats and dogs with CKD.

Discovery and Biochemistry

SDMA was first identified in urine in 1970.[28] SDMA and related asymmetric dimethylarginine (ADMA) are methylated amino acids generated intracellularly during protein turnover.[28,29] Protein arginine methyltransferases (PRMTs) produce SDMA and ADMA precursors through methylation of protein-bound L-arginine residues; SDMA and ADMA are released through protein degradation. Type I PRMTs are primarily responsible for the generation of ADMA and type II PRMTs (primarily PRMT5) generate SDMA. Almost all SDMA undergoes renal excretion[28,30] while only approximately 20% of ADMA is excreted by the kidneys and the rest is metabolized. Increased SDMA was initially identified in people with advanced kidney disease.[31] A meta-analysis of human patients found significant correlations between SDMA, GFR, and sCr.[32] Studies in cats and dogs have similarly reported a good correlation between SDMA and GFR (Supplemental Tables).[18–20,33–39]

IDENTIFYING DECREASED KIDNEY EXCRETORY FUNCTION
Glomerular Filtration Rate

Measurement of GFR is the recognized gold standard for quantitative assessment of kidney excretory function. However, it is not routinely performed on cats and dogs and is not specifically included in guidelines for diagnosing or staging CKD. Measuring GFR is complicated, time-consuming, requires administration of a suitable filtration marker, and obtaining timed blood samples and/or urine samples.[40] There is no single protocol or methodology for measurement of GFR; rather, there are multiple different protocols, filtration markers, and calculations that can be performed and each yield slightly different results. Methodology can affect the results and can cause substantial differences in measured GFR; published, estimated mean GFR for different methodologies can range from 1.38 to 4.85 mL/min/kg for dogs and 0.85 to 3.05 mL/min/kg for cats (Supplemental Tables).[18–20,33,41–45] Inulin clearance is generally considered the "ideal" method for measuring GFR because inulin is safe and inert, freely filtered through the glomerulus, not bound to any plasma proteins, and neither reabsorbed nor secreted by the renal tubules.[46,47] Nevertheless, inulin clearance is rarely performed because it is not widely available, is technically challenging and requires 24-h collection of all urine produced in a metabolic cage or with urethral catheterization.[47,48] Scintigraphy using radiolabeled markers, including ^{125}I sodium iothalamate, ^{131}I sodium iodohippurate, ^{51}Cr-EDTA, and ^{99}Tc-DTPA can measure either global GFR or GFR of individual kidneys, but requires handling of radioactive waste and animals.

Cr clearance (endogenous or exogenous) techniques to measure GFR are easier to perform in clinical practice. Comparisons of exogenous Cr clearance have generally found a good correlation with inulin clearance in dogs, but results may underestimate GFR.[49–51] Although early studies suggested exogenous Cr clearance with continuous infusion may not be a good indicator of GFR in cats,[52,53] more recent feline studies suggest that bolus creatinine injections may yield a reasonable measurement of GFR.[51,54,55] Creatinine clearance measurements are susceptible to overestimation of creatinine if Jaffe methods are used to measure sCr.[56,57]

Plasma iohexol clearance is also commonly used to measure GFR in cats and dogs. Iohexol is an iodinated contrast agent that is excreted unchanged in urine with a half-life of 74 minutes.[58] Unlike many contrast agents, iohexol is not believed to damage the kidneys.[41] Two stereoisomers, endo- and exo-iohexol, can produce different results[59–61] and the use of exo-iohexol has higher reproducibility.[54,55,62,63] Published protocols use widely varying numbers of plasma samples with different timing to measure iohexol clearance.[41,64,65] These differences in the type of iohexol and protocols should be accounted for when comparing results across published studies. Iohexol clearance has not been compared directly to inulin clearance in cats and dogs; rather, it has primarily been validated through comparison with exogenous Cr clearance.[60,61]

GFR can vary within individuals due to a variety of factors, including hydration, diet, medications, and diurnal variation.[52,66–69] Factors contributing to variation within the population are still poorly defined for cats and dogs. Estimated GFR for human samples is routinely calculated from sCr normalized to body surface area (rather than weight) and corrected for age, sex, and race, but the ideal standardization method(s) for measured GFR across dogs is still under investigation.[41] Body weight is often used to standardize GFR across dogs of different sizes, but metabolic scaling in very large and small dogs may result in nonlinear relationships between GFR and body weight (**Fig. 1**).[34,41] Age and sex do not seem to substantially impact GFR in dogs.[41] There have not been thorough investigations of the impact of breed on GFR for either dogs or cats. McKenna et al. (2019) recently published a strategy for estimating the degree of reduction in GFR for dogs with confirmed or suspected CKD by comparing individual GFR to mean GFR of the appropriate body weight category. Only dogs with a clinical indication for measuring GFR were used to generate the mean GFR for the groups. Estimated decreases in GFR greater than 20% identified some dogs without increased sCr that were later diagnosed with CKD or other kidney pathologies.[45] Further evaluation will be needed to understand the applicability of this strategy to a wider population and which normalization technique(s) are best for estimating individual GFR and comparing with the population.

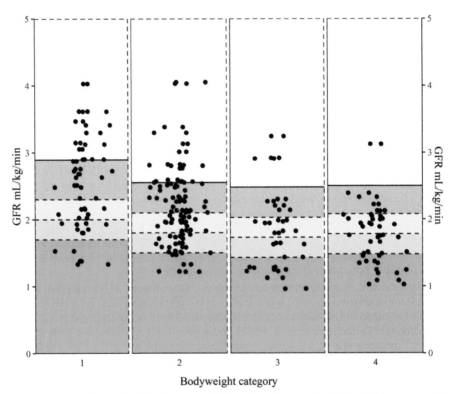

Fig. 1. Canine glomerular filtration rate (GFR) estimation results (mL/kg/min) represented graphically, separated by body weight Categories 1 (1.8–12.4 kg), 2(13.2–25.5 kg), 3 (25.7–31.6 kg), and 4 (32.0–70.3 kg). Each dot represents the GFR result from a patient. The area on each chart with a green background represents a GFR decrease of less than 20% from the mean GFR of the body weight category, the yellow background represents a GFR decrease of ≥ 20% but less than 30% from mean GFR, the orange background represents a ≥ 30% but less than 40% decrease in GFR from mean GFR, and the red background represents a ≥ 40% decrease in GFR from the mean GFR. (Recreated with data from Mckenna and colleagues 2020 https://doi.org/10.1111/jvim.15561).

Relationship of symmetric dimethylarginine and serum creatinine to decreased glomerular filtration rate

SCr and SDMA are the most common surrogate markers for GFR in veterinary medicine. Both sCr and SDMA inversely correlate with GFR, but do not perfectly correlate with each other.[18–20,35,36,45,70] SCr has an exponential relationship with GFR such that at low sCr small changes can represent large changes in GFR, and then at higher sCr, large changes in sCr represent small changes in GFR.[6] SDMA, on the other hand, has a linear relationship with GFR.[33] SDMA increases above the reference interval (RI) with an average of 40% reduction in GFR, while SCr does not increase above the RI until approximately 75% reduction in GFR.[18–20,33,50] Trending of sCr over time can detect smaller changes in GFR with relatively small changes in sCr when sCr remains within the RI; however this approach requires historical baseline data for the individual dog or cat as there can be inter-individual variability in the homeostatic set point for creatinine.

Methodological differences can contribute to analytical variability when comparing results generated using different methodologies. Differences between sCr measured with Jaffe, modified Jaffe, and enzymatic reactions have been described.[71] Less is known about methodologic differences in SDMA. Veterinary research and publications have primarily used IDEXX Laboratories, Inc., proprietary methods to measure SDMA in the Reference Laboratories and on Catalyst analyzers. These methods are highly correlated with liquid chromatography-mass spectrometry, which is the gold standard methodology.[19,20,72,73] Recent research has investigated differences between results generated by IDEXX methodologies,[74–76] and between other commercially available methodologies.[77,78] As expected, differences were found between results from the reference laboratory methodologies and in-house module Catalyst analyzers. While these differences are often expected to be subtle it would be recommended to use the same platform for measurements whereby patient trending of SDMA concentration is clinically indicated. This would extend to exercising consistency in laboratory choice given the variety of methodologies used to measure SDMA in the current commercial market.

Comparisons of different studies around the sensitivity and specificity of sCr and SDMA for specific GFR cutoffs are complicated by differences in GFR measurement, analytical methods, concurrent diseases in the population, patient population selection, and varying GFR cutoffs (Supplemental Tables).[34–37] Most studies have found good sensitivity and specificity for both sCr and SDMA at different GFR cutoffs.[18–20,34–37,70]

Extrarenal contributors to symmetric dimethylarginine and serum creatinine

As a variety of extrarenal factors can impact the serum or plasma concentration of kidney biomarkers, including dehydration and changes in food and water consumption, and production or loss of biomarkers or their precursors, evaluation of kidney function should always include clinical history and physical examination, urinalysis, and relevant imaging findings. Evaluation of the appropriateness of the USG is important for the evaluation of kidney function.[17,21] Dehydration can increase both sCr and SDMA by temporarily decreasing plasma volume and GFR. As sCr correlates positively with muscle mass, it can provide inaccurate estimates of GFR in cats and dogs with muscle loss or heavy muscling.[19,79] Use of the World Small Animal Veterinary Association Global Nutrition Committee muscle condition scoring system (MCS),[80] or other MCS protocols, can help practitioners identify animals with poor muscle condition even if they are overweight or obese.[81,82] Diet is an often overlooked extrarenal contributor to sCr and ingestion of meat (raw or cooked) can cause a transient postprandial increase in sCr.[12,46] There are fewer known extrarenal influences on SDMA.[20,43,83–85] *In vitro* increases in SDMA production have been found in cells with alanine-glyoxylate aminotransferase 2 variants and in cells with upregulation of PRTM5.[84–86] Increased serum SDMA has been reported in people with a variety of cancers, although the mechanism of these increases remains unclear and could relate to kidney function due to infiltration, paraneoplastic effects, or increased cellular production.[87,88] There seem to be some breed-associated differences in SDMA and sCr concentrations in cats and dogs.[89–92] Greyhounds have higher homeostatic concentrations of both SDMA and sCr.[90,91,93,94] SDMA is higher in Greyhounds of all ages than in non-Greyhound breeds[90,91]; sCr is only increased in adult Greyhounds, likely due to high muscle mass.[93] Boxers appear to have a higher frequency of increased SDMA and/or sCr in puppies through adulthood but whether this is due to increased development of kidney pathology or other mechanisms is unclear.[89,95,96] Birman cats have a higher frequency of increased sCr and SDMA than other cat breeds.[92,97]

Analytical and biological variability of kidney biomarkers

There is inherent variability between measurements of any analyte due to preanalytical, analytical, and biological factors. Preanalytical variability could arise from differences affecting blood collection, storage, shipment, etc. Analytical variability arises from inherent imprecision within an instrument, between instruments, and between methodologies. Biological variability arises within an individual animal or population of animals. A robust quality management program is necessary to minimize preanalytical and analytical variability in samples measured on either reference laboratory or in-clinic analyzers. Although all analyzers need routine quality control and maintenance, there are different recommendations for quality management in reference/academic laboratories and for in-clinic analyzers. There are published recommendations for establishing robust management programs for in-clinic analyzers.[98–100]

Biological variability can occur within an individual (eg, diurnal, seasonal, hormonal, diet, aging, etc.) or between individuals within a population (eg, genetics, environment, age distribution, etc.). Biological variability is presented as the variability within an individual (CV_I) and the variability within the population (CV_G).[101] The index of individuality (IOI) and reference change value (RCV) are common ways to express clinically relevant information about the interaction of biological and analytical variability.

The IOI uses the CV_I, CV_A, and CV_G to provide information about how the amount of variability expected for an individual relates to the amount of variability expected in the population. A low IOI indicates that for a particular individual, the range of repeated measurements around the animal's homeostatic set point would fall within a narrow band of population RI (ie, there is more population variation than within-individual variation) (**Fig. 2**). For analytes with a high IOI, the range of repeated measurements around an animal's homeostatic set point may exceed the width of the population RI (ie, there is more within-individual variation than population variation) (see **Fig. 2**). Although analytes with a higher IOI have a wider range of possible results for a particular "true" value, it does not indicate that results are equally likely across that entire range; most repeated measurements would be clustered around the individual's "true" value. For cats and dogs, sCr has a low IOI and SDMA has a moderate IOI (**Table 1**).[102–106] The IOI also influences how much additional information can be gained by repeating measurements following an unexpectedly increased concentration. Assuming the patient has relatively stable kidney function over the recheck period, a second SDMA concentration is more helpful at identifying the "true" SDMA concentration and identifying false positives than a second sCr is at identifying false positives (see **Fig. 2**).[107]

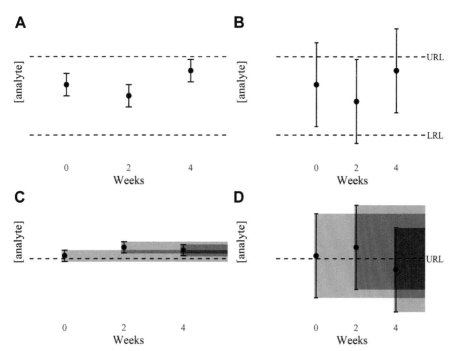

Fig. 2. Relationship of the index of individuality (IOI) to the reference interval (RI). The measured concentration is shown as a dot and the 95% confidence interval (*lines*) shows the range of possible concentrations that could be "true value" associated with this measurement. (*A,B*) Show an animal with 3 measurements over time of a hypothetical analyte whereby the concentrations at each measurement fall between the upper reference limit (URL) and lower reference limit (LRL) of the reference interval. If the hypothetical analyte has a low IOI (*A*), all measured concentrations for these "true" values should fall between the URL and LRL. However, if the analyte has a high IOI (*B*), the measured concentrations for the same "true" values could potentially fall above the URL or below the LRL. (*C,D*) Assuming stable analyte concentrations in the animal, repeated measurements of analytes can help identify false-positive increases in the analyte concentration and provide additional information about the patient's "true" value. If the analyte has a low IOI (*C*), repeated concentrations should cluster closely and minimal additional information about the likely "true" value is added. For analytes with a high IOI (*D*), more variation in measured concentrations is expected, and the repeated measurements help to narrow the range of likely "true" value.

Additionally, if there is no historical data available for comparison, it is also possible to misinterpret an sCr within the RI as representing "normal" GFR even though it is increased for the individual's homeostatic setpoint.

The RCV uses the CV_I and CV_A to identify the difference needed between 2 concentrations to determine if they are statistically different. Measuring RCV is sometimes recommended to detect a clinically significant change in analyte concentration for analytes with low IOI (<0.6) instead of using population RIs or cut-offs to detect "abnormal" results. However, the putative advantage of using RCV over population RIs to identify patients with significant changes is highly dependent on the IOI and the desired statistical power.[108] The RCV may be helpful for identifying clinically important changes for some analytes, but, similar to clinical decision points, the clinical goals and desired statistical power influence the RCV the study generates. Several

Table 1
Index of individuality (IOI) for symmetric dimethylarginine (SDMA) and serum creatinine (sCr) for cats and dogs

| | Index of Individuality (IOI) | | | |
| | Dogs | | Cats | |
Article	SDMA	sCr	SDMA	sCr
Kopke et al,[103] 2018	0.87	0.28	—	—
Hillaert et al,[102] 2021	0.73	—	—	—
Falkenö et al,[104] 2016	—	0.30	—	—
Trumel et al,[105] 2016	—	—	—	0.50
Prieto et al,[106] 2020	—	—	0.91[a]	0.45[a]

[a] Converted from inverse IOI in the original article.

studies have recently calculated RCVs for SDMA and sCr in cats and dogs based on the available biological and analytical variability for those analytes (Supplemental Tables).[75,103,106,109]

Reference intervals and clinical cutoffs

RIs for a given analyte are determined statistically by laboratories to provide a representation of the range of analyte values observed in a characterized, healthy population. In the United States, guidelines for RI generation are set out by Clinical Laboratory Standards Institute[110] and American Society for Veterinary Clinical Pathology.[111] Ideally, a minimum of 120 clinically healthy animals are prospectively selected for the purpose of generating the RI. As prospective selection and large populations are not always feasible or possible, guidelines also contain statistical guidance for smaller sample populations. RIs reflect the reference population and method used to generate that RI, so RIs may vary between laboratories, methodologies, and populations. Statistically, the RI represents the central 95% of the reference population, so 5% of the values from the RI population fall outside of the newly established RI. This indicates that some healthy animals will also have "normal" concentrations that fall outside of the RI and investigation of whether a concentration is "normal" or "abnormal" for the individual may require additional testing. As discussed above, some analytes may benefit more from individual baseline values than population RIs.

Clinical decision points, or cutoffs, serve a fundamentally different purpose from RIs. Cutoffs are intended to separate populations of animals (eg, diagnosis of disease, staging, treatment guidance, etc.) rather than define the range of results expected in a healthy population. Although cutoffs are sometimes referred to as "upper reference limits," that term refers specifically to RIs and should not be used for cutoffs. Therefore, cutoffs can, but do not necessarily, align with RIs; they may overlap with RIs, be clearly distinct from the RI, or be separated by a clinical "gray area" without a clear interpretation. Like RIs, cutoffs reflect the population and population size used to generate the cutoff; they should be applied with caution to broader populations or populations dissimilar to the study population.

Several recent studies have evaluated possible clinical decision limits for SDMA and sCr in cats and dogs. IDEXX Laboratories recommends the same SDMA cutoff of greater than 14 μg/dL for recognizing an average of 40% decrease in GFR for cats and dogs.[18] These cutoffs were generated using colony cats and dogs with and without CKD to understand the relationship between the mean decrease in GFR and the number of subjects identified by an increased SDMA above the RI.[18,19] IRIS uses a similar cutoff

Table 2
Symmetric dimethylarginine and serum creatinine in International Renal Interest Society (IRIS) chronic kidney disease staging guidelines (2019 update)

IRIS Stage	Dogs		Cats	
	SDMA (μg/dL)	sCr (mg/dL)	SDMA (μg/dL)	sCr (mg/dL)
1	< 18	< 1.4	< 18	< 1.6
2	18–35	1.4–2.8	18–25	1.6–2.8
3	36–54	2.9–5.0	26–38	2.9–5.0
4	>54	>5.0	>38	>5.0

of at least 2 SDMA concentrations greater than 14 μg/dL to diagnose CKD and different cutoffs to stage previously diagnosed CKD (**Table 2**). Two recent publications describing client-owned dogs, and one with client-owned cats, have suggested other SDMA cutoffs to identify cats and dogs with CKD. [34] [35] McKenna et al.(2020)[34] proposed clinical cutoffs of 18 μg/dL for SDMA and 1.34 mg/dL for sCr to identify subjects with at least a 40% decrease in GFR in a retrospective study of diagnostic samples submitted by referring veterinarians using a concurrently published method for estimating percentage decreased GFR[455] The population used to develop the estimated GFR included only dogs with diagnostic GFR testing. As the primary reason for clinical GFR measurement is a concern for decreased kidney excretory function, this population may have had decreased GFR compared with a healthy population which may result in lower mean values for healthy dogs and inaccurate estimates of the reduction in GFR for some patients. Pelander and colleagues (2018) prospectively enrolled dogs with a diagnosis or suspicion of stable CKD and a small number of healthy dogs to evaluate the sensitivity and specificity of SDMA, sCr, and cystatin C for identifying GFR less than 30.8 mL/min/L and suggested cutoffs of 16 μg/dL for SDMA and 1.4 mg/dL for sCr for detecting GFR at this level. These suggested cutoffs for dogs are consistent with biomarker concentrations at the border between IRIS stage 1 and 2 CKD but may not be appropriate for identifying many dogs with stage 1 CKD. Brans and colleagues (2021) proposed an SDMA cutoff of 18 μg/dL and an sCr cutoff of 1.76 mg/dL for differentiating between healthy, diabetic, and CKD cats (defined as single sCr > 1.83 mg/dL with USG <1.035) using GFR determined by iohexol. The CKD definition in this study is consistent with IRIS Stage 2 in cats, so the cutoff is not designed to differentiate healthy cats from cats with IRIS Stage 1 CKD. These dog and cat SDMA and sCr cutoffs would primarily identify cats and dogs with IRIS stage 2 and should not be confused with the upper limit of the RI.

Differences in populations, GFR methodologies, and classification of CKD underlie differences in suggested cutoffs. Ideally, further studies to identify if differences between suggested clinical decision points are due to differences in methodology, definitions of CKD, and/or decreased GFR, or populations would be valuable. Clinical decision points should always be evaluated with careful attention to the population and methodologies used to generate them and to the desired clinical goals.

CLINICAL UTILITY OF SYMMETRIC DIMETHYLARGININE
Clinical Presentation of Chronic Kidney Disease

The frequency of abnormal physical examination findings and the severity of clinical signs increase with the severity of CKD. In Stage 1 and Stage 2, clinical signs and

Table 3
Common clinical signs and physical examination findings in cats and dogs with CKD

Clinical Signs	Physical Examination Findings
Polyuria and polydipsia	Palpable kidney abnormalities
Decreased appetite	Evidence of weight loss
Weight loss	Evidence of muscle loss
Lethargy	Dehydration
Bad breath	Pallor
	Oral ulcers
	Hypertensive retinopathy

physical examination findings are often absent, although they become more common or more pronounced with later-stage CKD (**Table 3**).

Clinical biochemistry and imaging findings are particularly important in assessing kidney health in the early stages of CKD as clinical signs and examination findings are inconsistent. USG often shows adequate or appropriate urine concentration early in the disease when there are more functional nephrons. USG should always be interpreted in the context of the patient's hydration status as a wide range of USGs can be appropriate in well-hydrated healthy cats and dogs (**Table 4**). Making a diagnosis of CKD based on the IRIS CKD guidelines requires at least one of the specific findings including: increasing sCr or SDMA within the RI, persistently increased SDMA, sCr and/or BUN, inappropriate USG for the hydration status, structural kidney abnormalities identified on imaging, persistent renal proteinuria, or documented renal tubular dysfunction.

Role of Symmetric Dimethylarginine in International Renal Interest Society Guidelines for the Diagnosis and Staging of Chronic Kidney Disease

IRIS was created in 1998 to help veterinary practitioners better understand, diagnose, stage, and treat renal disease in cats and dogs. Once there is a diagnosis of CKD, the IRIS staging guidelines provide a standardized method for assessing severity and recommendations for monitoring and management of CKD. SDMA was provisionally included in the IRIS CKD staging guidelines and fully incorporated in 2019 (see **Table 2**).[9] For staging, animals should have at least 2 stably increased kidney biomarker concentrations without clinical dehydration.[9] The inclusion of SDMA in the recommendations for diagnosis and staging help identify CKD in animals with minimal to absent clinical signs or physical examination findings, have retained urine concentrating ability, or have sCr within the RI and lack historical data for trending of sCr.[9,18,19] In cases whereby SDMA indicates a higher stage than sCr, the guidelines suggest staging and treating the patient at the higher stage indicated by SDMA.[9] Evaluating SDMA and sCr together, therefore, can provide better clinical information to guide therapeutic recommendations for cats and dogs with CKD, and may be particularly beneficial in animals with muscle loss or poor body condition.[19,43]

Clinical Value of Earlier Identification of Chronic Kidney Disease

CKD is an active process and most cats and dogs experience both recognized and unrecognized active kidney injury events in the course of their disease. It is, therefore, imperative to have a diverse and robust approach to evaluating kidney function. At the time of writing, biomarkers for active kidney injury are a topic of research but

Table 4
Interpretation of urine specific gravity (USG) in evaluating urine concentrating ability adapted from Watson et al,[122] 2015

USG	Classification	Interpretation
>1.030 (dog) >1.035 (cat)	Concentrated	Indicates adequate functioning nephrons (>33% functional nephrons) Suggests potential dehydration in azotemic animals
1.013–1.029 (dog) 1.013–1.034 (cat)	Moderately concentrated	May be appropriate in well-hydrated animals Inappropriate in dehydrated animals Suggests kidney disease in azotemic animals
1.008–1.013	Isosthenuric	Inappropriate in dehydrated animals Substantial kidney disease in azotemic animals
< 1.008	Dilute	May be appropriate in overhydrated animals Suggests retention of urine diluting ability (>33% functional nephrons)

Data from Watson ADJ, Lefebvre HP, Elliot J. Using urine specific gravity. Published 2015. Accessed October 5, 2929. http://www.iris-kidney.com/education/urine_specific_gravity.html.

biomarkers of GFR are still the most available tests for functional kidney injuries.[112] SDMA has made it easier to identify cats and dogs experiencing mild declines in GFR while sCr is within the RI or corroborate animals under suspicion of early disease. Long-term serial evaluation of GFR or surrogate markers can also inform diagnosis and management recommendations for cats and dogs with CKD, though this is still an area with rapid and on-going development.[113–115] Specifically in dogs, using SDMA as part of the parameters to identify CKD is particularly supported in dogs with previous positive tests results for *Borrelia* spp., *Anaplasma* spp., *Ehrlichia* spp., or *Leishmania* spp.[116–118]

Management recommendations for IRIS Stage 1 and Stage 2 CKD focus on discontinuing nephrotoxic medications, preventing dehydration, identifying and treating concurrent diseases, and monitoring and treating hypertension and proteinuria.[10,11] Identification of Stage 1 and Stage 2 CKD may increase the likelihood of finding treatable causes of kidney disease (including pyelonephritis, borreliosis, ehrlichiosis, leishmaniasis, obstructive urolithiasis, or chronic toxicities) and preventing or slowing further kidney damage.[116–118] Even if no treatable underlying conditions are identified, earlier diagnosis and management may slow the rate of progression of CKD and improve the quality and/or quantity of life for affected animals.[15] Prescription renal diets are recommended for cats and dogs with Stage 2 disease and total phosphorus concentrations of ^{3}4.6 mg/dL.[10,11] Preliminary studies have suggested that dietary management may also benefit animals with IRIS Stage 1 CKD and slow age-associated decreases in GFR.[16,119,120] Additional research is needed to identify effective therapies for cats and dogs with Stage 1 and early Stage 2 CKD or identify subsets of cats and dogs that would benefit from therapy.

Behavior of Symmetric Dimethylarginine and Serum Creatinine in Chronic Kidney Disease

Many cats and dogs with CKD have an initial acute kidney injury or small repetitive injuries that contribute to the development of CKD.[24,25,121] In some cases these acute kidney injuries lead to clinical signs and are recognized on biochemistry results, but others likely go undetected. Many cats and dogs go through a "compensatory" stage after initial active injury and biochemical parameters may return to within the RI.[25]

These "normal" parameters may complicate practitioner recognition of the kidney damage that has occurred. This compensatory period can last for several days or many months. When interpreting these fluctuations in renal parameters, it is important to recall that cats and dogs have significant biological variability in GFR and that this biological variability may be more pronounced in animals with disease. Therefore, it is not uncommon to see SDMA or sCr fluctuate around or across the upper reference limit or around clinical decision points before becoming persistently increased.[114,115] This potential for a compensatory period and changes in reported biomarker concentrations due to biological and analytical variation emphasizes the importance of consistent follow-up testing using the same methodology, and of trending kidney biomarkers in animals with suspected or known disease.

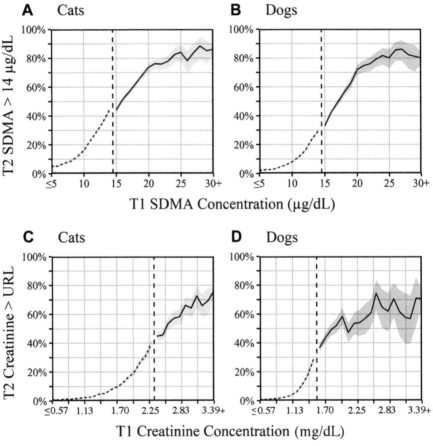

Fig. 3. Probability of an increased kidney biomarker concentration (T2) based on the biomarker concentration from the previous measurement (T1). (*A, B*) The probability of an SDMA ≥ 14 μg/dL at T2 increased with T1 SDMA concentration. (*C,D*) The probability of an sCr above the RI for cats and dogs at T2 increased with the T1 sCr value. A & B are reproduced from Mack and colleagues 2021 (https://doi.org/10.1016/j.tvjl.2021.105732) under a CC-BY copyright agreement. C & D are modified from the figures in Michael and colleagues 2021 (https://doi.org/10.1016/j.tvjl.2021.105729) to show sCr in mg/dL under a CC-BY copyright agreement.

Increased SDMA and sCr are relatively common laboratory findings. A recent study evaluated persistence or probability that the SDMA or sCr remained above the RI at the next measurement, and concordance, or agreement of increased SDMA and sCr, in more than 165,000 dogs and more than 90,000 cats.[114,115] The probabilities of persistently increased SDMA or sCr following an initial increase in SDMA or sCr concentration are shown in **Fig. 3**. Cats and dogs with an initial mild increase in SDMA (defined as 15–19 μg/dL) or any sCr above the species-specific RI had an approximately 50% probability of having persistently increased SDMA or sCr.[114,115] For animals whereby SDMA decreased to within the RI at the next measurement, approximately 50% would be expected to have at least one additional increased SDMA concentration within 12 months.[114] This study suggested that many cats and dogs with mild, persistent SDMA increases would not have increased sCr at the initial increase in SDMA but would develop increased sCr within 2 years.[114] On the other hand, cats and dogs with persistently increased sCr would be expected to already have increased SDMA at the initial increase.[115] There is, therefore, strong evidence that SDMA complements sCr, BUN, and USG in screening animals for early-stage CKD.[18–20,114,115]

SDMA and sCr do not perfectly correlate with each other and different degrees of reduction in GFR result in the biomarker concentration above their respective RIs. In some cases paired SDMA and sCr can seem discrepant, with one result within or below the RI and one above the RI. It is common for SDMA to be mildly increased in cats and dogs with sCr within or below the RI.[9,114] Increased sCr without increased SDMA is less common and occurs in approximately 2% to 4% of cat and dog results (data on file at IDEXX.). In Michael and colleagues (2021), the rate of discrepant results was higher because the cats and dogs with a prior increase in SDMA were excluded from the study, but discrepantly increased sCr usually resolved within 2 years due to an increase in SDMA or reduction in sCr.[115] Although the mechanisms of discrepantly increased sCr are unclear, differences in biomarker handling with individual kidney disease etiologies, extrarenal effects on sCr and/or SDMA, or inter-individual differences in homeostatic set points for these biomarkers are some potential contributors. IRIS staging guidelines indicate that when discrepant biomarkers affect the staging of CKD, animals should be staged and treated in accordance with stable values indicating the higher stage.[5]

SUMMARY

SDMA should be considered a staple surrogate marker of GFR for clinicians diagnosing, staging, and monitoring cats and dogs with CKD. Interpretation of SDMA concentration should be part of the total assessment of kidney function, including sCr, BUN, electrolytes, serum phosphorous and calcium, complete urinalysis, USG, UPC when indicated, complete blood count, and relevant imaging results. Adjunct tests such as infectious disease screening, blood pressure, and imaging should also be considered when clinically indicated to identify underlying diseases. Technological improvements in ultrasound imaging capability and the ability to visualize trends in analyte concentrations over time have also improved clinician's ability to diagnose patients with CKD. In addition to surrogate biomarkers for GFR (eg, SDMA and sCr), research into additional kidney biomarkers for acute kidney injury and for guiding personalized therapy recommendations will likely continue to transform diagnosis and management of CKD in the coming years.

As research into additional kidney biomarkers continues and imaging technology improves, there is a continued opportunity for recognition of patients at risk for progressive CKD or with early stages of CKD. This provides an opportunity for interventions and management to the slow progression of disease and for research into dietary interventions or targeted therapies for IRIS stage 1 and stage 2 CKD.

CLINICS CARE POINTS

- Optimal evaluation of kidney health would include SDMA alongside traditional kidney function biomarkers, urinalysis, and complete blood count.
- Establishing the nature of the kidney disease, as either acute, chronic, or acute on chronic will allow improved interpretation of SDMA and all kidney biomarkers.
- Inclusion of SDMA in pre-anesthetic, preventive care, and sick patient testing improves interpretation with trended values and individualized patient assessment.
- SDMA is available in multiple methodologies, both reference laboratory and point-of-care, while all measure SDMA given analytical variability it is suggested to trend SDMA on the same methodology for best results.

DISCLOSURE

All authors are employees of IDEXX Laboratories, Inc.

SUPPLEMENTARY DATA

Supplementary data related to this article can be found online at https://doi.org/10.1016/j.cvsm.2022.01.003. Correlation of symmetric dimethylarginine (SDMA) and serum creatinine (sCr) concentration to glomerular filtration rate (GFR) and methodology for measuring GFR in cats and dogs.

REFERENCES

1. O'Neill DG, Church DB, McGreevy PD, et al. Longevity and mortality of cats attending primary care veterinary practices in England. J Feline Med Surg 2015;17(2):125–33.
2. Conroy M, Brodbelt DC, O'Neill D, et al. Chronic kidney disease in cats attending primary care practice in the UK: a VetCompass [TM] study. Vet Rec 2019;184(17):526.
3. Fleming JM, Creevy KE, Promislow DEL. Mortality in North American Dogs from 1984 to 2004: an investigation into age-, size-, and breed-related causes of death: mortality of dogs in North America. J Vet Intern Med 2011;25(2):187–98.
4. Lulich JP, Osborne CA, O'Brien T, et al. Feline renal failure: questions, answers, questions. Compend Continuing Education Practicing Veterinarian 1992;14:127–52.
5. Marino CL, Lascelles BDX, Vaden SL, et al. Prevalence and classification of chronic kidney disease in cats randomly selected from four age groups and in cats recruited for degenerative joint disease studies. J Feline Med Surg 2014;16(6):465–72.
6. Sparkes AH, Caney S, Chalhoub S, et al. ISFM Consensus Guidelines on the Diagnosis and Management of Feline Chronic Kidney Disease. J Feline Med Surg 2016;18(3):219–39.
7. O'Neill DG, Elliott J, Church DB, et al. Chronic Kidney Disease in Dogs in UK veterinary practices: prevalence, risk factors, and survival. J Vet Intern Med 2013;27(4):814–21.

8. Perini-Perera S, Del-Ángel-Caraza J, Pérez-Sánchez AP, et al. Evaluation of Chronic Kidney Disease Progression in Dogs With Therapeutic Management of Risk Factors. Front Vet Sci 2021;8:621084.

9. International Renal Interest Society. IRIS Staging of CKD. 2019. Available at: http://www.iris-kidney.com/pdf/IRIS_Staging_of_CKD_modified_2019.pdf. Accessed April 2, 2021.

10. International Renal Interest Society. Treatment Recommendations for CKD in Dogs. 2019. Available at: http://www.iris-kidney.com/pdf/IRIS-DOG-Treatment_Recommendations_2019.pdf. Accessed October 5, 2021.

11. International Renal Interest Society. Treatment Recommendations for CKD in Cats. 2019. Available at: http://www.iris-kidney.com/pdf/IRIS_CAT_Treatment_Recommendations_2019.pdf. Accessed October 5, 2021.

12. Rudinsky AJ, Harjes LM, Byron J, et al. Factors associated with survival in dogs with chronic kidney disease. J Vet Intern Med 2018;32(6):1977–82.

13. Pedrinelli V, Lima DM, Duarte CN, et al. Nutritional and laboratory parameters affect the survival of dogs with chronic kidney disease. In: Clegg S, editor. PLoS One 2020;15(6):e0234712.

14. Boyd LM, Langston C, Thompson K, et al. Survival in Cats with Naturally Occurring Chronic Kidney Disease (2000-2002). J Vet Intern Med 2008;22(5):1111–7.

15. Grauer GF. Early Detection of Renal Damage and Disease in Dogs and Cats. Vet Clin North Am Small Anim Pract 2005;35(3):581–96.

16. Hall JA, MacLeay J, Yerramilli M, et al. Positive impact of nutritional interventions on serum symmetric dimethylarginine and creatinine concentrations in client-owned geriatric dogs. In: Aguilera AI, editor. PLoS one 2016;11(4):e0153653.

17. Paepe D, Daminet S, Feline CKD. Diagnosis, staging and screening – what is recommended? J Feline Med Surg 2013;15(1_suppl):15–27.

18. Hall JA, Yerramilli M, Obare E, et al. Serum Concentrations of Symmetric Dimethylarginine and Creatinine in Dogs with Naturally Occurring Chronic Kidney Disease. J Vet Intern Med 2016;30(3):794–802.

19. Hall JA, Yerramilli M, Obare E, et al. Comparison of serum concentrations of symmetric dimethylarginine and creatinine as kidney function biomarkers in cats with Chronic Kidney Disease. J Vet Intern Med 2014;28(6):1676–83.

20. Nabity MB, Lees GE, Boggess MM, et al. Symmetric dimethylarginine assay validation, stability, and evaluation as a marker for the early detection of Chronic Kidney Disease in dogs. J Vet Intern Med 2015;29(4):1036–44.

21. Doit H, Dean RS, Duz M, et al. What outcomes should be measured in feline chronic kidney disease treatment trials? Establishing a core outcome set for research. Prev Vet Med 2021;192:105348.

22. Dunaevich A, Chen H, Musseri D, et al. Acute on chronic kidney disease in dogs: Etiology, clinical and clinicopathologic findings, prognostic markers, and survival. J Vet Intern Med 2020;34(6):2507–15.

23. Chen H, Dunaevich A, Apfelbaum N, et al. Acute on chronic kidney disease in cats: Etiology, clinical and clinicopathologic findings, prognostic markers, and outcome. J Vet Intern Med 2020;34(4):1496–506.

24. Cowgill LD, Polzin DJ, Elliott J, et al. Is Progressive Chronic Kidney Disease a Slow Acute Kidney Injury? Vet Clin North Am Small Anim Pract 2016;46(6):995–1013.

25. Brown CA, Elliott J, Schmiedt CW, et al. Chronic Kidney Disease in aged cats: clinical features, morphology, and proposed pathogeneses. Vet Pathol 2016;53(2):309–26.

26. Debruyn K, Haers H, Combes A, et al. Ultrasonography of the feline kidney: Technique, anatomy and changes associated with disease. J Feline Med Surg 2012;14(11):794–803.

27. Hokamp JA, Cianciolo RE, Boggess M, et al. Correlation of urine and serum biomarkers with renal damage and survival in dogs with naturally occurring Proteinuric Chronic Kidney Disease. J Vet Intern Med 2016;30(2):591–601.

28. Kakimoto Y, Akazawa S. Isolation and Identification of N,N- and N,N' -Dimethylarginine, Nε-Mono-, Di-, and Trimethyllysine, and Glucosylgalactosyl- and Galactosyl-δ-hydroxylysine from Human Urine. J Biol Chem 1970;245(21): 5751–8.

29. McDermott JR. Studies on the catabolism of NG-methylarginine, NG, NG-dimethylarginine and NG, NG-dimethylarginine in the rabbit. Biochem J 1976; 154(1):179–84.

30. Schwedhelm E, Böger RH. The role of asymmetric and symmetric dimethylarginines in renal disease. Nat Rev Nephrol 2011;7(5):275–85.

31. Leone A, Moncada S, Vallance P, et al. Accumulation of an endogenous inhibitor of nitric oxide synthesis in chronic renal failure. The Lancet 1992;339(8793): 572–5.

32. Kielstein JT, Salpeter SR, Bode-Boeger SM, et al. Symmetric dimethylarginine (SDMA) as endogenous marker of renal function—a meta-analysis. Nephrol Dial Transplant 2006;21(9):2446–51.

33. Braff J, Obare E, Yerramilli M, et al. Relationship between serum symmetric dimethylarginine concentration and glomerular filtration rate in cats. J Vet Intern Med 2014;28(6):1699–701.

34. McKenna M, Pelligand L, Elliott J, et al. Relationship between serum iohexol clearance, serum SDMA concentration, and serum creatinine concentration in non-azotemic dogs. J Vet Intern Med 2020;34(1):186–94.

35. Pelander L, Häggström J, Larsson A, et al. Comparison of the diagnostic value of symmetric dimethylarginine, cystatin C, and creatinine for detection of decreased glomerular filtration rate in dogs. J Vet Intern Med 2019;33(2):630–9.

36. Brans M, Daminet S, Mortier F, et al. Plasma symmetric dimethylarginine and creatinine concentrations and glomerular filtration rate in cats with normal and decreased renal function. J Vet Intern Med 2021;35(1):303–11.

37. Hall JA, Yerramilli M, Obare E, et al. Comparison of serum concentrations of symmetric dimethylarginine and creatinine as kidney function biomarkers in healthy geriatric cats fed reduced protein foods enriched with fish oil, L-carnitine, and medium-chain triglycerides. The Vet J 2014;202(3):588–96.

38. Tatematsu S, Wakino S, Kanda T, et al. Role of nitric oxide–producing and –degrading pathways in coronary endothelial dysfunction in Chronic Kidney Disease. JASN 2007;18(3):741–9.

39. Hall JA, Yerramilli M, Obare E, et al. Serum concentrations of symmetric dimethylarginine and creatinine in cats with kidney stones. In: Aguilera AI, editor. PLoS one 2017;12(4):e0174854.

40. Pressler BM. Clinical approach to advanced renal function testing in dogs and cats. Vet Clin North Am Small Anim Pract 2013;43(6):1193–208.

41. Von Hendy-Willson VE, Pressler BM. An overview of glomerular filtration rate testing in dogs and cats. The Vet J 2011;188(2):156–65.

42. Paepe D, Lefebvre HP, Concordet D, et al. Simplified methods for estimating glomerular filtration rate in cats and for detection of cats with low or borderline glomerular filtration rate. J Feline Med Surg 2015;17(10):889–900.

43. Hall JA, Yerramilli M, Obare E, et al. Relationship between lean body mass and serum renal biomarkers in healthy dogs. J Vet Intern Med 2015;29(3):808–14.

44. Bexfield NH, Heiene R, Gerritsen RJ, et al. Glomerular Filtration Rate Estimated by 3-Sample Plasma Clearance of Iohexol in 118 Healthy Dogs. J Vet Intern Med 2008;22(1):66–73.

45. McKenna M, Pelligand L, Elliott J, et al. Clinical utility of estimation of glomerular filtration rate in dogs. J Vet Intern Med 2020;34(1):195–205.

46. Haller M, Müller W, Estelberger W, et al. Single-injection inulin clearance — a simple method for measuring glomerular filtration rate in dogs. Res Vet Sci 1998;64(2):151–6.

47. Kukanich B, Coetzee JF, Gehring R, et al. Comparative disposition of pharmacologic markers for cytochrome P-450 mediated metabolism, glomerular filtration rate, and extracellular and total body fluid volume of Greyhound and Beagle dogs. J Vet Pharmacol Ther 2007;30(4):314–9.

48. Moe L, Heiene R. Estimation of glomerular filtration rate in dogs with 99M-Tc-DTPA and iohexol. Res Vet Sci 1995;58(2):138–43.

49. Finco DR, Coulter DB, Barsanti JA. Simple, accurate method for clinical estimation of glomerular filtration rate in the dog. Am J Vet Res 1981;42(11):1874–7.

50. Finco DR, Brown SA, Crowell WA, et al. Exogenous creatinine clearance as a measure of glomerular filtration rate in dogs with reduced renal mass. Am J Vet Res 1991;52(7):1029–32.

51. Watson ADJ, Lefebvre HP, Concordet D, et al. Plasma Exogenous Creatinine Clearance Test in Dogs: Comparison with Other Methods and Proposed Limited Sampling Strategy. J Vet Intern Med 2002;16(1):22–33.

52. Ross LA, Finco DR. Relationship of selected clinical renal function tests to glomerular filtration rate and renal blood flow in cats. Am J Vet Res 1981;42(10):1704–10.

53. Uribe D, Krawiec DR, Twardock AR, et al. Quantitative renal scintigraphic determination of the glomerular filtration rate in cats with normal and abnormal kidney function, using 99mTc-diethylenetriaminepentaacetic acid. Am J Vet Res 1992;53(7):1101–7.

54. van Hoek I, Vandermeulen E, Duchateau L, et al. Comparison and Reproducibility of Plasma Clearance of Exogenous Creatinine, Exo-iohexol, Endo-iohexol, and 51Cr-EDTA in Young Adult and Aged Healthy Cats. J Vet Int Med 2007;21(5):950.

55. van Hoek I, Lefebvre HP, Kooistra HS, et al. Plasma clearance of exogenous creatinine, exo-iohexol, and endo-iohexol in hyperthyroid cats before and after treatment with radioiodine. J Vet Intern Med 2008;22(4):879–85.

56. IFCC Scientific Division. Enzymatic assays for creatinine: time for action. Clin Chem Lab Med 2008;46(4):567–72.

57. Drion I, Cobbaert C, Groenier KH, et al. Clinical evaluation of analytical variations in serum creatinine measurements: why laboratories should abandon Jaffe techniques. BMC Nephrol 2012;13(1):133.

58. Mützel W, Speck U. Pharmacokinetics and biotransformation of iohexol in the rat and the dog. Acta Radiol Suppl 1980;362:87–92.

59. Miyamoto K. Use of plasma clearance of iohexol for estimating glomerular filtration rate in cats. Am J Vet Res 2001;62(4):572–5.

60. Brown SA, Finco DR, Boudinot FD, et al. Evaluation of a single injection method, using iohexol, for estimating glomerular filtration rate in cats and dogs. Am J Vet Res 1996;57(1):105–10.

61. Finco DR, Braselton WE, Cooper TA. Relationship between plasma iohexol clearance and urinary exogenous creatinine clearance in dogs. J Vet Intern Med 2001;15(4):368–73.

62. Le Garreres A, Laroute V, De La Farge F, et al. Disposition of plasma creatinine in non-azotaemic and moderately azotaemic cats. J Feline Med Surg 2007;9(2):89–96.

63. van Hoek I, Lefebvre HP, Peremans K, et al. Short- and long-term follow-up of glomerular and tubular renal markers of kidney function in hyperthyroid cats after treatment with radioiodine. Domest Anim Endocrinol 2009;36(1):45–56.

64. Pocar P, Scarpa P, Berrini A, et al. Diagnostic potential of simplified methods for measuring glomerular filtration rate to detect chronic kidney disease in dogs. J Vet Intern Med 2019;33(5):2105–16.

65. Baklouti S, Concordet D, Borromeo V, et al. Population Pharmacokinetic Model of Iohexol in Dogs to Estimate Glomerular Filtration Rate and Optimize Sampling Time. Front Pharmacol 2021;12:634404.

66. Koopman MG, Koomen GCM, Krediet RT, et al. Circadian Rhythm of Glomerular Filtration Rate in Normal Individuals. Clin Sci 1989;77(1):105–11.

67. Calcagno PL, Rubin MI. Effect of dehydration produced by water deprivation, diarrhea and vomiting on renal function in infants. Pediatrics 1951;7(3):328–40.

68. Anastasio P, Cirillo M, Spitali L, et al. Level of hydration and renal function in healthy humans. Kidney Int 2001;60(2):748–56.

69. Finco DR, Cooper TL. Soy Protein Increases Glomerular Filtration Rate in Dogs with Normal or Reduced Renal Function. The J Nutr 2000;130(4):745–8.

70. El-Khoury JM, Bunch DR, Hu B, et al. Comparison of symmetric dimethylarginine with creatinine, cystatin C and their eGFR equations as markers of kidney function. Clin Biochem 2016;49(15):1140–3.

71. Braun JP, Lefebvre HP, Watson ADJ. Creatinine in the Dog: A Review. Vet Clin Pathol 2003;32(4):162–79.

72. El-Khoury JM, Bunch DR, Reineks E, et al. A simple and fast liquid chromatography–tandem mass spectrometry method for measurement of underivatized l-arginine, symmetric dimethylarginine, and asymmetric dimethylarginine and establishment of the reference ranges. Anal Bioanal Chem 2012;402(2):771–9.

73. Prusevich P, Patch D, Obare E, et al. Validation of a novel high throughput immunoassay for the quantification of symmetric dimethylarginine (SDMA). Am Assoc Clin Chem Ann Mtg 2015;S152.

74. Baral RM, Freeman KP. Variability of symmetric dimethylarginine in apparently healthy dogs. J Vet Intern Med 2019;33(1):7–8.

75. Baral RM, Freeman KP, Flatland B. Comparison of serum and plasma SDMA measured with point-of-care and reference laboratory analysers: implications for interpretation of SDMA in cats. J Feline Med Surg 2021;23(10):906–20.

76. Brans M, Marynissen S, Mortier F, Daminet S, Duchateau L, Paepe D. Effect of storage conditions and measurement device on serum symmetric dimethylarginine in cats and dogs. In: European College of Veterinary Internal Medicine 31st Annual Congress; 2021.

77. Ogeer J, Aucoin D, Andrews J. Antech SDMA ELISA performs well in comparison with IDEXX SDMA and liquid chromatography mass spectrometry (LCMS). 2020. Available at: https://www.antechdiagnostics.com/assets/site/downloads/AM-200-01-01_SDMA_Abstract_08-04-20_Digital.pdf. Accessed September 14, 2021.

78. Ernst R, Ogeer J, McCrann D, et al. Comparative performance of IDEXX SDMA Test and the DLD SDMA ELISA for the measurement of SDMA in canine and feline serum. In: Thamm DH, editor. PLoS One 2018;13(10):e0205030.

79. Lefebvre HP, Laroute V, Concordet D, et al. Effects of renal impairment on the disposition of orally administered enalapril, benazepril, and their active metabolites. J Vet Intern Med 1999;13(1):21–7.

80. World Small Animal Veterinary Association. Muscle Condition Score. 2013. Available at: https://wsava.org/wp-content/uploads/2020/01/Muscle-Condition-Score-Chart-for-Dogs.pdf. Accessed October 12, 2021.

81. Chandler ML, Takashima G. Nutritional Concepts for the Veterinary Practitioner. Vet Clin North Am Small Anim Pract 2014;44(4):645–66.

82. Watson AD, Church DB, Fairburn AJ. Postprandial changes in plasma urea and creatinine concentrations in dogs. Am J Vet Res 1981;42(11):1878–80.

83. Yu L, Lacorcia L, Finch S, et al. Assessment of serum symmetric dimethylarginine and creatinine concentrations in hyperthyroid cats before and after a fixed dose of orally administered radioiodine. J Vet Intern Med 2020;34(4):1423–31.

84. Lüneburg N, Lieb W, Zeller T, et al. Genome-Wide Association Study of l -Arginine and Dimethylarginines Reveals Novel Metabolic Pathway for Symmetric Dimethylarginine. Circ Cardiovasc Genet 2014;7(6):864–72.

85. Sloan SL, Renaldo KA, Long M, et al. Validation of protein arginine methyltransferase 5 (PRMT5) as a candidate therapeutic target in the spontaneous canine model of non-Hodgkin lymphoma. In: Thamm DH, editor. PLoS One 2021;16(5): e0250839.

86. Sun L, Xia WY, Zhao SH, et al. An asymmetrically dimethylarginated nuclear 90 kDa protein (p90aDMA) induced by interleukin (IL)-2, IL-4 or IL-6 in the tumor microenvironment is selectively degraded by autophagy. Int J Oncol 2016;48(6): 2461–71.

87. Bednarz-Misa I, Fleszar MG, Zawadzki M, et al. L-Arginine/NO pathway metabolites in colorectal cancer: relevance as disease biomarkers and predictors of adverse clinical outcomes following surgery. JCM 2020;9(6):1782.

88. Chachaj A, Wiśniewski J, Rybka J, et al. Asymmetric and symmetric dimethylarginines and mortality in patients with hematological malignancies—a prospective study. In: Gallyas F, editor. PLoS one 2018;13(5):e0197148.

89. Coyne M, Szlosek D, Clements C, et al. Association between breed and renal biomarkers of glomerular filtration rate in dogs. Vet Rec 2020 [Epub ahead of print].

90. Couto CG, Murphy R, Coyne M, et al. Serum symmetric dimethylarginine concentration in greyhound pups and adults. Top Companion Anim Med 2021;45: 100558.

91. Liffman R, Johnstone T, Tennent-Brown B, et al. Establishment of reference intervals for serum symmetric dimethylarginine in adult nonracing Greyhounds. Vet Clin Pathol 2018;47(3):458–63.

92. Paltrinieri S, Giraldi M, Prolo A, et al. Serum symmetric dimethylarginine and creatinine in Birman cats compared with cats of other breeds. J Feline Med Surg 2018;20(10):905–12.

93. Feeman WE, Couto CG, Gray TL. Serum Creatinine Concentrations in Retired Racing Greyhounds. Vet Clin Pathol 2003;32(1):40–2.

94. Martinez J, Kellogg C, Iazbik MC, et al. The Renin-Angiotensin-Aldosterone System in Greyhounds and Non-Greyhound Dogs. J Vet Intern Med 2017;31(4): 988–93.

95. Pelander L, Ljungvall I, Egenvall A, et al. Incidence of and mortality from kidney disease in over 600,000 insured Swedish dogs. Vet Rec 2015;176(25):656.

96. Cavalera MA, Gernone F, Uva A, et al. Clinical and histopathological features of renal maldevelopment in boxer dogs: a retrospective case series (1999–2018). Animals 2021;11(3):810.

97. Gunn-Moore D, Dodkin S, Sparkes A. Letter to the editor. J Feline Med Surg 2002;4(3):165–6.

98. Gunn-Christie RG, Flatland B, Friedrichs KR, et al. ASVCP quality assurance guidelines: control of preanalytical, analytical, and postanalytical factors for urinalysis, cytology, and clinical chemistry in veterinary laboratories. Vet Clin Pathol 2012;41(1):18–26.

99. Flatland B, Freeman KP, Vap LM, et al. ASVCP guidelines: quality assurance for point-of-care testing in veterinary medicine. Vet Clin Pathol 2013;42(4):405–23.

100. Cook JR, Hooijberg EH, Freeman KP. Quality management for in-clinic laboratories: the total quality management system and quality plan. J Am Vet Med Assoc 2021;258(1):55–61.

101. Fraser CG. Biological variation: from principles to practice. Washington, DC: AACC Press; 2013.

102. Hillaert A, Liu DJX, Daminet S, et al. Serum symmetric dimethylarginine shows a relatively consistent long-term concentration in healthy dogs with a significant effect of increased body fat percentage. In: Clegg S, editor. PLoS One 2021; 16(2):e0247049.

103. Kopke MA, Burchell RK, Ruaux CG, et al. Variability of symmetric dimethylarginine in apparently healthy Dogs: IOI of SDMA. J Vet Intern Med 2018;32(2): 736–42.

104. Falkenö U, Hillström A, von Brömssen C, et al. Biological variation of 20 analytes measured in serum from clinically healthy domestic cats. J VET Diagn Invest 2016;28(6):699–704.

105. Trumel C, Monzali C, Geffré A, et al. Hematologic and biochemical biologic variation in Laboratory Cats. J Am Assoc Lab Anim Sci 2016;55(5):503–9.

106. Prieto JM, Carney PC, Miller ML, et al. Biologic variation of symmetric dimethylarginine and creatinine in clinically healthy cats. Vet Clin Pathol 2020;49(3): 401–6.

107. Petersen PH, Sandberg S, Fraser CG, et al. Influence of index of individuality on false positives in repeated sampling from healthy individuals. Clin Chem Lab Med 2001;39(2):106–65.

108. Iglesias N, Petersen PH, Ricós C. Power function of the reference change value in relation to cut-off points, reference intervals and index of individuality. Clin Chem Lab Med (CCLM) 2005;43(4):441–8.

109. Baral RM, Freeman KP, Flatland B. Analytical quality performance goals for symmetric dimethylarginine in cats. Vet Clin Pathol 2021;50(1):57–61.

110. Clinical and Laboratory Standards Institute. Defining, establishing and verifying reference intervals in the clinical laboratory: approved guideline. 3rd edition. Pennsylvania: Clinical and Laboratory Standards Institute; 2010. p. 1–76.

111. Friedrichs KR, Harr KE, Freeman KP, et al. ASVCP reference interval guidelines: determination of de novo reference intervals in veterinary species and other related topics. Vet Clin Pathol 2012;41(4):441–53.

112. Gordin E, Gordin D, Viitanen S, et al. Urinary clusterin and cystatin B as biomarkers of tubular injury in dogs following envenomation by the European adder. Res Vet Sci 2021;134:12–8.

113. Finch NC, Syme HM, Elliott J. Repeated measurements of renal function in evaluating its decline in cats. J Feline Med Surg 2018;20(12):1144–8.
114. Mack RM, Hegarty E, McCrann DJ, et al. Longitudinal evaluation of symmetric dimethylarginine and concordance of kidney biomarkers in cats and dogs. Vet J 2021;276:105732.
115. Michael HT, Mack RM, Hegarty E, et al. A longitudinal study of the persistence of increased creatinine and concordance between kidney biomarkers in cats and dogs. Vet J 2021;276:105729.
116. Drake C, Coyne M, McCrann DJ, et al. Risk of development of Chronic Kidney Disease After Exposure to Borrelia burgdorferi and Anaplasma spp. Top Companion Anim Med 2021;42:100491.
117. Burton W, Drake C, Ogeer J, et al. Association Between Exposure to Ehrlichia spp. and Risk of Developing Chronic Kidney Disease in Dogs. J Am Anim Hosp Assoc 2020;56(3):159–64.
118. Giapitzoglou S, Saridomichelakis MN, Leontides LS, et al. Evaluation of serum symmetric dimethylarginine as a biomarker of kidney disease in canine leishmaniosis due to Leishmania infantum. Vet Parasitol 2020;277:109015.
119. Hall JA, Yerramilli M, Obare E, et al. Nutritional interventions that slow the age-associated decline in renal function in a canine geriatric model for elderly humans. J Nutr Health Aging 2016;20(10):1010–23.
120. Hall JA, Fritsch DA, Yerramilli M, et al. A longitudinal study on the acceptance and effects of a therapeutic renal food in pet dogs with IRIS-Stage 1 chronic kidney disease. J Anim Physiol Anim Nutr 2018;102(1):297–307.
121. Jepson RE. Current understanding of the pathogenesis of progressive Chronic Kidney Disease in Cats. Vet Clin North Am Small Anim Pract 2016;46(6):1015–48.
122. Watson ADJ, Lefebvre HP, Elliot J. Using urine specific gravity. 2015. Available at. http://www.iris-kidney.com/education/urine_specific_gravity.html. Accessed October 5, 2929..

Pyometra in Small Animals 2.0

Ragnvi Hagman, DVM, PhD

KEYWORDS

- Endometritis • Cystic endometrial hyperplasia • Sepsis • Aglepristone
- Prostaglandin • Cabergoline • Bromocriptine • Epidemiology

KEY FACTS

- Pyometra is a potentially life-threatening illness in middle-aged to older female pets. It is common in bitches and queens and usually diagnosed within 4 months of estrus.

- Hormones and bacteria are involved in the disease development, and progesterone plays a key role. Disorders of the endometrium such as cystic endometrial hyperplasia (CEH) are considered predisposing factors, but pyometra and CEH can develop independently.

- There are considerable age- and breed-related differences in the occurrence of pyometra, and genetic factors may contribute to an increased vulnerability in high-risk breeds.

- The diagnosis is based on case history, clinical signs and findings on physical examination, hematology and biochemistry laboratory tests, and diagnostic imaging identifying intrauterine fluid.

- Peritonitis, endotoxemia, and systemic inflammatory response syndrome are common complications of pyometra and are associated with more severe illness. Several biomarkers and inflammatory variables have been identified that may be valuable for diagnosis, prognostication, and treatment evaluation.

- The safest and most effective treatment of pyometra is surgical ovariohysterectomy, which directly removes the source of infection and prevents recurrence. Purely medical (pharmacologic) treatment can be an alternative in younger and otherwise healthy breeding animals with open cervix pyometra and without other uterine or ovarian pathologies.

 Video content accompanies this article at http://www.vetsmall.theclinics.com.

INTRODUCTION

Pyometra, literally meaning "pus-filled uterus," is a common illness in adult intact female dogs and cats and a less frequent diagnosis in other small animal species.[1,2] The disease is characterized by an acute or chronic suppurative bacterial infection of the uterus after estrum with accumulation of inflammatory exudate in the uterine lumen

Department of Clinical Sciences, Swedish University of Agricultural Sciences, PO Box 7054, Uppsala SE-75007, Sweden
E-mail address: Ragnvi.Hagman@slu.se

Vet Clin Small Anim 52 (2022) 631–657
https://doi.org/10.1016/j.cvsm.2022.01.004   **vetsmall.theclinics.com**
0195-5616/22/© 2022 The Author(s). Published by Elsevier Inc. This is an open access article under the CC BY license (http://creativecommons.org/licenses/by/4.0/).

and a variety of clinical and pathologic manifestations, locally and systemically.[3] The disease develops during the luteal phase, and progesterone plays a key role for the establishment of infection with ascending opportunistic bacteria. The pathogen most often isolated from pyometra uteri is *Escherichia coli (E. coli)*.[4–6] A wide range of clinical signs are associated with the disease, which can be life-threatening in severe cases. It is important to seek immediate veterinary care when pyometra is suspected because a patient's status may deteriorate rapidly and early intervention increases chances of survival. The diagnosis is generally straightforward but can be challenging when there is no vaginal discharge and obscure clinical signs. Surgical ovariohysterectomy (OHE) is the safest and most efficient treatment, but purely medical alternatives may be an option in some cases.

EPIDEMIOLOGY AND RISK FACTORS

Pyometra is an important disease, particularly in countries where elective neutering of healthy dogs and cats is not generally performed.[1,2,7] In Sweden, an average 20% of all bitches are diagnosed before 10 years of age and more than 50% in certain high-risk breeds. The disease generally affects middle-aged to older bitches, with a mean age at diagnosis of 7 years, and has been reported in dogs from 4 months to 18 years of age. The overall incidence rate is 199 per 10,000 dog-years at risk.[7] In cats, pyometra is not as common, which is believed to depend on less progesterone dominance due to seasonality and induced ovulation. In queens, 2.2% are diagnosed with the disease before 13 years of age, with an incidence rate of 17 cats per 10,000 cat-years at risk.[2] The mean age at diagnosis is 5.6 years, with an age range of 10 months to 20 years, and the incidence increases with age and markedly over 7 years of age.[2,8,9] There are age- and breed-related differences in the occurrence of pyometra in dogs, *i.e.* some breeds develop the illness at an earlier age and in a larger proportion than other breeds.[1,7] Breed differences have also been reported in cats diagnosed with pyometra.[2] The clear breed predisposition suggests that genetic risk factors are involved in disease development (**Tables 1** and **2**).[1,2,7,9–12] In the golden retriever, a breed that has increased risk of pyometra, a genome-wide significant association to a region on chromosome 22, localized in the *ABCC4* gene, was recently identified.[10] The findings suggests a potential causal function of this gene, which encodes a prostaglandin transporter, to the development of pyometra, but that the complex disease likely is promoted by several genetic risk factors.

Exogenous treatments with steroid hormones, such as progestogens, or estrogen compounds that increase the response to progesterone are associated with increased risk of the disease.[12,13] Pregnancy is slightly protective in dogs, an effect that is also influenced by breed.[14] Cystic endometrial hyperplasia (CEH) is believed to increase the uterine susceptibility for infection.[15,16] In cats, little is known about risk factors and protective factors but previous hormone therapy (ie, exogenous progesterone) is associated with an increased risk.[17].

CAUSE AND PATHOGENESIS

The complex pathogenesis of pyometra is not yet completely understood but involves both hormonal and bacterial factors. Although most studies have been done in dogs, the development is believed similar in cats. The uterine environment during the luteal phase is suitable for pregnancy but also for microbial growth. Progesterone stimulates growth and proliferation of endometrial glands, increased secretion, cervical closure, and suppression of myometrial contractions.[15] The local leukocyte response and uterine resistance to bacterial infection also become decreased.[18–20] Circulating

Table 1
The 10 dog breeds with highest and lowest risk of developing pyometra, expressed as proportion of bitches per breed that had developed the disease before the age of 10 years, out of the total number of bitches in that breed, as investigated in Swedish insurance data

Dog Breed at High Risk at < 10 y of Age	Proportion (%)
Bernese Mountain Dog	66
Great Dane	62
Leonberger	61
Rottweiler	58
Irish Wolfhound	58
Staffordshire Bull Terrier	54
Keeshond	52
Bull Terrier	52
Bouvier des Flandres	50
Newfoundland	50
Dog Breed at Low Risk at < 10 y of Age	
Finnish Spitz	3
Norrbotten Spitz	4
Coton de Tulear	5
Maltese	8
Gordon Setter	8
Laika	8
Saluki	10
Tibetan Terrier	10
Lancashire Bull Terrier	10
Norwich Terrier	11

Adapted from Jitpean S, Hagman R, Strom Holst B, et al. Breed variations in the incidence of pyometra and mammary tumours in Swedish dogs. Reprod Domest Anim 2012; 47(Suppl 6):347-350; with permission.

Table 2
Proportion of queens diagnosed with pyometra before the age of 10 years in different breeds/breed groups, as investigated in Swedish insurance data

Cat Breed/Breed Group and Risk at < 10 y of Age	Pyometra (%)
All breeds	2.2
Norwegian Forest cat	14.8
Birman	3.1
Persian group	3.4
Siamese group	8.8
Domestic cat	0.9

Adapted from Hagman R, Strom Holst B, Moller L, et al. Incidence of pyometra in Swedish insured cats. Theriogenology 2014;82:114-120; with permission.

concentrations of estrogen and progesterone are not usually abnormally elevated in pyometra, and increased numbers and sensitivity of hormone receptors are believed to initiate an amplified response.[21,22] Simultaneous corpora lutea and follicular cysts are more often found in bitches with pyometra, supporting a synergistic hormonal effect.[23]

Progesterone-mediated pathologic proliferation and growth of endometrial glands and formation of cysts (ie, CEH) is believed to predispose for pyometra but the 2 disorders can develop independently (**Fig. 1**).[24] Sterile fluid may accumulate in the uterine lumen, with or without CEH, which is defined as hydrometra or mucometra or, more rarely, hemometra, depending on the type of fluid and its mucin content. Clinical signs are generally subclinical or mild when there is no bacterial infection of the uterus.[3,25,26] Pseudoplacentational endometrial hyperplasia, with the endometrium organized in a placenta-like pattern, has been associated with pyometra, but its role in the development is not precisely known.[27,28]

E coli is the predominant pathogen isolated from pyometra uteri, but other species may also occur (**Table 3**).[4,29–32] More than one bacterial species can be involved, and cultures are sometimes negative.[31,32] Emphysematous pyometra is caused by gas-producing bacteria.[33] A healthy uterus eliminates bacteria that have entered during cervical opening, but the clearance capacity varies depending on the estrus cycle stage. Experimental *E coli* infection during the luteal phase more often leads to CEH/pyometra compared with other estrus cycle stages.[34] The infection is most likely ascending because the same strains are present in the gastrointestinal tract, but hematogenic spread could possibly also occur.[6,35,36] *E coli* are natural inhabitants of the vaginal flora[37] and have an increased ability to adhere to specific receptors in a progesterone-stimulated endometrium.[5] The glycosylation of the endometrium may also facilitate bacterial attachment.[38] Certain serotypes of *E coli* are more common and often exhibit the same virulence traits as isolates from urinary tract infections.[39–41] The ability to produce biofilm may be important for *E coli* in pyometra.[42,43] The same bacterial clone can frequently be isolated from the uterus and the urinary bladder in pyometra.[5,6,36]

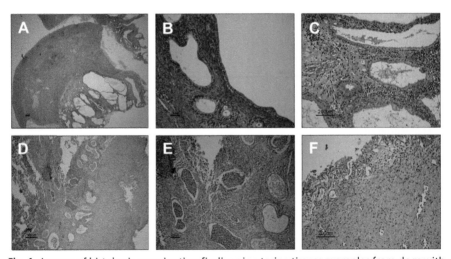

Fig. 1. Images of histologic examination findings in uterine tissues examples from dogs with CEH/pyometra. (*A*) CEH; (*B*) larger magnification of (*A*); (*C*) CEH-endometritis; (*D*) pyometra; (*E*) larger magnification of (*D*); (*F*) pyometra-atrophic endometrium.

Table 3
Bacterial species isolated from the uterus in bitches and queens with pyometra

Organism	Proportion in Bitches (%)	Proportion in Queens (%)
Escherichia coli	65–90	71
Staphylococcus spp	2–15	8
Streptococcus spp	4–23	19
Pseudomonas spp	1–8	—
Proteus spp	1–4	—
Enterobacter spp	1–3	—
Nocardia spp	1	0
Pasteurella spp	1–2	<1
Klebsiella spp	2–14	<1
Mixed culture	4–16	—
No growth	10–26	20
Mycoplasma spp, Enterococcus spp, Clostridium perfringens, Corynebacterium spp, Citrobacter spp, Moraxella spp, Edwardsiella spp, and others	<1	<1

Data from Refs.[4,5,8,9,11,31,33,54,60–62,102].

Bacteria and bacterial products are potent inducers of local and systemic inflammation. Endotoxins, lipopolysaccharide component of gram-negative bacteria such as E coli, are released into the circulation during bacterial disintegration and induce fever, lethargy, tachycardia, and tachypnea.[44–46] Higher endotoxin concentrations may cause fatal shock, disseminated intravascular coagulation, and generalized organ failure.[46,47] Pyometra has been associated with endotoxemia[47,48] and bacteremia,[49] and disseminated infection may affect various organs.[50,51] Approximately 60% of bitches and 86% of queens with pyometra suffer from sepsis (ie, life-threatening organ dysfunction caused by a dysregulated host response to an infectious process).[52,53] The illness is considered a medical emergency, and it is important to seek immediate veterinary care because a patient's health status may deteriorate rapidly.

CLINICAL PRESENTATION

Typically, middle-aged to older animals are presented up to 2 months to 4 months after estrus with a history of various signs associated with the genital tract and systemic illness (**Table 4**). A continuous or intermittent mucopurulent to hemorrhagic vaginal discharge is often present but can be absent if the cervix is closed.[54] The systemic illness is often more severe if the cervix is closed, and the uterus may become severely distended.[55] Classic systemic signs are anorexia, depression/lethargy, polydipsia, polyuria, tachycardia, tachypnea, weak pulse quality, and abnormal visible mucous membranes. Fever, dehydration, vomiting, abdominal pain on palpation, anorexia, gait abnormalities, and diarrhea are present in approximately 15% to 30% of bitches with the disease.[54,56] The most common clinical signs in queens are vaginal discharge, lethargy, and gastrointestinal disturbances, such as anorexia, vomiting, and diarrhea

Table 4
History data and clinical signs in bitches with pyometra

Case History and Clinical Signs	In Percentage (%)
Vaginal discharge[a]	57–88
Lethargy/depression[a]	63–100
Inappetence/anorexia[a]	42–87
Polydipsia[a]	28–89
Polyuria[a]	34–73
Vomiting	13–38
Diarrhea	0–27
Abnormal mucous membranes	16–76
Dehydration	15–94
Palpable enlarged uterus	19–40
Pain on abdominal palpation	23–80
Lameness	16
Distended abdomen	5
Fever	32–50
Hypothermia	3–10
Tachycardia	23–28
Tachypnea	32–40
Systemic inflammatory response syndrome	57–61

[a] Usually in greater than 50% of the bitches.
Data from Refs.[25,26,55,56,61,102,118]

(**Fig. 2**).[8,11] Vaginal discharge may be absent or concealed by fastidious cleaning habits in up to 40% of affected queens.[9] Weight loss, dehydration, polydipsia/polyuria, tachycardia, tachypnea, abdominal pain on palpation, abnormal mucous membranes (pale, hyperemic, or toxic), and unkept appearance are other findings associated with feline pyometra.

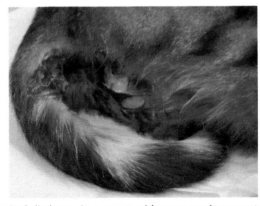

Fig. 2. Purulent vaginal discharge in a queen with open cervix pyometra.

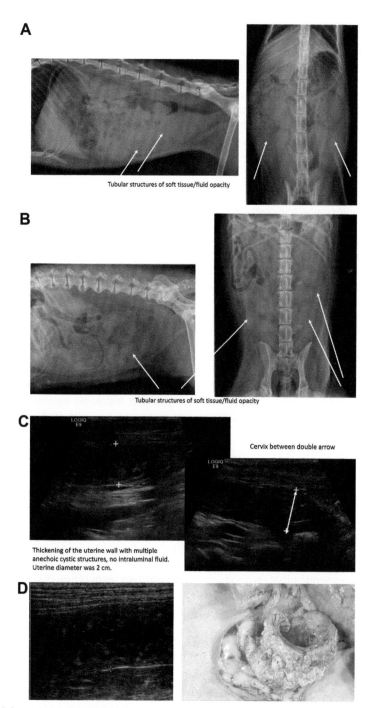

Fig. 3. (*A*) Uterine enlargement in a cat; diagnosis: pyometra. Tubular structures of soft tissue/fluid opacity (*arrows*). (*B*) Uterine enlargement in a dog; diagnosis: CEH. Tubular structures of soft tissue/fluid opacity (*arrows*). (*C*) Ultrasound images of CEH in a dog. Thickening of the uterine wall with multiple anechoic cystic structures, no intraluminal fluid. Uterine

DIAGNOSIS

The disease is easy to recognize in classic cases but can be more challenging when there is no vaginal discharge (ie, closed cervix), and the history and clinical picture are obscure. Pyometra should be a differential diagnosis in bitches and queens admitted with signs of illness after estrus, but the disease can occur at any time during the estrus cycle. The preliminary diagnosis is based on history and findings on physical and gynecologic examinations, hematology and blood biochemistry analyses, and ultrasonography and/or radiography of the abdomen. Bacteriologic culturing of the vaginal discharge is not helpful for the diagnosis because the same microbes are present in the vagina in healthy animals.[57] Careful abdominal palpation, to avoid rupture of a fragile uterus, may identify an enlarged uterus. Diagnostic imaging is valuable for determining the uterine size and to rule out other causes of uterine enlargement (**Fig. 3**). Radiography frequently identifies a large tubular structure in the caudoventral abdomen. Ultrasonography has the advantage of detecting intrauterine fluid, even when the uterine diameter is within the normal range, and of revealing additional pathologic changes of the uterine tissue and ovaries, such as ovarian cysts or CEH, which may affect the outcome of medical treatment negatively (**Fig. 4**, Video 1). In emphysematous pyometra, the gas-filled uterus is visible on diagnostic imaging (**Fig. 5**).[33,58] More advanced diagnostic imaging techniques are seldom necessary. Differential diagnoses include mucometra, hydrometra, and hemometra that may have similar clinical presentation and ultrasonography findings.[59] Vaginal cytology usually shows severe leukocyte degeneration, neutrophils and some macrophages, plasmacytes, and lymphocytes but bacterial phagocytosis is not always visible.[60] Vaginoscopy is helpful for determining the origin of a vaginal discharge and to exclude other pathologies but is usually not performed in the emergent clinical setting. The diagnosis pyometra is verified by postoperative macroscopic and histologic examination of the uterus and ovaries and microbiological examination of the uterine content.

CLINICOPATHOLOGIC TESTING—LABORATORY PARAMETERS

Hematology and biochemistry parameter abnormalities are generally investigated,[56,61] with additional tests performed depending on the health status (**Table 5**). Leukocytosis, with neutrophilia and left shift, and monocytosis are characteristic findings in pyometra together with normocytic and normochromic regenerative anemia. Renal dysfunction is common, to which endotoxemia, glomerular dysfunction, renal tubular damage, and decreased response to antidiuretic hormone contribute.[62,63] Concomitant cystitis and proteinuria usually resolve after treatment of the pyometra, but severe proteinuria that remains may predispose for renal failure.[62] Circulating inflammatory mediators and acute phase proteins are generally increased.[64,65] A hypercoagulable state is usually present.[66]

---

diameter was 2 cm. Cervix located between double-headed arrow. (*D*) CEH and pyometra—thickening of the uterine wall with multiple anechoic cystic structures; the intraluminal fluid was purulent. Both images in (*D*) are of the same uterus. The uterine diameter was 2 cm. (*E*) CEH in a rabbit. (*F*) Atrophic wall pyometra: enlarged uterus with a thin wall and echogenic intraluminal fluid. (*G*) Uterus or small intestines of the same diameter (radiograph to the left). Uterus between white double-headed arrow, CEH. Small intestine with typical layered appearance between black double-headed arrow.

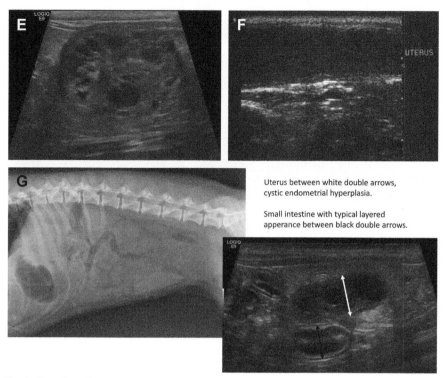

Uterus between white double arrows, cystic endometrial hyperplasia.

Small intestine with typical layered apperance between black double arrows.

Fig. 3. (*continued*).

TREATMENT ALTERNATIVES

Surgical treatment, OHE, is safest and most effective because the source of infection and bacterial products are removed and recurrence prevented.[61] Laparoscopically assisted techniques have been developed but are not commonly used and only in

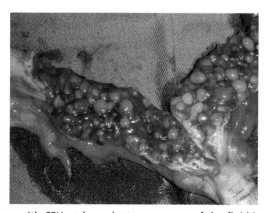

Fig. 4. Canine uterus with CEH and purulent appearance of the fluid in some cysts.

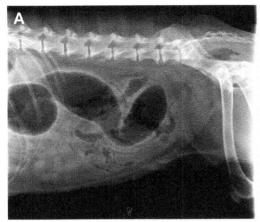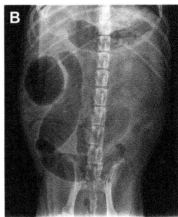

Fig. 5. (*A*, *B*) Canine emphysematous pyometra, radiography images.

mild cases.[67] Medical management (solely pharmacologic) may be possible in young and otherwise healthy breeding animals or in a patient for whom anesthesia and surgery are hazardous. In patients with serious illness or when complications, such as peritonitis or organ dysfunctions, are present or the cervix is closed, medical treatment is not recommended and surgery is the treatment of choice. Candidates for medical treatment need to be carefully selected for best prognosis for recovery and subsequent fertility.[68] Microbiological culturing and sensitivity testing are prerequisites for optimal selection of antimicrobial therapy, for which samples are obtained from the cranial vagina or postoperatively from the uterus.

SURGICAL TREATMENT

Before surgery, the patient is stabilized with adequate intravenous fluid therapy to correct hypotension, hypoperfusion, shock, dehydration, acid-base balance and electrolyte abnormalities, coagulation disturbances, and organ dysfunctions.[69] Monitoring and intervention in critically ill patients following parameters according to the "rule of 20" is recommended.[70] In moderately to severely and severely ill patients, or if sepsis or serious complications are identified, intravenous broad-spectrum bactericidal antimicrobials are administered to prevent systemic effects of bacteremia and sepsis.[71] The initial choice of antimicrobial drug should be effective against the most common pathogen *E coli* and adjusted after culture and sensitivity results to a narrow-spectrum alternative.[71] The drug should not be nephrotoxic, and the dose, route, and frequency of administration are adjusted to ascertain optimal effect. In one study, 90% of *E coli* pyometra isolates were sensitive to ampicillin.[4] The frequency of antimicrobial resistance, however, may differ by geographic location, which needs to be considered, and national regulations concerning restriction of antimicrobial usage in pets should be followed.[30,35] In life-threatening peritonitis, severe sepsis, or septic shock, a combination of antimicrobials is usually recommended for covering a wider range of pathogens.[71] If the health status is close to normal or only mildly depressed and without complications or concurrent diseases, OHE is curative for pyometra per se and antimicrobials not included in the perioperative supportive treatment.

Removal of the infection is key, and surgery should not be unnecessarily delayed due to the risk of endotoxemia and sepsis when the uterus remains in situ. Anesthesia and perioperative management are focused on maintaining hemodynamic function,

Table 5
Laboratory findings in bitches with pyometra

Abnormality	In No. of Bitches (%)
Leukopenia	4
Leukocytosis	61
Neutropenia	4
Neutrophilia	55
Monocytopenia	3
Monocytosis	60
Anemia	55
Band neutrophils	40
Band neutrophils >3%	83
Trombocytopenia	37
Toxic changes present	9
Increased ALAT	22
Hypoalbuminemia	33
Decreased ALP	49
Increased ALP	37
Increased AST	64
Cholesterolemia	74
Hypernatremia	29
Hypochloremia	2
Hypochloremia	33
Azotemia	5
BUN decreased	10
BUN increased	5
Bile acids increased	21
Hypoglycemia	6
Hyperglycemia	4
Hypokalemia	4
Hypercalcemia	6
Hypokalemia	25
Hyperlactatemia	10
Urine enzymes increased	42
Bacteriuria	25

Abbreviations: ALAT, alanine aminotransferase; ALP, alkaline phosphatase; AST, aspartate transaminase; BUN, blood urea nitrogen.
Data from Refs.[25,56,62].

gastrointestinal function and protection, pain management, cellular oxygenation, nutrition, and nursing care.[72] Certain drugs may alleviate the inflammatory response.[73] A standard OHE is performed with some modifications.[17,74] The uterus may be large, friable, and prone to rupture, and it is important to handle the tissues carefully (**Figs. 6–11**). The abdominal cavity should be protected from accidental leakage of pus via uterine

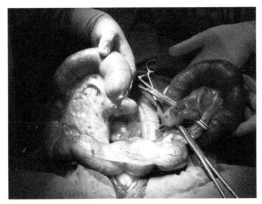

Fig. 6. Canine pyometra uterus.

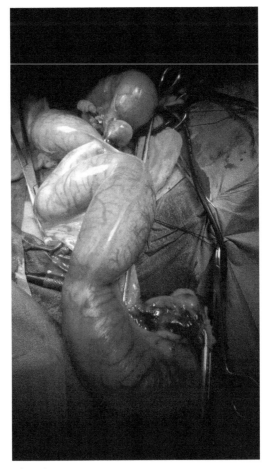

Fig. 7. Canine pyometra uterus.

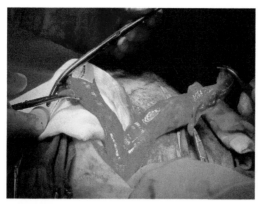

Fig. 8. Feline pyometra uterus.

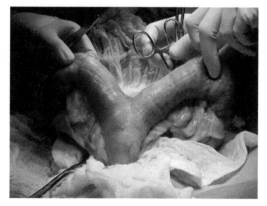

Fig. 9. Canine pyometra uterus.

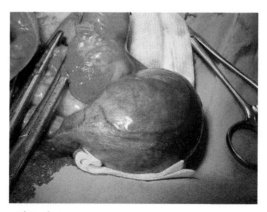

Fig. 10. Canine pyometra uterus.

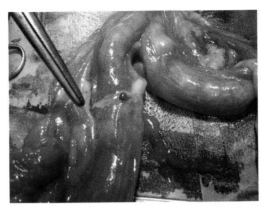

Fig. 11. Canine pyometra uterus with rupture and leakage of pus showing at the tip of the clamp.

laceration or the fallopian tubes/ovarian bursa opening by packing off the uterus with moistened laparotomy swabs (see **Fig. 11**). Vessels in the broad ligament are usually ligated. Purulent material is completely removed from the remaining cervical tissue stump, which is not oversewn. Urine for bacterial culturing can be obtained by cystocentesis when the bladder is exposed. The abdomen is routinely closed but if contaminated with pus this should be removed and the abdomen rinsed with several liters of warmed physiologic saline solution and a closed suction (or open) drainage considered.[72,74] Samples for bacterial culturing are acquired before abdominal closure if needed. For verification of the diagnosis, macroscopic and histopathologic examination of the uterus and ovaries is performed.

Intensive postoperative monitoring is essential, and in uncomplicated cases 1 day to 2 days of postoperative hospitalization is usually sufficient. The need for continued supportive care and antimicrobial therapy is evaluated several times daily on a case-by-case basis.[64] Antimicrobial therapy is discontinued as soon as possible. The overall health status and most laboratory abnormalities improve rapidly after surgery and often normalize within 2 weeks.[64,75]

Considering the seriousness of pyometra, the prognosis for survival is good and mortality rates relatively low, 3% to 20%.[1,9,56,76] If more severe systemic illness or complications, such as uterine rupture, peritonitis, or septic shock, develop, however, mortality rates can be considerably higher.[9,71,77] In queens with pyometra and uterine rupture, a mortality rate of 57% has been reported.[8] Complications develop in approximately 20% of patients with pyometra, the most common peritonitis, in 12%.[9,50,51,56,78] Other reported complications include uveitis, urinary tract infection, intracranial thromboemboli, bacterial osteomyelitis, pericarditis, myocarditis, septic arthritis, incisional swelling, dehiscence, urethral trauma, recurrent estrus, uterine stump pyometra, fistulous tracts, and urinary incontinence.[50,51,62]

MEDICAL (NONSURGICAL) TREATMENT

For purely medical (pharmacologic) management, careful patient selection is central to ensure the best possible outcome (ie, resolution of clinical illness and maintained fertility). Suitable candidates are young and otherwise healthy breeding bitches and queens with open cervix and that have no ovarian cysts. It is important that the patients are stable and not critically ill, because it may take up to 48 hours until treatment effect for some drugs used.[79] Contraindications include systemic illness, fever or hypothermia, intrauterine fetal remains, organ dysfunctions, or complications, such as peritonitis or sepsis. Adverse drug effects may occur, and endotoxemia and sepsis can quickly transform a clinically stable pyometra to an emergency. Hospitalization is therefore recommended to allow close monitoring, supportive treatments, and rapid intervention. Clinical signs, reduction, and clearing of the vaginal discharge; the uterine size; and laboratory abnormalities gradually normalize in 1 to 3 weeks.[80] OHE may be necessary without delay if complications arise or the general health status deteriorates and in refractory cases. Antimicrobials alone for treatment of pyometra may reduce the disease and prevent its progression but does not result in uterine healing.

The strategies of medical treatment are to minimize effects of progesterone by preventing its production and/or action, eliminate the uterine infection, promote relaxation of the cervix and expulsion of the intraluminal pus, and facilitate uterine healing. Commonly used drugs are natural prostaglandin $F_{2\alpha}$ ($PGF_{2\alpha}$) or its synthetic analogue cloprostenol, dopamine agonists (cabergoline and bromocriptine), or progesterone-receptor blockers (aglepristone)[81] (**Tables 6** and **7**). The available protocols for purely medical treatment of pyometra include systemic antimicrobial therapy, often recommended for 2 weeks or more.[82] The shortest effective duration of adjunctive antimicrobial therapy, however, has not been determined, and 5 days and 6 days were sufficient in 2 studies using aglepristone.[79,83] The antimicrobial drug and administration protocol should be based on bacterial culturing, sensitivity tests, and pharmacokinetics/pharmacodynamics for achieving optimal effect. Additional supportive treatment, including intravenous fluids and electrolyte supplementation, is provided depending on physical examinations and laboratory tests results.

$PGF_{2\alpha}$ is luteolytic and uterotonic and stimulates smooth musculature. Side effects, such as hypothermia, frequent defecation, diarrhea, salivation, vomiting, restlessness, shivering, and depression, are common and dose dependent and may last for approximately 1 hour after administration.[84] PGF_{2a} should be administrated far from feeding to reduce the risk of vomiting. Treatment with metoclopramide or walking the bitch for 15 minutes to 20 minutes after administration has been suggested to lessen nausea and vomiting.[81,85] Serious adverse effects of the drug ($PGF_{2\alpha}$), such as death, shock, and ventricular tachycardia, have been reported and the therapeutic window is narrow, which is why dosage calculations should be done meticulously. It is therefore very important to choose the lowest possible effective dose and hospitalize patients during treatment of monitoring and immediate intervention if severe side-effects develop. Brachycephalic breeds may be predisposed to bronchospasm, making $PGF_{2\alpha}$ contraindicated.[83,85] Owner consent, with information of potential risks, is necessary to obtain before extralabel drug usage. Several protocols are still considered experimental, because efficiency and optimal dosages have not yet been established. For natural $PGF_{2\alpha}$, i.e. dinoprost tromethamine, subcutaneous administration of 0.1 mg/kg every 12 hours to 24 hours until resolution is the dose generally recommended in bitches and queens. Despite at the lower end of the recommended range and administered once daily, this dose is associated with many undesired side effects (the recommended range includes higher doses, following evaluation of the effect of a lower dose), which is why other lower dose alternatives and drug combinations are becoming more commonly used.[84,86] Other investigators suggest starting by giving 10 µg/kg subcutaneously 5 times on the first day, gradually increasing the dose to 25µg/kg 5 times on the second day, and reaching 50 µg/kg by day 3. Doses of 50 µg/kg were then given 3 times to 5 times daily from day 3 and onward over the treatment period, a regime resulting in side effects in 15% of treated bitches.[81] A dose of 100 µg/kg natural $PGF_{2\alpha}$ administered subcutaneously once daily for 7 days resulted

Table 6
Examples of studies of medical treatment protocols for open cervix pyometra in dogs

Drug	N	Protocol and Dosage	Outcome and Side Effects	Reference
Aglepristone	24	Aglepristone 10 mg/kg SC q 24 h on day 2, 7 and 14	Recovery in 100%; recurrence after up to 54 mo 12%; fertility in 12% of 17 bitches mated	Jurka et al,[93] 2010
Aglepristone	28	Aglepristone 10 mg/kg SC q 24 h on days 1, 2, 7, 15, and 23, 29 if not cured	Recovery in 75% (resolution of clinical signs); recurrence: 48% after up to 6 y; fertility in 69% of 13 mated bitches	Ros et al,[94] 2014
Aglepristone	52	Aglepristone 10 mg/kg SC q 24 h on days 1, 2, and 7	Recovery in 92%; recurrence: 10% after 3 mo, 19% in 37 bitches followed-up to 1 y; fertility in 83% (5/6 mated bitches)	Trasch et al,[92] 2003
Aglepristone	13	Aglepristone 10 mg/kg SC q 24 h on days 1, 2, 7, and 14	Recovery in 46%	Gurbulak et al,[91] 2005
Aglepristone	20	Aglepristone 10 mg/kg SC q 24 h on days 1, 2, and 8 and if not cured on day 15	Recovery in 60%	Fieni,[79] 2006
Aglepristone + cloprostenol	32	Aglepristone 10 mg/kg SC q 24 h on days 1, 2, and 8 and if not cured on days 14 and 28 + cloprostenol: 1 µg/kg SC q 24 h on days 3–7	Recovery in 84%; no side effect of cloprostenol in 45% of the bitches; in 56% some side effects were noted: loss of appetite, lethargy, vomiting, nausea; 19% recurrence; in closed cervix pyometra cases: recovery in 76.5%, in open cervix pyometra recovery in 74.3%; 1 euthanasia due to declining health, 1 death; Follow-up time: 90 d and up to 2 y in 23 bitches; fertility in 80% (4/5 mated bitches)	Fieni,[79] 2006

Drug	N	Protocol and Dosage	Outcome and Side Effects	Reference
Aglepristone	73	Traditional protocol: aglepristone 10 mg/kg SC q 24 h on days 1, 2, and 7 (26 bitches). Modified protocol: aglepristone 10 mg/kg SC q 24 h on days 1, 3, 6, and 9 (47 bitches)	Recovery with traditional protocol in 88%; recurrence: 17%; fertility in 86% Resolution of clinical signs of pyometra with modified protocol, in 100%; recurrence: 0%; fertility in 78%; follow-up after 2 y	Contri et al,[83] 2015
Aglepristone + cloprostenol	15	Aglepristone 10 mg/kg SC q 24 h on days 1, 3, 8, and 15 (if not cured) + cloprostenol: 1 μg/kg SC q 24 h on days 3 and 8 (N = 8) or 1 μg/kg, SC q 24 h on days 3, 5, 8 10, 12, and 15 (N = 7)	Recovery in 100%, recurrence: 20% by the next estrus cycle (in all 15 bitches); fertility in 100% (1 bitch mated); no side effects reported	Gobello et al,[100] 2003
Cabergoline + cloprostenol	29	Cabergoline 5 μg/kg PO q 24 h + cloprostenol 1 μg/kg SC q 24 h for 7–14 d	Recovery in 83% by day 14, recurrence: 21%; fertility in 1/2 mated bitches. Mild side effects noted.	Corrada et al,[90] 2006
Cabergoline + cloprostenol	22	Cabergoline 5 μg/kg PO q 24 h + cloprostenol 5 μg/kg every third day SC for 7–13 d	Recovery in 90.5% by day 13; recurrence: 20%; fertility in 64% of 11 bitches mated; side effects: retching, vomiting, mild abdominal straining, diarrhea, and panting up to 60 min after administration	England et al,[80] 2007

All protocols combined with and systemic antimicrobial therapy. See the original reference for the most accurate information and more details.
Abbreviations: N, number of bitches; PO, per os; PG, prostaglandin; recovery, resolution of pyometra; SC, subcutaneous.

Table 7
Selected studies of medical treatment protocols for open cervix pyometra in cats

Drug	N	Protocol and Dosage	Outcome and Side Effects	Reference
PGF$_{2\alpha}$ (natural)	21	0.1 mg/kg SC q 12–24 h for 3–5 d (6 queens); 0.25 mg/kg was used in 15 queens but was not more effective	Resolution of signs of pyometra and return to cyclicity in 95%; treatment was repeated in 1 queen; fertility in 81%; no difference between the 2 different dosages (ie, the lower dosage recommended); transient side effects observed in 76%: vocalization, panting, restlessness, grooming, tenesmus, salivation, diarrhea, kneading, mydriasis, emesis, urination, and lordosis lasting up to 60 min. Recurrence of pyometra in 14% (3 cats)	Davidson et al,[8] 1992
Prostaglandin F$_{2\alpha}$ (synthetic analogue cloprostenol)	5	5 μg/kg SC q 24 h for 3 consecutive days	Resolution of signs of pyometra in 100%; no recurrence after 1 y; fertility in 40%; transient side effects: diarrhea, vomiting, vocalization	Garcia Mitacek et al,[101] 2014
Progesterone receptor blocker (aglepristone)	10	10 mg/kg SC q 24 h on days 1, 2, and 7 and on day 14 (if not cured)	Resolution of signs of pyometra in 90%; no recurrence after 2 y follow-up; no side effects observed	Nak et al,[96] 2009

See the original reference for the most accurate information and more details.
Abbreviations: IM, intramuscular administration; q, every; N, number of cats; PO, oral administration; SC, subcutaneous administration.

in recovery in 7 bitches, but many side effects were observed and lower doses are preferable.[87] Natural PGF$_{2\alpha}$, 20 μg/kg, was given intramuscularly 3 times daily up to 8 consecutive days in 1 study, and 30 μg/kg was given subcutaneously twice daily for 8 days in another study, resulting in resolution of the illness in 70% of 10 bitches and 100% of 7 bitches, respectively, and no side effects.[88,89] More recent low-dose protocols recommend subcutaneous administration of natural PGF$_{2\alpha}$ at a dose of 10 to 50 μg/kg every 4 to 6 hours.[82] The synthetic PGF$_{2\alpha}$ analogue cloprostenol is administered at a notably lower dose than for natural PGF$_{2\alpha}$,[87] and accurate calculations are crucial to avoid serious side effects or fatalities. For cloprostenol, subcutaneous administration of 1 μg/kg to 3 μg/kg every 12 hours to 24 hours to resolution/effect is the recommended dose for bitches and queens.[84] Subcutaneous administration of low-dose cloprostenol, 1 μg/kg, once daily was effective in 100% of 7 bitches in one study but with a high recurrence rate, 85%, and subsequent fertility rate of 14%.[87]

The dopamine agonists cabergoline and bromocriptine are effectively luteolytic from day 25 after estrus because of their antiprolactin effects and have been used together with $PGF_{2\alpha}$ for augmented treatment of pyometra.[80,81] Cabergoline usually causes less vomiting than bromocriptine, which is an advantage.[81,82,85] Cabergoline combined with a low dose of cloprostenol led to resolution of the illness in 90.5% of 22 treated bitches with pyometra in one study.[80] In another study using cabergoline and cloprostenol, 83% of 29 bitches recovered from the illness.[90] This combination was also shown the most effective compared with only low-dose cloprostenol or natural $PGF_{2\alpha}$.[86] For treatment of pyometra in cats, no clinical studies have been published on cabergoline and bromocriptine, but similar doses and regimes as for dogs have been suggested.[17]

The progesterone blocker aglepristone is commonly used in Europe for treatment of pyometra (see **Tables 6** and **7**) but is not currently approved for use in North America. Aglepristone binds to progesterone receptors effectively and competitively and without stimulating any of the hormone's effects. Side effects are usually rare and not severe and cervical relaxation induced within 48 hours.[79,83,91–94] According to the recommended protocol, 10 mg/kg aglepristone is administered subcutaneously once daily on days 1, 2, and 7 or 8 and on days 14 and 28 if not cured. This protocol results in success rates of 46% to 100%, recurrence rates 0% to 48%, and subsequent fertility rates of 69% to 85%.[95] Aglepristone was administered more frequently (on days 1, 3, 6, and 9) in a modified protocol, which resulted in resolution of the illness in all 47 treated bitches and with no reported recurrence for up to 2 years.[83] Treatment with aglepristone resulted in resolution of pyometra in 9 of 10 queens, with no recurrence reported after 2 years and no side effects observed (see **Table 7**).[96]

Local treatment methods of pyometra have been shown effective but are not yet commonly used in clinical practice in bitches and have not been reported in cats.[97] Intravaginal infusion of prostaglandins and antimicrobials yielded successful result in 15 of 17 treated bitches, without side effects or recurrence after 12 months.[98] Aglepristone, in combination with intrauterine antimicrobials, was successful in 9 of 11 bitches.[91] Intrauterine drainage through transcervical catheters may facilitate recovery in refractory cases.[97] Surgical drainage and intrauterine lavage resulted infertility in 100% of 8 treated bitches.[99] Whether prostaglandin E_2, administered intravaginally or orally, gives a cervical relaxation that is beneficial in medical treatment protocols remains to be studied.[82,85]

PROGNOSIS AFTER MEDICAL TREATMENT

The prognosis for survival and fertility is considered guarded to good. Breeding on the subsequent estrus cycle is consistently recommended after medical treatment, to avoid recurrence. The mean reported long-term success (resolution of clinical illness) of medical treatment is approximately 86% (range 46%–100%) in dogs[76,79,80,83,87,90–92,94,100] and 95% (range 90%–100%) in cats[8,96,101] (see **Tables 6** and **7**). The prognosis for fertility after medical treatment is generally considered good, with a mean fertility rate of 70% (range 14%–100%) reported in dogs and of 60% in cats. The mean recurrence rate reported in dogs is 29% (range 0%–85%) and 0% to 14% in cats. Fertility rates after aglepristone treatment are higher in younger (<5 years) bitches and those that have no other uterine or ovarian pathology.[93,94]

PREDICTIVE MARKERS

Of clinical and laboratory parameters investigated, leukopenia has been associated with both presence of peritonitis and increased postoperative hospitalization in surgically treated bitches with pyometra.[56] Concentrations of the acute-phase proteins, C-reactive protein, and serum amyloid A are increased in sepsis.[78,102] Concentrations of C-reactive protein and $PGF_{2\alpha}$ have been linked with length of postoperative hospitalization.[25,78] Acute-phase proteins concentrations decrease gradually during postoperative recovery, and maintained or increased concentrations may indicate complications.[64,65] Persistent proteinuria and urinary protein-creatinine indicate renal disease that requires special attention.[62] Central venous oxygen saturation and base deficit and lactate levels were valuable for determining outcome in bitches with pyometra and sepsis.[103] Band neutrophil concentrations, lymphopenia and monocytosis, blood urea nitrogen greater than 30 mg/dL, and creatinine concentrations greater than 1.5 mg/dL have been associated with death.[104] Certain inflammatory variables, proteins, and measurement of cell-free DNA may be clinically useful for prognostication if cage-side tests become available.[105–107] In queens, white blood cell counts, neutrophils, band neutrophils, monocytes, and the percentage band neutrophils were positively, and albumin concentrations negatively, associated with postoperative hospitalization.[11]

DIFFERENTIATION OF PYOMETRA AND MUCOMETRA OR HYDROMETRA

Fluid in the uterine lumen is present in both pyometra and mucometra/hydrometra, and their clinical manifestations can be similar. In pyometra, however, life-threatening complications may develop because of the bacterial infection, and differentiation of these disorders is thus important to optimize treatments. Ultrasonographic examination of the uterus illustrating the fluid echogenicity and hemodynamic parameters may be helpful in some cases but is not diagnostic.[59] The health status is more depressed and lethargy and gastrointestinal disturbances more frequently observed in pyometra. More than 3 clinical signs of illness and a more pronounced inflammatory response also indicate pyometra as opposed to mucometra/hydrometra.[25,26]

PREVENTION

To diagnose and treat CEH and pyometra early is favorable, and noninvasive diagnostic methods are warranted.[108,109] Elective OHE has the advantage of being performed in a healthy animal and preventing pyometra and other uterine diseases. Because there are many negative side effects of spaying, all pros and cons of such intervention need to be thoroughly evaluated in each individual.[7,110] If breeding on the first estrus after medical treatment is not possible, close monitoring is advisable to rule out abnormalities that may emerge during the luteal phase. Progesterone receptor blockers or prostaglandins may prevent the development of pyometra in high-risk patients.[108] Some investigators recommend postponing the subsequent estrus after medical treatment of pyometra, to promote uterine healing.[81]

STUMP PYOMETRA

A stump pyometra is when pyometra develops in residual uterine tissue in incompletely spayed bitches and queens, most often because of hormone-producing ovarian remnants.[111] The clinical presentation is similar, except for a history of previous spay. Ultrasonography usually shows areas of local fluid accumulation at the tissue stump, but it may be difficult to localize the ovarian remnant tissue unless follicles

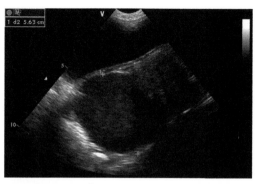

Fig. 12. Stump pyometra due to ovarian remnant.

are present (**Fig. 12**). Incomplete resection is the leading cause, but ectopic or revascularized ovarian tissue separated from the ovary during surgery have also been proposed.[111] Treatment includes surgical resection of remaining uterine and ovarian tissue, in combination with supportive treatments and antimicrobials, if indicated.

In addition to dogs and cats, pyometra has been described in many small animals such as rabbits (see **Fig. 3**), rodents, guinea pigs, hamsters, gerbils, ferrets, and chipmunks.[112–115] In other pets, the causative microbes often differ from the bacteria isolated in dogs and cats with the disease. Ultrasonography and cytology are helpful to confirm a presumptive diagnosis based on clinical signs and physical examination, and the preferred treatment is OHE. Aglepristone, combined with antibiotics, has been used successfully for medical treatment in a golden hamster and a guinea pig.[116,117]

ACKNOWLEDGMENTS

The author is very grateful for the following experts' contributions: Dr Fredrik Södersten, DVM, PhD, Swedish University of Agricultural Sciences, performed histopathology examinations and provided the images in **Fig. 1**. Dr George Mantziaras, DVM, PhD, VetRepro, Athens, Greece, provided the ultrasonography Video 1 supplementary files and the stump pyometra ultrasonography image for **Fig. 12**. Associate Professor, Kerstin Hansson, DVM, PhD, Diplomate ECVDI, Swedish University of Agricultural Sciences (SLU) and the University Animal Hospital, SLU, provided the diagnostic imaging and text in **Fig. 3**. The University Animal Hospital, SLU, is acknowledged for the radiography images in **Fig. 5**A and B.

DISCLOSURE

The author has nothing to disclose.

SUPPLEMENTARY DATA

Supplementary data related to this article can be found online at https://doi.org/10.1016/j.cvsm.2022.01.004.

REFERENCES

1. Egenvall A, Hagman R, Bonnett BN, et al. Breed risk of pyometra in insured dogs in Sweden. J Vet Intern Med 2001;15:530–8.

2. Hagman R, Strom Holst B, Moller L, et al. Incidence of pyometra in Swedish insured cats. Theriogenology 2014;82:114–20.
3. Dow C. The cystic hyperplasia-pyometra complex in the bitch. J Comp Pathol 1959;69:237–50.
4. Hagman R, Greko C. Antimicrobial resistance in Escherichia coli isolated from bitches with pyometra and from urine samples from other dogs. Vet Rec 2005;157:193–6.
5. Sandholm M, Vasenius H, Kivisto AK. Pathogenesis of canine pyometra. J Am Vet Med Assoc 1975;167:1006–10.
6. Wadas B, Kuhn I, Lagerstedt AS, et al. Biochemical phenotypes of Escherichia coli in dogs: comparison of isolates isolated from bitches suffering from pyometra and urinary tract infection with isolates from faeces of healthy dogs. Vet Microbiol 1996;52:293–300.
7. Jitpean S, Hagman R, Strom Holst B, et al. Breed variations in the incidence of pyometra and mammary tumours in Swedish dogs. Reprod Domest Anim 2012; 47(Suppl 6):347–50.
8. Davidson AP, Feldman EC, Nelson RW. Treatment of pyometra in cats, using prostaglandin F2 alpha: 21 cases (1982-1990). J Am Vet Med Assoc 1992; 200:825–8.
9. Kenney KJ, Matthiesen DT, Brown NO, et al. Pyometra in cats: 183 cases (19791984). J Am Vet Med Assoc 1987;191:1130–2.
10. Arendt M, Ambrosen A, Fall T, Kierczak M, Tengvall K, Meadows JRS, Karlsson Å, Lagerstedt AS, Bergström T, Andersson G, Lindblad-Toh K, Hagman R. The ABCC4 gene is associated with pyometra in golden retriever dogs. Sci Rep 2021;11:16647.
11. Hagman R, Karlstam E, Persson S, et al. Plasma PGF 2 alpha metabolite levels in cats with uterine disease. Theriogenology 2009;72:1180–7.
12. Niskanen M, Thrusfield MV. Associations between age, parity, hormonal therapy and breed, and pyometra in Finnish dogs. Vet Rec 1998;143:493–8.
13. Von Berky AG, Townsend WL. The relationship between the prevalence of uterine lesions and the use of medroxyprogesterone acetate for canine population control. Aust Vet J 1993;70:249–50.
14. Hagman R, Lagerstedt AS, Hedhammar A, et al. A breed-matched case-control study of potential risk-factors for canine pyometra. Theriogenology 2011;75: 1251–7.
15. Cox JE. Progestagens in bitches: a review. J Small Anim Pract 1970;11:759–78.
16. England GC, Moxon R, Freeman SL. Delayed uterine fluid clearance and reduced uterine perfusion in bitches with endometrial hyperplasia and clinical management with postmating antibiotic. Theriogenology 2012;78:1611–7.
17. Hollinshead F, Krekeler N. Pyometra in the queen: to spay or not to spay? J Feline Med Surg 2016;18:21–33.
18. Wijewardana V, Sugiura K, Wijesekera DP, et al. Effect of ovarian hormones on maturation of dendritic cells from peripheral blood monocytes in dogs. J Vet Med Sci 2015;77:771–5.
19. Rowson LE, Lamming GE, Fry RM. Influence of ovarian hormones on uterine infection. Nature 1953;171:749–50.
20. Hawk HW, Turner GD, Sykes JF. The effect of ovarian hormones on the uterine defense mechanism during the early stages of induced infection. Am J Vet Res 1960;21:644–8.
21. Chaffaux S, Thibier M. Peripheral plasma concentrations of progesterone in the bitch with pyometra. Ann Rech Vet 1978;9:587–92.

22. Prapaiwan N, Manee-In S, Olanratmanee E, et al. Expression of oxytocin, progesterone, and estrogen receptors in the reproductive tract of bitches with pyometra. Theriogenology 2017;89:131–9.

23. Strom Holst B, Larsson B, Rodriguez-Martinez H, et al. Prediction of the oocyte recovery rate in the bitch. J Vet Med A Physiol Pathol Clin Med 2001;48:587–92.

24. De Bosschere H, Ducatelle R, Vermeirsch H, et al. Cystic endometrial hyperplasia-pyometra complex in the bitch: should the two entities be disconnected? Theriogenology 2001;55:1509–19.

25. Fransson BA, Karlstam E, Bergstrom A, et al. C-reactive protein in the differentiation of pyometra from cystic endometrial hyperplasia/mucometra in dogs. J Am Anim Hosp Assoc 2004;40:391–9.

26. Hagman R, Kindahl H, Fransson BA, et al. Differentiation between pyometra and cystic endometrial hyperplasia/mucometra in bitches by prostaglandin F2alpha metabolite analysis. Theriogenology 2006;66:198–206.

27. Santana CH, Santos DO, Trindade LM, Moreira LGA, Paixao TA, Santos R. Association of pseudoplacentational endometrial hyperplasia and pyometra in dogs. J Comp Path 2020;180:79–85.

28. Schlafer DH, Gillford AT. Cystic endometrial hyperplasia, pseudo-placentational endometrial hyperplasia, and other cystic conditions of the canine and feline uterus. Theriogenology 2008;70:349–58.

29. Borresen B, Naess B. Microbial immunological and toxicological aspects of canine pyometra. Acta Vet Scand 1977;18:569–71.

30. Coggan JA, Melville PA, de Oliveira CM, et al. Microbiological and histopathological aspects of canine pyometra. Braz J Microbiol 2008;39:477–83.

31. Fransson B, Lagerstedt AS, Hellmen E, et al. Bacteriological findings, blood chemistry profile and plasma endotoxin levels in bitches with pyometra or other uterine diseases. Zentralbl Veterinarmed A 1997;44:417–26.

32. Grindlay M, Renton JP, Ramsay DH. O-groups of Escherichia coli associated with canine pyometra. Res Vet Sci 1973;14:75–7.

33. Hernandez JL, Besso JG, Rault DN, et al. Emphysematous pyometra in a dog. Vet Radiol Ultrasound 2003;44:196–8.

34. Nomura K, Yoshida K, Funahashi H, et al. The possibilities of uterine infection of Escherichia coli inoculated into the vagina and development of endometritis in bitches. Jpn J Reprod 1988;34:199–203.

35. Agostinho JM, de Souza A, Schocken-Iturrino RP, et al. Escherichia coli strains isolated from the uteri horn, mouth, and rectum of bitches suffering from pyometra: virulence factors, antimicrobial susceptibilities, and clonal relationships among strains. Int J Microbiol 2014;2014:979584.

36. Hagman R, Kuhn I. Escherichia coli strains isolated from the uterus and urinary bladder of bitches suffering from pyometra: comparison by restriction enzyme digestion and pulsed-field gel electrophoresis. Vet Microbiol 2002;84:143–53.

37. Watts JR, Wright PJ, Whithear KC. Uterine, cervical and vaginal microflora of the normal bitch throughout the reproductive cycle. J Small Anim Pract 1996;37:54–60.

38. Szczubial M, Kankofer M, Wawrykowski, et al. Activity of the glycosidases β-galactosidase, α-L-fucosidase, β-N-acetyl-hexosaaminidase, and sialidase in uterine tissues from female dogs in diestrus with and without pyometra. Therigenology 2021;177:133–9.

39. Mateus L, Henriques S, Merino C, et al. Virulence genotypes of Escherichia coli canine isolates from pyometra, cystitis and fecal origin. Vet Microbiol 2013;166:590–4.

40. Siqueira AK, Ribeiro MG, Leite Dda S, et al. Virulence factors in Escherichia coli strains isolated from urinary tract infection and pyometra cases and from feces of healthy dogs. Res Vet Sci 2009;86:206–10.

41. Chen YM, Wright PJ, Lee CS, et al. Uropathogenic virulence factors in isolates of Escherichia coli from clinical cases of canine pyometra and feces of healthy bitches. Vet Microbiol 2003;94:57–69.

42. Fiamengo TE, Runcan EE, Premanandan C, Blawut B, Coutinho da Silva MA. Evaluation of Biofilm Production by Escherichia coli Isolated From Clinical Cases of Canine Pyometra. Top Companion Anim Med 2020;39:100429.

43. Lopes CE, De Carli S, Imperico Riboldi C, de Lorenzo C, Panziera W, Driemeier D, Maboni Siquiera F. Pet pyometra: correlating bacteria pathogenicity to endometrial histological changes. Pathogens 2021;10:833.

44. Pugliese M, La Maestra R, Passantino A, Cristarella S, De Majo M, Biondi V, Quartuccio M. Electrocardiographic findings in bitches affected by closed cervix pyometra. Vet Sci 2020;7:183.

45. Van Miert ASJ, Frens J. The reaction of different animal species to bacterial pyrogens. Zentralbl Veterinarmed A 1968;15:532–43.

46. McAnulty JF. Septic shock in the dog: a review. J Am Anim Hosp Assoc 1983;19: 827–36.

47. Okano S, Tagawa M, Takase K. Relationship of the blood endotoxin concentration and prognosis in dogs with pyometra. J Vet Med Sci 1998;60:1265–7.

48. Hagman R, Kindahl H, Lagerstedt AS. Pyometra in bitches induces elevated plasma endotoxin and prostaglandin F2alpha metabolite levels. Acta Vet Scand 2006;47:55–67.

49. Karlsson I, Wernersson S, Ambrosen A, et al. Increased concentrations of C-reactive protein but not high-mobility group box 1 in dogs with naturally occurring sepsis. Vet Immunol Immunopathol 2013;156:64–72.

50. Marretta SM, Matthiesen DT, Nichols R. Pyometra and its complications. Probl Vet Med 1989;1:50–62.

51. Wheaton LG, Johnson AL, Parker AJ, et al. Results and complications of surgical treatment of pyometra: a review of 80 cases. J Am Anim Hosp Assoc 1987; 25:563–8.

52. Singer M. The new sepsis consensus definitions (Sepsis-3): the good, the not-so-bad, and the actually-quite-pretty. Intensive Care Med 2016;42:2027–9.

53. Brady CA, Otto CM, Van Winkle TJ, et al. Severe sepsis in cats: 29 cases (19861998). J Am Vet Med Assoc 2000;217:531–5.

54. Børresen B. Pyometra in the dog. II.-A pathophysiological investigation. II. Anamnestic, clinical and reproductive aspects. Nord Vet Med 1979;31:251–7.

55. Jitpean S, Ambrosen A, Emanuelson U, et al. Closed cervix is associated with more severe illness in dogs with pyometra. BMC Vet Res 2017;13:11.

56. Jitpean S, Strom-Holst B, Emanuelson U, et al. Outcome of pyometra in female dogs and predictors of peritonitis and prolonged postoperative hospitalization in surgically treated cases. BMC Vet Res 2014;10:6.

57. Bjurstrom L. Aerobic bacteria occurring in the vagina of bitches with reproductive disorders. Acta Vet Scand 1993;34:29–34.

58. Mattei C, Fabbi M, Hansson K. Radiographic and ultrasonographic findings in a dog with emphysematous pyometra. Acta Vet Scand 2018;60:67.

59. Bigliardi E, Parmigiani E, Cavirani S, et al. Ultrasonography and cystic hyperplasia- pyometra complex in the bitch. Reprod Domest Anim 2004;39:136–40.

60. Vandeplassche M, Coryn M, De Schepper J. Pyometra in the bitch: cytological, bacterial, histological and endocrinological characteristics. Vlaams Diergeneeskd Tijdschr 1991;60:207–11.
61. Hardy RM, Osborne CA. Canine pyometra: pathophysiology, diagnosis and treatment of uterine and extra-genital lesions. J Am Anim Hosp Assoc 1974;10:245–67.
62. Maddens B, Heiene R, Smets P, et al. Evaluation of kidney injury in dogs with pyometra based on proteinuria, renal histomorphology, and urinary biomarkers. J Vet Intern Med 2011;25:1075–83.
63. Asheim A. Renal function in dogs with pyometra. 8. Uterine infection and the pathogenesis of the renal dysfunction. Acta Pathol Microbiol Scand 1964;60:99–107.
64. Dabrowski R, Kostro K, Lisiecka U, et al. Usefulness of C-reactive protein, serum amyloid A component, and haptoglobin determinations in bitches with pyometra for monitoring early post-ovariohysterectomy complications. Theriogenology 2009;72:471–6.
65. Vilhena H, Figueiredo M, Cerón JJ, Pastor J, Miranda S, Craveiro H, Pires MA, Tecles F, Rubio CP, Dabrowski R, Duarte S, Silvestre-Ferreira AC, Tvarijonaviciute A. Acute phase proteins and antioxidant responses in queens with pyometra. Theriogenology 2018;115:30–7.
66. Dorsey TI, Rozanski EA, Sharp CR, et al. Evaluation of thromboelastography in bitches with pyometra. J Vet Diagn Invest 2018;30(1):165-168.
67. Becher-Deichsel A, Aurich JE, Schrammel N, et al. A surgical glove port technique for laparoscopic-assisted ovariohysterectomy for pyometra in the bitch. Theriogenology 2016;86:619–25.
68. Fieni F, Topie E, Gogny A. Medical treatment for pyometra in dogs. Reprod Domest Anim 2014;49(Suppl 2):28–32.
69. Fantoni D, Shih AC. Perioperative fluid therapy. Vet Clin North Am Small Anim Pract 2017;47:423–34.
70. Kirby R. An introduction to SIRS and the rule of 20. In: Kirby R, Linklater A, editors. Monitoring and intervention for the critically ill small animal. Ames (IA): Wiley Blackwell; 2017. p. 1–8.
71. DeClue A. Sepsis and the systemic inflammatory response syndrome. In: Ettinger SJ, Feldman EC, Cote E, editors. Textbook of veterinary internal medicine: diseases of the dogs and cat. 8th edition. St Louis (MO): Elsevier; 2016. p. 554–60.
72. Devey JJ. Surgical considerations in the emergent small animal patient. Vet Clin North Am Small Anim Pract 2013;43:899–914.
73. Liao PY, Chang SC, Chen KS, et al. Decreased postoperative C-reactive protein production in dogs with pyometra through the use of low-dose ketamine. J Vet Emerg Crit Care (San Antonio) 2014;24:286–90.
74. Tobias KM, Wheaton LG. Surgical management of pyometra in dogs and cats. Semin Vet Med Surg (Small Anim 1995;10:30–4.
75. Bartoskova A, Vitasek R, Leva L, et al. Hysterectomy leads to fast improvement of haematological and immunological parameters in bitches with pyometra. J Small Anim Pract 2007;48:564–8.
76. Feldman EC, Nelson RW. Cystic endometrial hyperplasia/pyometra complex. In: Feldman EC, Nelson RW, editors. Endocrinology and reproduction. 3rd edition. St Louis (MO): Saunders; 2004. p. 852–67.
77. Fantoni DT, Auler Junior JO, Futema F, et al. Intravenous administration of hypertonic sodium chloride solution with dextran or isotonic sodium chloride solution for treatment of septic shock secondary to pyometra in dogs. J Am Vet Med Assoc 1999;215:1283–7.

78. Fransson BA, Lagerstedt AS, Bergstrom A, et al. C-reactive protein, tumor necrosis factor alpha, and interleukin-6 in dogs with pyometra and SIRS. J Vet Emerg Crit Care 2007;17:373–81.

79. Fieni F. Clinical evaluation of the use of aglepristone, with or without cloprostenol, to treat cystic endometrial hyperplasia-pyometra complex in bitches. Theriogenology 2006;66:1550–6.

80. England GC, Freeman SL, Russo M. Treatment of spontaneous pyometra in 22 bitches with a combination of cabergoline and cloprostenol. Vet Rec 2007;160:293–6.

81. Verstegen J, Dhaliwal G. Verstegen-Onclin K. Mucometra, cystic endometrial hyperplasia, and pyometra in the bitch: advances in treatment and assessment of future reproductive success. Theriogenology 2008;70:364–74.

82. Lopate C. Pyometra, cystic endometrial hyperplasia (hydrometra, mucometra, hematometra). In: Greco DS, Davidson AP, editors. Blackwell's five-minute veterinary consult clinical companion, small animal endocrinology and reproduction. Hoboken (NJ): Wiley-Blackwell; 2017. p. 53–62.

83. Contri A, Gloria A, Carluccio A, et al. Effectiveness of a modified administration protocol for the medical treatment of canine pyometra. Vet Res Commun 2015;39:1–5.

84. Davidson A. Female and male infertility and subfertility. In: Nelson RW, Couto CG, editors. Small animal internal medicine. 5th edition. St Louis (MO): Elsevier; 2014. p. 951–65.

85. Greer M. Canine reproduction and neonatology - a practical guide for veterinarians, veterinary staff and breeders. Jackson (WY): Teton Newmedia; 2015.

86. BSAVA small animal formulary. 8th edition. Gloucester (United Kingdom): British Small Animal Veterinary Association; 2014.

87. Jena B, Rao KS, Reddy KCS, et al. Comparative efficacy or various therapeutic protocols in the treatment of pyometra in bitches. Vet Med 2013;58:271–6.

88. Arnold S, Hubler M, Casal M, et al. Use of low dose prostaglandin for the treatment of canine pyometra. J Small Anim Pract 1988;29:303–8.

89. Sridevi P, Balasubramanian S, Devanathan T, et al. Low dose prostaglandin F2 alpha therapy in treatment of canine pyometra. Indian Vet J 2000;77:889–90.

90. Corrada Y, Arias D, Rodriguez R, et al. Combination dopamine agonist and prostaglandin agonist treatment of cystic endometrial hyperplasia-pyometra complex in the bitch. Theriogenology 2006;66:1557–9.

91. Gurbulak K, Pancarci M, Ekici H, et al. Use of aglepristone and aglepristone + intrauterine antibiotic for the treatment of pyometra in bitches. Acta Vet Hung 2005;53:249–55.

92. Trasch K, Wehrend A, Bostedt H. Follow-up examinations of bitches after conservative treatment of pyometra with the antigestagen aglepristone. J Vet Med A Physiol Pathol Clin Med 2003;50:375–9.

93. Jurka P, Max A, Hawrynska K, et al. Age-related pregnancy results and further examination of bitches after aglepristone treatment of pyometra. Reprod Domest Anim 2010;45:525–9.

94. Ros L, Holst BS, Hagman R. A retrospective study of bitches with pyometra, medically treated with aglepristone. Theriogenology 2014;82:1281–6.

95. Gogny A, Fieni F. Aglepristone: a review on its clinical use in animals. Theriogenology 2016;85:555–66.

96. Nak D, Nak Y, Tuna B. Follow-up examinations after medical treatment of pyometra in cats with the progesterone-antagonist aglepristone. J Feline Med Surg 2009;11:499–502.

97. Lagerstedt A-S, Obel N, Stavenborn M. Uterine drainage in the bitch for treatment of pyometra refractory to prostaglandin F2α. J Small Anim Pract 1987;28:215–22.

98. Gabor G, Siver L, Szenci O. Intravaginal prostaglandin F2 alpha for the treatment of metritis and pyometra in the bitch. Acta Vet Hung 1999;47:103–8.
99. De Cramer KG. Surgical uterine drainage and lavage as treatment for canine pyometra. J S Afr Vet Assoc 2010;81:172–7.
100. Gobello C, Castex G, Klima L, et al. A study of two protocols combining aglepristone and cloprostenol to treat open cervix pyometra in the bitch. Theriogenology 2003;60:901–8.
101. Garcia Mitacek MC, Stornelli MC, Tittarelli CM, et al. Cloprostenol treatment of feline open-cervix pyometra. J Feline Med Surg 2014;16:177–9.
102. Jitpean S, Pettersson A, Hoglund OV, et al. Increased concentrations of Serum amyloid A in dogs with sepsis caused by pyometra. BMC Vet Res 2014;10:273.
103. Conti-Patara A, de Araujo Caldeira J, de Mattos-Junior E, et al. Changes in tissue perfusion parameters in dogs with severe sepsis/septic shock in response to goal-directed hemodynamic optimization at admission to ICU and the relation to outcome. J Vet Emerg Crit Care (San Antonio) 2012;22:409–18.
104. Kuplulu S, Vural MR, Demirel A, et al. The comparative evaluation of serum biochemical, haematological, bacteriological and clinical findings of dead and recovered bitches with pyometra in the postoperative process. Acta Veterinaria-Beograd 2009;59:193–204.
105. Hagman R. Diagnostic and prognostic markers for uterine diseases in dogs. Reprod Domest Anim 2014;49(Suppl 2):16–20.
106. Kuleš J, Horvatić A, Guillemin N, Ferreira RF, Mischke R, Mrljak V, Chadwick CC, Eckersall PD. The plasma proteome and the acute phase protein response in canine pyometra. J Proteomics 2020;223:103817.
107. Ahn S, Bae H, Kim J, et al. Comparison of clinical and inflammatory parameters in dogs with pyometra before and after ovariohysterectomy. Can J Vet Res 2021;85: 271–8.
108. Mir F, Fontaine E, Albaric O, et al. Findings in uterine biopsies obtained by laparotomy from bitches with unexplained infertility or pregnancy loss: an observational study. Theriogenology 2013;79:312–22.
109. Christensen BW, Schlafer DH, Agnew DW, et al. Diagnostic value of transcervical endometrial biopsies in domestic dogs compared with full-thickness uterine sections. Reprod Domest Anim 2012;47(Suppl 6):342–6.
110. Artl S, Wehrend A, Reichler IM. Kastration der Hundin - neue und alte Erkenntnisse zu Vor- und nachteilen. Tierärztliche Praxis Kleintiere 2017;45:253–63.
111. Ball RL, Birchard SJ, May LR, et al. Ovarian remnant syndrome in dogs and cats: 21 cases (2000-2007). J Am Vet Med Assoc 2010;236:548–53.
112. Kondert L, Mayer J. Reproductive medicine in guinea pigs, chinchillas and degus. Vet Clin North Am Exot Anim Pract 2017;20:609–28.
113. Martorell J. Reproductive disorders in pet rodents. Vet Clin North Am Exot Anim Pract 2017;20:589–608.
114. Mancinelli E, Lord B. Urogenital system and reproductive disease. Glouchester (United Kingdom): BSAVA; 2016.
115. Heap RB. Prostaglandins in pyometrial fluid from the cow, bitch and ferret. Br J Pharmacol 1975;55:515–8.
116. Engelhardt AB. Behandlung des Endometritis/Pyometrakomplexes eines Meerschweinchens - ein Fallbericht. Prakt Tierarzt 2006;87:14–6.
117. Pisu MC, Andolfatto A, Veronesi MC. Pyometra in a six-month-old nulliparous golden hamster (Mesocricetus auratus) treated with aglepristone. Vet Q 2012;32:179–81.
118. Nelson RW, Feldman EC. Pyometra. Vet Clin North Am Small Anim Pract 1986; 16:561–76.

Acute Kidney Injury in Dogs and Cats

Linda Ross, DVM, MS

KEYWORDS

- Acute kidney injury • Ischemia • Nephrotoxin • Azotemia • Oliguria

KEY POINTS

- Acute kidney injury has 4 clinical phases: initiation, extension, maintenance, and recovery.
- Various pathophysiologic mechanisms contribute to renal cellular damage and death, including degradation of ATP, cytoskeletal alterations, changes in nitric oxide, and inflammation.
- Appropriate fluid administration is key to therapy.
- The prognosis varies according to the cause of renal injury.

INTRODUCTION

Acute kidney injury (AKI) is defined as an abrupt decrease in kidney function. Categories of AKI include prerenal (hemodynamic), renal (intrinsic renal disease), and postrenal (obstructive nephropathy or rupture of the urine collecting system). Only renal AKI is discussed in this article.

The clinical course of AKI can be divided into 4 phases. The first, or initiation phase, occurs during and immediately after the insult to the kidneys when pathologic damage to the kidney occurs. The second is the extension phase, during which ischemia, hypoxia, inflammation, and cellular injury continue. Clinical and laboratory abnormalities may not be evident during the first 2 phases. The third, or maintenance phase, is usually characterized by azotemia, uremia, or both and may last for days to weeks. Oliguria (<0.5 mL urine per kilogram body weight per hour) or anuria (no urine production) may occur during this stage, although urine production is highly variable. The fourth phase is recovery, during which time renal tubular repair occurs and azotemia improves. Marked polyuria may occur during this stage as the result of partial restoration of renal tubular function and of osmotic diuresis of accumulated solutes. Renal function may return to normal, or the animal may be left with residual renal dysfunction. Milder renal pathologic conditions can result in nonazotemic renal failure and are

Department of Clinical Sciences, Cummings School of Veterinary Medicine, Tufts University, 200 Westboro Road, North Grafton, MA 01536, USA
E-mail address: linda.ross@tufts.edu

characterized by abnormalities similar to those seen during the polyuric recovery phase of AKI.[1–4]

There are many causes of AKI in dogs and cats, and the prognosis for each can vary considerably (**Box 1**). Therefore, every attempt should be made to identify the cause as early as possible in case management.[3–5]

Grading schemes for AKI have been developed for people and animals. In people, several systems have been used: the RIFLE system (risk, injury, failure, loss and end-stage disease), AKIN (acute kidney injury network), and KDIGO (kidney disease: improving global outcomes).[6] In animals, the International Renal Interest Society has developed a similar grading system (**Table 1**).[7]

PATHOPHYSIOLOGY

AKI causes decreased renal function through several mechanisms, which include decreased intrarenal blood flow and tubular cell damage. Ischemia causes rapid degradation of intracellular adenosine triphosphate (ATP), which in turns leads to damage to the renal tubular cytoskeleton. Microvillar actin cores disassemble, resulting in loss of apical microvilli. Cells lose their polarity, resulting in altered solute trafficking. In proximal tubular cells, Na^+K^+-ATPase dissociates from its normal location on the basolateral plasma membrane and is redistributed to the apical cell membrane. This redistribution results in transport of sodium and water across the apical membrane into the tubular lumen and is one of the major mechanisms causing the increased fractional excretion of sodium in ischemic AKI. Actin cytoskeleton damage also results in loss of tight and adherens junctions, resulting in a back leak of glomerular filtrate from the tubular lumen to the interstitium. Integrins are heterodimeric glycoproteins that mediate cell-cell adhesion. With ischemia, they redistribute from the basal to the apical tubular cell membrane. This results in loss of anchorage of tubular cells to the basement membrane and cell desquamation, contributing to back leak. Expression of integrin receptors may result in clumping of desquamated cells and adherence to the apical cell membrane of intact tubular cells, contributing to cast formation and tubular obstruction.[2,3,8,9]

Nitric oxide (NO) plays a variety of roles in the kidney, including regulation of local circulation and directing fluid and electrolyte reabsorption in tubules. During AKI, inducible NO increases, whereas endothelial NO decreases. This imbalance results in a loss of antithrombogenic properties of the endothelium that increases susceptibility to microvascular thrombosis, enhances neutrophil motility, and induces tubular epithelial cell injury. NO can react with superoxide to form peroxynitrite, which in turn is cytotoxic and can cause lipid peroxidation and DNA damage. Peroxynitrite and other reactive oxygen species can destabilize the cytoskeletal proteins and integrins necessary to maintain cell-cell adhesion.[8,9]

Tubular cell death in AKI can be the result of either necrosis or apoptosis. Necrosis results in cell rupture and the release of proteolytic enzymes, which then incite inflammation. Apoptosis usually occurs without inciting tissue injury or inflammation. Whether necrosis or apoptosis occurs in AKI is primarily dependent on the severity of the insult.[8,9]

The inflammatory response is now recognized as playing a major role in AKI. Neutrophils are the first cells to accumulate at the site of ischemic injury, where they release toxic granules that can induce further tissue damage. Monocytes are then recruited from the bloodstream; M1 monocytes, which release cytokines, and M2 monocytes, which differentiate into macrophages and assist in tissue repair.[10] Activated interstitial dendritic cells produce cytokines that can recruit inflammatory cells.

Box 1
Selected causes of acute kidney injury in the dog and cat

Nephrotoxins

Organic compounds
  Ethylene glycol
  Solvents
  Pesticides

Heavy metals
  Lead
  Mercury
  Arsenic
  Bismuth

Drugs
  Antibacterials
    Aminoglycosides
    Cephalosporins
    Tetracyclines
    Sulfonamides
    Penicillins
    Vancomycin
    Fluoroquinolones
  Amphotericin B
  Chemotherapeutics
    Cisplatin and carboplatin
    Doxorubicin
    Methotrexate
  Cyclosporine
  Azathioprine
  Angiotensin-converting enzyme inhibitors
  Allopurinol
  Cimetidine
  Methoxyflurane
  Lipid-lowering drugs
  Nonsteroidal anti-inflammatory drugs
  Penicillamine
  Vitamin D analogues
  Thiacetarsamide

Plants
  Grapes/raisins
  Lily plant[a]

Other toxins
  Envenomation (eg, snake, bee)
  Hemoglobin/myoglobin

Melamine/cyanuric acid

Radiographic contrast agents

Superphosphate fertilizer

Vitamin D–containing rodenticides

Infectious

Bacterial pyelonephritis

Leptospirosis

Babesiosis

Leishmaniasis
Borreliosis

Ischemia

Volume depletion

Hypotension (eg, deep anesthesia)

Hyperviscosity
   Hyperglobulinemia
   Polycythemia

Disseminated intravascular coagulation

Renal vessel thrombosis

Shock
   Hemorrhagic
   Septic

Decreased cardiac output

Other

Systemic inflammatory response syndrome

Hypercalcemia

Pancreatitis

Sepsis

Neoplasia (lymphoma)

[a] Cats only.

Table 1
International Renal Interest Society classification system for acute kidney injury

AKI Blood	Blood Creatinine (mg/dL)	Clinical Description
Grade I	<1.6	Nonazotemic AKI: a. Documented AKI: (Historical, clinical, laboratory, or imaging evidence of AKI, clinical oliguria/anuria, volume responsiveness[a]) and/or b. Progressive nonazotemic increase in blood creatinine; ≥0.3 mg/dL (≥26.4 μmol/L) within 48 h c. Measured oliguria (<1 mL/kg/h) or anuria over 6 h
Grade II	1.7–2.5	Mild AKI: a. Documented AKI and static or progressive azotemia b. Progressive azotemic increase in blood creatinine; ≥0.3 mg/dL (≥26.4 μmol/L) within 48 h, or volume responsiveness[a] c. Measured oliguria (<1 mL/kg/h) or anuria over 6 h
Grade III	2.6–5.0	Moderate to severe AKI:
Grade IV	5.1–10.0	a. Documented AKI and increasing severities of azotemia and
Grade V	>10.0	functional renal failure

[a] Volume responsive is an increase in urine production to greater than 1 mL/kg/h over 6 h and/or decrease in serum creatinine to baseline over 48 h.

Lymphocytes, especially T lymphocytes, contribute to inflammation in AKI, as does altered endothelial cell function. Many of these mechanisms are being investigated as potential therapeutic targets for prevention and/or treatment of AKI. However, this is complicated by the fact that some of these cells also participate in the repair of renal tissue in the recovery phase.[8,11]

AKI can cause distant organ injury (organ cross-talk), which can contribute to or be the cause of death. AKI is associated with increased serum levels of proinflammatory cytokines, which is consistent with systemic inflammatory response syndrome. The end result of cytokine release is inflammation, neutrophil accumulation, endothelial injury, increased lung capillary permeability, and noncardiogenic pulmonary edema.[12] Cardiac changes, such as cellular apoptosis, cardiac hypertrophy, increased cardiac macrophages, and mitochondrial damage, have been found in experimental models of AKI.[13] Acute uremia can be associated with encephalopathy, although the exact mechanism is unknown. Experimental studies in rodents have found increased neuronal pyknosis and microgliosis and elevated levels of proinflammatory cytokines (keratinocyte-derived chemoattractant and granulocyte colony-stimulating factor) in the brain. Other possible mechanisms of neurologic dysfunction include AKI-induced changes in the blood-brain barrier.[8]

DIAGNOSIS

The clinical signs of AKI are nonspecific except for a short duration of illness (hours to days). Signs may include lethargy, anorexia, vomiting, diarrhea, polydipsia/polyuria, or oliguria/anuria. Physical abnormalities are also nonspecific and may include dehydration, oral ulceration, and tongue tip necrosis. Renomegaly and renal pain can be clues to AKI as the cause of illness.

Examination of the animal with AKI should include a clinical estimate of hydration, assessment of cardiovascular status, evaluation of renal or abdominal pain, and measurement of arterial blood pressure. Radiographs can aid in the assessment of renal size and shape and the presence of uroliths, but abdominal ultrasonography is more helpful in that it allows more precise measurement of renal size, determination of the echogenicity of the renal parenchyma, and identification of cysts or masses in the kidneys. Pyelectasia may be seen with pyelonephritis, and renal hyperechogenicity with ethylene glycol (EG), grape/raisin, or lily toxicity. Subcapsular fluid accumulation may be seen with various conditions, including leptospirosis and lymphoma in cats. Intravenous (IV) urography is usually not beneficial in identifying causes of AKI because animals with an elevated serum creatinine concentration lack sufficient renal function to excrete and concentrate the contrast medium. In addition, iodinated contrast media are potentially nephrotoxic. Computerized tomography and MRI do not usually provide more information than ultrasonography and have the disadvantage of requiring general anesthesia.

Initial laboratory evaluation should include a complete blood count, serum biochemistry profile, assessment of acid-base status, urinalysis, and urine culture. Additional serum and urine should be saved in the event further tests are indicated. Leukocytosis may indicate an infectious cause of AKI. Blood urea nitrogen (BUN) and creatinine may be elevated, but AKI should not be ruled out if azotemia is not present.[2,3] Sodium concentration may be low, normal, or high depending on the disease process, degree of vomiting and/or diarrhea, and any prior therapy. Hyperkalemia occurs primarily in animals that are in the oliguric or anuric phase of AKI. Serum calcium levels are normal to low in the absence of hypercalcemia-induced AKI; hypocalcemia may occur in animals with EG toxicity. Hyperphosphatemia may be present, the degree of which reflects the severity of renal dysfunction. Metabolic acidosis is often present. Urinalysis shows isosthenuria with AKI, whereas a prerenal cause of the azotemia may be suspected with an increased urine specific gravity. Mild to moderate glucosuria may be seen with acute tubular damage. Urine pH is usually acidic, although it may be alkaline in the presence of some bacterial urinary tract infections. The urine sediment should be carefully examined for the presence of casts, white blood cells, bacteria, and crystals.

Tests to identify specific causes of AKI should be performed as appropriate to the historical findings and physical examination. Bacterial urine culture should be performed in all cases to assess for the presence of pyelonephritis. Serum EG levels can be measured using a point-of-care test, or through human medical laboratories. Available test kits measure the intact EG molecule and therefore are accurate only within the first few hours after ingestion. In the absence of blood levels, severe metabolic acidosis with an elevated anion gap or large numbers of calcium oxalate crystals in the urine sediment suggest a diagnosis of EG toxicity. Serum cholecalciferol levels should be measured in animals with hypercalcemia suspected to be due to ingestion of rodenticides containing cholecalciferol (vitamin D). Newer rodenticides are formulated with cholecalciferol instead of vitamin K antagonists, resulting in potential increases of hypercalcemic-induced AKI cases.

All dogs with AKI living in endemic areas should be tested for leptospirosis.[1,5] Microscopic agglutination titers for the most common infecting serovars can be determined. Titers may be negative or low early in the course of disease, and convalescent titers should be measured 7 to 14 days later. A 4-fold increase in titer is consistent with leptospirosis.[5,14] Acute and convalescent titers should ideally be measured by the same laboratory because there can be considerable variation in results from different laboratories.[15] Point-of-care tests are available to detect antibodies to leptospires, and polymerase chain reaction (PCR) tests to detect leptospiral DNA. None of these tests differentiate serovars, and recent Leptospira vaccination can cause false positives. False negative results can occur if testing is done early in the course of the disease before antibodies are detectable. For PCR testing, false negatives can occur if the animal has been receiving antibiotics.[14]

Histopathologic examination of renal tissue yields the most definitive information about the chronicity of the disease process but does not necessarily identify a specific cause. Because much of the therapy for AKI is the same regardless of cause, renal biopsy is indicated only when the results would change therapy or prognosis. The benefit should also be weighed against the risks of biopsy. An ultrasound-guided biopsy performed under injectable anesthesia may be the safest for the animal, although biopsies obtained via laparoscopy or laparotomy are also options. A renal aspirate is useful only when lymphoma is suspected, although false negative results may still occur.[1,3]

THERAPEUTIC OPTIONS

Treatment of AKI consists of specific therapy for the cause, in addition to supportive therapy based on the stage of acute renal failure and the animal's fluid, electrolyte, and acid-base status.

Specific Therapy

Specific therapy to correct or eliminate the cause of AKI should be instituted if the cause is known or suspected. Administration of any nephrotoxic drugs should be discontinued. Vomiting should be induced in animals with known recent toxin ingestion, such as EG, rodenticides, or lilies in cats. Animals that have been exposed to toxins should receive an antidote if available. Those that have ingested EG should receive 4-methylpyrazole (4-MP) or ethanol to prevent the metabolism of EG to its toxic components. It should be noted that cats require a higher dose of 4-MP than dogs.[16,17] The renal excretion of intact EG can be enhanced by IV fluid diuresis. Hemodialysis or therapeutic plasma exchange can also remove some toxins.[18–20] In geographic areas where leptospirosis occurs, all dogs with presumed AKI should receive antibiotics effective against leptospires (penicillin, amoxicillin, or doxycycline). Empiric therapy with an antibiotic that is primarily excreted by the kidneys is indicated for suspect pyelonephritis cases.

Supportive Therapy

Fluid therapy
Correction and maintenance of the animal's hydration, acid-base, and electrolyte status are the cornerstones of treatment for AKI. IV fluid therapy is indicated for all hospitalized patients with a diagnosis of AKI. Frequent monitoring of various parameters is key to making appropriate adjustments in therapy. These parameters include clinical assessment of hydration, body weight, mucous membrane capillary refill time, heart and respiratory rate, arterial blood pressure, packed cell volume and plasma total solids, and serum chemistry parameters, including BUN, creatinine, sodium, potassium, chloride, and phosphorus.

The initial volume of fluid to be administered should be calculated based on the animal's body weight and degree of hydration. The formula used is:

$$\text{Body weight (kg)} \times \text{estimated \% dehydration} \times 1000 = \text{fluid deficit in milliliters}$$

Fluid deficits should be replaced within 4 to 6 hours to restore normal renal blood flow (RBF). Maintenance fluid requirements must be met (44–66 mL/kg/d), in addition to estimated fluid losses from causes such as vomiting and diarrhea. An isotonic, polyionic fluid, such as lactated Ringer solution (LRS) or Plasma-Lyte A (Baxter, Deerfield, IL, USA), may be administered initially. If hyperkalemia is present or suspected because of oliguria or anuria, a potassium-free fluid, such as 0.9% sodium chloride, should be administered. Following rehydration, the type of fluid should be adjusted based on the animal's fluid and electrolyte status.[3,4] Continued administration of fluids high in sodium relative to maintenance needs may lead to hypernatremia, especially in cats. Fluids containing less sodium, such as half-strength LRS with 2.5% dextrose or 0.45% NaCl in 2.5% dextrose, may be indicated for longer maintenance therapy.[3] Traditionally, IV fluids were administered at as high a rate as the animal could tolerate without adverse signs, with the goal of maximizing glomerular filtration rate (GFR) and RBF. However, increasing fluid administration does not necessarily equate to improved renal function and survival outcomes. It has the potential to worsen AKI as the result of venous congestion and edema within the encapsulated kidney, compressing intrarenal vessels and tubules. In addition, there may be adverse effects on cardiopulmonary function, especially given the increase in pulmonary capillary permeability seen with AKI. Recent studies have found that fluid overload is associated with adverse consequences and decreased survival, especially because dialysis to remove excess fluid is not readily available to many practices.[21–24]

Measuring urine output is one of the most important and likely the most neglected aspect of monitoring animals with AKI. It is essential to accurately assess the animal's fluid balance, in addition to other fluid balance parameters (body weight, hydration status). Placement of an indwelling urinary catheter is the most accurate method for monitoring urine volume. However, the benefits of an indwelling catheter must be weighed against the risks of ascending infection, and the need for sedation or anesthesia to place the catheter. The risk of infection can be reduced by scrupulous attention to sterile placement of the catheter, maintenance of a closed collection system, and daily cleaning of the visible portions of the catheter with disinfectant. Because the incidence of catheter-induced infections increases rapidly after 3 days, changing the urinary catheter every 2 to 3 days may be beneficial.[25] For very small animals or those in which a urinary catheter cannot be placed, absorbent pads can be used to estimate urine volume. These pads are weighed before placement and after use, and the urine volume is calculated from the difference (1 kg equals approximately 1000 mL).

Management of oliguria or anuria

Once hydration has been achieved, urine flow should rapidly increase to 2 to 5 mL/kg/h, depending on the rate of IV fluid administration. If urine production is not sufficient, the clinician should first reassess the animal's hydration status. Decreased circulating blood volume can result in decreased GFR and an appropriate decrease in urine volume. If the animal is normally hydrated or volume overloaded, the rate of fluid administration should be slowed to prevent further fluid overload and associated adverse effects. An indwelling urinary catheter should be placed if not already present. Calculation of the "ins and outs" can then be used to determine appropriate quantities of IV fluids (note: this method should not be used if the animal is dehydrated). The fluid requirement for insensible losses (estimated at 22 mL/kg/d) is calculated for a short interval of time, typically 4 hours. An estimate of the amount of fluid lost owing to vomiting, diarrhea, or other loss is added. The volume of urine produced during the previous time interval is added to this amount, giving the volume of IV fluids to be administered over the subsequent 4-hour period. This regimen helps maintain hydration while minimizing the risk of fluid overload.[4,21,26]

Specific therapy to increase urine flow is the next step in the treatment of patients with oliguria/anuria. Furosemide, a loop diuretic, is the initial drug of choice. Although furosemide may increase urine output by its action on renal tubules, it does not increase GFR or improve outcome. Its value lies in increasing urine output so that IV fluid therapy to correct acid-base and electrolyte imbalances can continue. An initial dose of 2 mg/kg IV is suggested; if effective, an increase in urine production should be seen within 20 to 40 minutes. If the initial dose fails to increase urine production, escalating doses to 4 to 6 mg/kg can be administered at hourly intervals. The effective dose can continue to be given at 6- to 8-hour intervals as needed. However, studies have shown that a loading dose of 0.66 mg/kg followed by continuous rate infusion (CRI) at 0.66 mg/kg/h has been shown to be more effective than intermittent dosing in producing diuresis in normal dogs.[27] A CRI of 0.5 to 1.0 mg/kg/h is the currently recommended protocol.[3,4]

In the past, mannitol has been recommended as an option to increase urine output by osmotic diuresis. However, studies have not shown mannitol to be any more effective than volume expansion alone, and this author no longer recommends its use.[3,28]

Dopamine as a low-dose CRI was used in the past to increase urine production in oliguric or anuric animals. Dopamine stimulates 2 types of dopamine receptors (DA-1 and DA-2) in addition to α- and β-adrenergic receptors. In normal dogs, it causes an increase in RBF and urine volume; GFR increases or is unchanged. Higher doses of dopamine can result in serious adverse effects, including tachyarrhythmias, vasoconstriction, and hypertension.[29] Dopamine is no longer considered to have a role in the prevention or treatment of AKI in humans based on several meta-analyses that failed to show a clinical benefit in survival or need for dialysis.[30,31] There is little documentation on the efficacy of dopamine in dogs and cats with AKI, and its use to increase urine production in oliguric or anuric AKI is no longer recommended.

Fenoldopam is a selective DA-1 agonist that has been found to be renoprotective in humans. However, most human studies have shown that its main benefit is reduction of the risk of AKI, rather than as therapy after it occurs.[32] Some studies in healthy experimental dogs and cats found that fenoldopam infusion increased urine production.[2,33] However, one study of critically ill cats and dogs with AKI that received fenoldopam showed no improvement in survival to discharge, length of hospital stay, or improvement in renal biochemical parameters when compared with patients with AKI not receiving fenoldopam.[34] Another prospective study of dogs with heatstroke that received fenoldopam found that it had no beneficial effects on urine production, GFR, fractional excretion of sodium, or the occurrence and severity of AKI. It was not, however, associated with any observable adverse effects.[35] These clinical studies suggest that fenoldopam may not be beneficial in improving renal function or urine output in dogs and cats with AKI.

If pharmacologic measures fail to increase urine output or improve azotemia and uremia, renal replacement therapy (RRT) is indicated. A discussion of RRT is beyond the scope of this article. A partial list of veterinary centers providing RRT is available online.[36]

Management of polyuria

Animals that recover from the oliguric or anuric phase of AKI or those that have milder renal injury and do not become azotemic often have profound polyuria for days to weeks. These animals can develop electrolyte abnormalities, especially hyponatremia and hypokalemia, that need to be corrected with IV or, sometimes, oral therapy. Frequent monitoring of serum electrolytes and adjustment of therapy should be performed until urine output decreases and renal function and serum electrolyte concentrations stabilize.

Correction of acid-base and electrolyte abnormalities

Metabolic acidosis is common in animals with AKI. Alkalinizing therapy can result in significant complications, including paradoxic cerebrospinal fluid acidosis, decreased ionized serum calcium level, and hypernatremia. It is therefore not recommended unless the blood pH level is less than 7.1 or the serum bicarbonate level is less than 12 mEq/L, after correcting fluid deficits. If necessary, the bicarbonate deficit is calculated as follows:

$$\text{Body weight (kg)} \times 0.3 \times (24 - \text{animal bicarbonate}) = \text{mEq bicarbonate deficit}$$

One-half of the deficit is administered IV over 30 minutes, and acid-base status is reassessed. If the arterial blood pH is not ≥ 7.2, the remainder is given in IV fluids over the next 2 to 4 hours at which time acid-base status is again reassessed.[2]

Moderate to severe, life-threatening hyperkalemia may occur if the animal is oliguric or anuric. The first and most important step in therapy for hyperkalemia is to ensure urine production and excretion. Animals with severe hyperkalemia or those with persisting oliguria may benefit from additional specific therapy, such as with sodium bicarbonate, regular insulin, and glucose, or, in life-threatening situations, calcium gluconate, which helps protect the heart against the effects of severe hyperkalemia.[26]

Drug dosage adjustment

The dose and/or frequency of administration of drugs excreted by the kidneys may need to be adjusted in animals with AKI. This is especially true for those drugs that have a low margin of safety.[37] Formulas that use GFR can be used to calculate an adjusted dose. Serum creatinine can be substituted as an approximation for GFR, although their relationship becomes nonlinear after the creatinine exceeds 4 mg/dL:

Patient interval (h) = Normal interval (h) × serum creatinine concentration

Patient dose = Normal dose ÷ serum creatinine concentration

Treatment of other uremic complications

Vomiting. Vomiting is one of the most common signs of uremia in animals with AKI. The cause of vomiting is multifactorial and can be both centrally and locally mediated. Drugs that inhibit gastric acid production may be beneficial, including histamine receptor antagonists, such as famotidine (0.5–1 mg/kg IV, intramuscularly [IM], or subcutaneously [SC] every 12–24 hours), and proton-pump inhibitors, such as pantoprazole (1 mg/kg IV every 12–24 hours) or esomeprazole (1 mg/kg IV or SC every 12 hours). Centrally acting antiemetics may also be beneficial. Maropitant (1 mg/kg IV or SC for up to 5 days) is a neurokinin-1 receptor antagonist that has efficacy against peripheral and centrally mediated vomiting. Metoclopramide, a dopamine antagonist, may be given as intermittent therapy at a dose of 0.2 to 0.5 mg/kg every 8 hours IV, IM, or SC or as a CRI at 1 to 2 mg/kg/d IV. Another centrally acting drug is ondansetron (0.1–0.2 mg/kg every 8 hours SQ or 0.5 mg/kg IV loading dose, then 0.5 mg/kg/h CRI).

Hypertension. Arterial hypertension is common in animals with AKI and may be exacerbated by IV fluid therapy. One study found that 37% of dogs with AKI had hypertension at admission, increasing to more than 80% (62% severe) during hospitalization.[38] Another found an incidence of 75% at admission or during hospitalization with 56% severe.[39] Pharmacologic treatment consists of amlodipine (0.2–0.4 mg/kg orally every 24 hours in dogs, 0.18–0.3 mg/kg orally every 24 hours in cats). Angiotensin converting enzyme inhibitors may decrease renal perfusion and are best avoided. If the animal is overhydrated, judicious reduction of the rate of IV fluid administration is indicated.

Nutritional management

Animals with AKI usually have anorexia, and this, combined with the catabolic state of AKI, can contribute to increased morbidity and mortality. Placement of a feeding tube allows administration of enteral nutrition. If enteral nutrition is not an option (eg, significant vomiting or regurgitation) and rapid improvement seems unlikely, parenteral nutrition can be instituted. Detailed information on enteral and parenteral nutrition can be found elsewhere.[40,41]

PROGNOSIS AND DURATION OF TREATMENT

The prognosis for dogs and cats with AKI varies with the cause and with certain clinical parameters.[3,42–46] Overall, the reported mortality in dogs with AKI is 41% to 66%, and in cats, is 58% to 73%.[3] Dogs with leptospirosis have a relatively good prognosis, with reported survival of 83%.[44] Conversely, dogs with EG toxicity that are already azotemic when diagnosed have been shown to have a poor to grave prognosis, even with therapy.[45,46] Survival rates for dogs with AKI owing to raisins or grapes were 88% in one study[47] and 53% in another in which clinical signs were more severe[48]; 30% when associated with acute pancreatitis[49]; and 31% when due to pit viper envenomation.[50] Degree of azotemia is not predictive of outcome, whereas decreased urine production is a poor prognostic indicator.[3,42,43,46] Other criteria that confer a poor prognosis for dogs with AKI include hypocalcemia, anemia, hyperphosphatemia, lack of improvement or worsening of azotemia with appropriate fluid and supportive therapy, and comorbid disorders, such as pancreatitis or sepsis.[42,45,46] For cats with AKI, hyperkalemia, lower body temperature, hypoalbuminemia, and decreased serum bicarbonate levels at presentation were associated with decreased survival.[43,51]

Supportive and specific treatment should be continued until one of the following occurs: (1) renal function returns to normal; (2) renal function improves and stabilizes, and the animal is doing well clinically; (3) renal function worsens, fails to improve, or does not improve sufficiently for the animal to be managed medically at home. In the first 2 scenarios, fluid therapy can be tapered, and other supportive medications can be adjusted in response to the animal's clinical signs. In the third scenario, RRT may be considered for a period of time to see if renal function improves.

SUMMARY

AKI is characterized by the rapid loss of nephron function, resulting in azotemia and/or fluid, electrolyte, and acid-base abnormalities. The decrease in renal function that occurs with AKI is multifactorial and includes decreased intrarenal blood flow and cellular damage. There are many potential causes of AKI in dogs and cats, and the prognosis varies with the cause. Therapy consists of specific treatment of the cause and supportive therapy that includes IV fluids. Overall, the reported mortality in dogs with AKI is 41% to 66%, and in cats, 58% to 73%.[3] If medical management fails to increase urine output or improve azotemia, RRT is indicated.

CLINICS CARE POINTS

- Every effort should be made to determine the cause of acute kidney injury to aid in determining the prognosis for the animal.
- Intravenous fluid therapy should be adjusted by frequent monitoring of the animal and various clinical parameters.
- Fluid overload is detrimental and should be avoided.
- Measuring urine output is important for appropriate calculation of fluid requirements.
- If the cause of acute kidney injury has not been determined, "treat for the treatable," that is, doxycycline for leptospirosis.

DISCLOSURE

The author has no conflicts of interest.

REFERENCES

1. Eatroff AE. Acute kidney injury. In: Bruyette DS, editor. Clinical small animal internal medicine vol. II. Hoboken (NJ): Wiley–Blackwell; 2020. p. 1089–99.
2. Cowgill LD, Langston C. Acute kidney insufficiency. In: Bartges J, Polzin DJ, editors. Nephrology and urology of small animals. Ames (IA): Wiley-Blackwell; 2011. p. 472–523.

3. Langston C. Acute kidney injury. In: Ettinger SJ, Feldman EC, Cote, editors. Textbook of veterinary internal medicine: diseases of the dog and cat. 8th edition. St Louis (MO): Elsevier; 2017. p. 4650–85.

4. Ross LA. Medical management of acute kidney injury. In: Bonagura JD, Twedt DC, editors. Current veterinary therapy XV. Philadelphia: Elsevier Saunders; 2014. p. 868–71.

5. Ross LA. Acute kidney injury in dogs and cats. Vet Clin Small Anim 2011;41:1–14.

6. Weisbord SD, Paul M, Palevsky PM. Prevention and management of acute kidney injury. In: Chertow GM, Marsden PA, Skorecki K, et al, editors. Brenner and Rector's the kidney. 11th edition. Elsevier; 2019. p. 940–77.

7. International Renal Interest Society. IRIS AKI grading criteria. Available at: http://www.iris-kidney.com/pdf/4_ldc-revised-grading-of-acute-kidney-injury.pdf. Accessed October 21, 2021.

8. Okusa MD, Portilla D. Pathophysiology of acute kidney injury. In: Chertow GM, Marsden PA, Skorecki K, et al, editors. Brenner and Rector's the kidney. 11th edition. Elsevier; 2019. p. 906–39.

9. Molitoris BA, Sharfuddin A. Pathophysiology of acute kidney injury. In: Alpern R, Moe O, editors. Caplan M Seldin and Giebisch's the kidney : physiology and pathophysiology. 5th edition. London: Elsevier Academic Press; 2013. p. 2527–75.

10. McWilliam SJ, Wright RD, Welsh GI, et al. The complex interplay between kidney injury and inflammation. Clin Kidney J 2021;14:780–8.

11. Han SJ, Lee HT. Mechanisms and therapeutic targets of ischemic acute kidney injury. Kidney Res Clin Pract 2019;38:427–40.

12. Faubel S, Edelstein CL. Mechanisms and mediators of lung injury after acute kidney injury. Nat Rev Nephrol 2016;12:48–60.

13. Doi K, Rabb H. Impact of acute kidney injury on distant organ function: recent findings and potential therapeutic targets. Kidney Int 2016;89:555–64.

14. Reagan KL, Sykes JE. Diagnosis of canine leptospirosis. Vet Clin North Am 2019; 49:719–31.

15. Miller MD, Annis KM, Lappin MR, et al. Variability in results of the microscopic agglutination test in dogs with clinical leptospirosis and dogs vaccinated against leptospirosis. J Vet Intern Med 2011;25:426–32.

16. Connally HE, Thrall MA, Hamar DW. Safety and efficacy of high-dose fomepizole compared with ethanol as therapy for ethylene glycol intoxication in cats. J Vet Emerg Crit Care (San Antonio) 2010;20:191–206.

17. Tart KM, Powell LL. 4-Methylpyrazole as a treatment in naturally occurring ethylene glycol intoxication in cats. J Vet Emerg Crit Care (San Antonio) 2011; 21:268–72.

18. Rosenthal MG, Labato MA. Use of therapeutic plasma exchange to treat nonsteroidal anti-inflammatory drug overdose in dogs. J Vet Intern Med 2019;33: 596–602.

19. Kicera-Temple K, Londoño L, Lanaux TM, et al. Treatment of a massive naproxen overdose with therapeutic plasma exchange in a dog. Clin Case Rep 2019;7: 1529–33.

20. Langston CA. Hemodialysis. In: Bartges J, Polzin DJ, editors. Nephrology and urology of small animals. Ames (IA): Wiley-Blackwell; 2011. p. 255–85.

21. Langston CA. Effects of IV fluids in dogs and cats with kidney failure. Front Vet Sci 2021;8:659960.

22. Yerram P, Karuparthi P, Misra M. Fluid overload and acute kidney injury. Hemodial Int 2010;14:348–54.

23. Cavanagh AA, Sullivan LA, Hansen BD. Retrospective evaluation of fluid overload and relationship to outcome in critically ill dogs. J Vet Emerg Crit Care 2016;26: 578–86.
24. Hansen B. Fluid overload. Front Vet Sci 2021;8:668688.
25. Barsant JA. Urinary tract catheterization and nosocomial infections in dos and casts. In: Proceedings of the ACVIM Forum. Anaheim CA 2010:445-447.
26. Langston C. Managing fluid and electrolyte disorders in kidney disease. Vet Clin North Am 2017;47:471–90.
27. Adin DB, Taylor AW, Hill RC, et al. Intermittent bolus injection versus continuous infusion of furosemide in normal adult greyhound dos. J Vet Intern Med 2003;17: 632–6.
28. McClellan JM, Goldstein RE, Erb HN, et al. Effects of administration of fluids and diuretics on glomerular filtration rate, renal blood flow, and urine output in healthy awake cats. Am J Vet Res 2006;67:715–22.
29. Sigrist NE. Use of dopamine in acute renal failure. J Vet Emerg Crit Care 2007;17: 117–26.
30. Kellum JA, Decker JM. Use of dopamine in acute renal failure: a meta-analysis. Crit Care Med 2001;29:1526–31.
31. Friedrich JO, Adhikari N, Herridge MS, et al. Meta-analysis: low-dose dopamine increases urine output but does not prevent renal dysfunction or death. Ann Intern Med 2005;142(7):510–24.
32. Noce A, Marrone G, Rovella V, et al. Fenoldopam mesylate: a narrative review of its use in acute kidney injury. Curr Pharm Biotechnol 2019;20:366–75.
33. Simmons JP, Wohl JS, Schwartz DD, et al. Diuretic effects of fenoldopam in healthy cats. J Vet Emerg Crit Care 2006;16(2):96–103.
34. Nielsen LK, Bracker K, Price LL. Administration of fenoldopam in critically ill small animal patients with acute kidney injury: 28 dogs and 34 cats (2008–2012). J Vet Emerg Crit Care 2015;25:396–404.
35. Segev G, Bruchim Y, Berl N, et al. Effects of fenoldopam on kidney function parameters and its therapeutic efficacy in the management of acute kidney injury in dogs with heatstroke. J Vet Intern Med 2018;32:1109–15.
36. American Society of Veterinary Nephrology and Urology. Hospitals offering advanced renal and urinary treatments. Available at: https://www.asvnu.org/facilities. Accessed October 20, 2021.
37. Boothe DM. Factors affecting drug disposition. In: Boothe DM, editor. Small animal pharmacology and therapeutics. 2nd edition. St Louis (MO): Elsevier Saunders; 2012. p. 34–70.
38. Geigy CA, Schweighauser A, Doherr M, et al. Occurrence of systemic hypertension in dogs with acute kidney injury and treatment with amlodipine besylate. J Small Anim Pract 2011;52:340–6.
39. Cole LP, Jepson R, Dawson C, et al. Hypertension, retinopathy, and acute kidney injury in dogs: a prospective study. J Vet Intern Med 2020;34:1940–7.
40. Marks SL. Nasoesophageal, esophagostomy, gastrostomy, and jejunal tube placement. In: Ettinger SJ, Feldman EC, Cote, editors. Textbook of veterinary internal medicine: diseases of the dog and cat. 8th edition. St Louis (MO): Elsevier; 2017. p. 938–51.
41. Chan D. Critical care nutrition. In: Ettinger SJ, Feldman EC, Cote, editors. Textbook of veterinary internal medicine: diseases of the dog and cat. 8th edition. St Louis (MO): Elsevier; 2017. p. 1987–96.
42. Behrend E, Grauer GF, Mani I, et al. Hospital-acquired acute renal failure in dogs: 29 cases (1983-1992). J Am Vet Med Assoc 1996;208:537–41.

43. Worwag S, Langston CE. Feline acute intrinsic renal failure: 32 cats (1997-2004). J Am Vet Med Assoc 2008;232:728–32.

44. Adin CA, Cowgill LD. Treatment and outcome of dogs with leptospirosis:36 cases (1990-1998). J Am Vet Med Assoc 2000;216:371–5.

45. Vaden SL, Levine J, Breitschwerdt EB. A retrospective case-control of acute renal failure in 99 dogs. J Vet Intern Med 1997;11:58–64.

46. Segev G, Kass PH, Francey T, et al. A novel clinical scoring system for outcome prediction in dogs with acute kidney injury managed by hemodialysis. J Vet Intern Med 2008;22:301–8.

47. Reich CF, Salcedo MC, Koenigshof AM, et al. Retrospective evaluation of the clinical course and outcome following grape or raisin ingestion in dogs (2005–2014): 139 cases. J Vet Emerg Crit Care 2020;30:60–5.

48. Schweighauser A, Henke D, Oevermann A, et al. Toxicosis with grapes or raisins causing acute kidney injury and neurological signs in dogs. J Vet Intern Med 2020;34:1957–66.

49. Gori E, Lippi I, Guidi G, et al. Acute pancreatitis and acute kidney injury in dogs. Vet J 2019;245:77–81.

50. Martinez J, Londoño LA, Schaer M. Retrospective evaluation of acute kidney injury in dogs with pit viper envenomation (2008-2017): 56 cases. J Vet Emerg Crit Care (San Antonio) 2020;30:698–705.

51. Lee Y-J, Chan JP-W, Hsu W-L, et al. Prognostic factors and a prognostic index for cats with acute kidney injury. J Vet Intern Med 2012;26:500–5.

Fluid and Electrolyte Therapy During Vomiting and Diarrhea

Luis H. Tello, MV, MS, DVM[a],*, Mariana A. Pardo, BVSc, MV, DACVECC[b,1]

KEYWORDS

- Dehydration • Vomiting/diarrhea • Fluid therapy • Small animals • Gastroenteritis

KEY POINTS

- Fluid therapy can be the most lifesaving and important therapeutic measure in a critical patient suffering from dehydration owing to gastrointestinal losses (vomiting and/or diarrhea).
- Fluid therapy should be tailored to the patient's history, presenting complaint, physical examination, and laboratory findings. It is specific to the patient's needs and modified based on the physical and laboratory findings until fluid therapy resuscitation end points are achieved.
- The selection of fluid replacement should be determined by electrolytes and blood gas analysis.

INTRODUCTION

Vomiting and diarrhea are among the most common presenting complaints seen at emergency veterinary hospitals around the world. A small animal general practice analysis of medical data from 2.5 million dogs and 500,000 cats revealed that gastrointestinal complaints constitute between 3% and 5% of overall cases.[1] Because of the varying causes of vomiting and diarrhea and their potential to be self-limiting, diagnostic approach will vary between patients. However, fluid therapy continues to be the mainstay treatment for the fluid and electrolyte abnormalities caused by gastrointestinal signs.

VOMITING

Vomiting is defined as a complex reflex that leads to the forceful expulsion of stomach contents through the mouth and requires the coordination of the gastrointestinal,

[a] Tigard Animal Hospital, National Veterinary Associates, Tigard, OR, USA; [b] White Plains Hospital, Veterinary Emergency Group, White Plains, NY, USA
[1] 201 Tarrytown Road, White Plains, NY 10607, USA
* Corresponding author. 15080 SW Gibraltar Court, Beaverton, OR, 97007.
E-mail address: drluistello@gmail.com

Vet Clin Small Anim 52 (2022) 673–688
https://doi.org/10.1016/j.cvsm.2022.01.011
0195-5616/22/© 2022 Elsevier Inc. All rights reserved.

musculoskeletal, and nervous system. Many structures are involved in the vomiting process. These include the vomiting center located in the reticular formation of the medulla oblongata, the chemoreceptor trigger zone (CRTZ) located on the floor of the fourth ventricle within the brain, and the vagal and sympathetic neurons stimulated by receptors in the abdominal viscera.[2] The CRTZ is located outside of the blood-brain barrier and may be stimulated by local or systemic inflammation, irritation, distension, hypertonicity, emetogenic substances such as toxins and medications, and disorders of the vestibular system.[3,4]

The color of vomitus will help the clinician locate its origin. Clear vomitus constitutes swallowed saliva from the stomach; yellow represents reflux of digested bile from the stomach; green coloration suggests undigested bile originating from the upper duodenum owing to an obstruction or ileus. A brown fluid with a fetid odor is most likely coming from the small intestines and suggests a total obstruction or generalized ileus. In the case of primary gastrointestinal disease, the presence of blood in the vomitus typically appears as a red-tinged fluid or as "coffee grounds." Streaks or flecks of blood within clear vomitus may come from gastric or esophageal irritation and is not of specific pathologic condition.[5]

Patients with profuse or prolonged vomiting will frequently present signs of dehydration and potentially hypovolemia owing to the significant volume loss through the gastrointestinal contents. A wide constellation of clinical signs that vary from vague to pathognomonic for a particular condition or cause can be seen (**Box 1**). The diagnostic dilemma is to unveil the inciting cause, treat and correct it, while at the same time treating all secondary complications related to the vomiting. In small animals, vomiting is a common and complex problem. Adult patients often have different and more chronic causes of vomiting than pediatric patients; nonetheless, the condition remains a common reason for dogs and cats to be presented for veterinary care.[6] Vomiting can be caused by both primary gastrointestinal diseases and extra-gastrointestinal diseases. Examples of primary disease include infectious, inflammatory, parasitic, obstructive (eg, foreign body, trichobezoar, worm impaction), drug-related, nutritional, and neoplastic. Extra-gastrointestinal causes include endocrinopathies (eg, hyperthyroidism, diabetes ketoacidosis, hypoadrenocorticism), metabolic disease (eg, renal and liver disease), inflammatory, toxicities, and other diseases processes, such as pancreatitis, sepsis, and/neoplasia (especially alimentary lymphoma). This wide spectrum of potential causes of vomiting increases the difficulty for the practitioner in making a definitive diagnosis.[7] The wide range of disease processes and severity can have major effects on fluid and electrolyte balance. Vomiting usually involves the loss of fluid containing Cl^-, K^+, Na^+, and HCO_3^-; this leads to electrolytes and acid-base derangements, with metabolic acidosis being the most common, followed by metabolic alkalosis.[8,9]

DIARRHEA

Diarrhea is the result of excess fecal water that may be from decreased intestinal absorption and/or increased intestinal secretion. Most cases of diarrhea are mild and self-limiting requiring minimal diagnostics and symptomatic care; however, for more severe cases, diagnostics and invasive therapy are warranted (**Box 2**). Small intestinal diarrhea typically results in a larger fecal volume and fluid content loss, electrolyte and protein loss, and acid-base abnormalities. Large bowel diarrhea is characterized by small volume, multiple depositions, with a soft consistency, and the presence of mucous or fresh blood. Tenesmus may or may not be present. It is important to differentiate small bowel versus large bowel because it has a significant impact on the

---

Box 1
Causesof vomiting in companion animals

Abdominal, alimentary disorders
- Infection
- Inflammation
- Malignancy
- Toxicity
- Obstruction
- Ulceration
- Intussusception
- Foreign bodies
- Motility disorders

Metabolic disorders
- Uremia
- Liver failure
- Electrolyte disorders
- Acid-base disorders

Systemic disorders
- Sepsis
- Endotoxemia
- Multiple organ failure

Exogenous medications
- Digitalis glycosides
- Erythromycin
- Chemotherapy
- Apomorphine
- Xylazine
- Nonsteroidal anti-inflammatory drugs

Abdominal extra-alimentary disorders
- Peritoneal disorders (eg, peritonitis)
- Urinary tract disorders (eg, bladder rupture)
- Reproductive disorders (eg, pyometra)
- Splenic disorders (eg, splenitis)
- Nutrition
- Dietary indiscretion
- Food hypersensitivity reactions

Endocrine disorders
- Diabetes mellitus (ketoacidosis)
- Hyperthyroidism
- Hypoadrenocorticism

Nervous system disorders
- Encephalitis/meningitis
- Hydrocephalus

Toxicity
- Ethylene glycol
- Heavy metals (copper, zinc, lead)
- Strychnine

Extracted from Washabau, RJ. Vomiting. In: Washabau, R.J. and Day, M. Canine & Feline Gastroenterology. Saunders, Elsevier Inc. 2013. p168.

---

diagnostic and treatment plan. Most commonly, the duration of the diarrhea is subjectively classified as acute (<14 days) or chronic (>14 days). The mechanisms of diarrhea, in the feline and canine patient, can be divided into 4 subcategories, and these can occur alone or in any combination. These are increased intestinal secretion;

Box 2
Common causes of diarrhea in dogs and cats

Alimentary disorders
- Food indiscretion
- Hypersensitivity
- Food allergy
- Food poison/toxicity
- Food change
- Excess of food
- Trash consumption

Metabolic/inflammatory disorders
- Stress
- Sepsis
- Inflammatory bowel disease
- Pancreatitis
- Lymphangiectasia
- Stress colitis
- Acute hemorrhagic diarrhea syndrome
- Hepatitis
- Cholangiohepatitis
- Chronic kidney disease
- Hyperthyroidism
- Hypoadrenocorticism
- Exocrine pancreatic insufficiency

Neoplastic disorders
- Carcinoma
- Lymphoma
- Intestinal stromal tumor

Medications
- Laxatives
- Chemotherapy
- Nonsteroidal anti-inflammatory drugs
- Antibiotics

Infectious
- Virus: parvovirus, coronavirus, distemper, rotavirus, feline leukemia, feline immunodeficiency
- Parasites: giardia, helminths
- Bacteria: campylobacter, clostridium, salmonella, *Escherichia coli*

---

decreased intestinal absorption; rapid transit of intestinal contents; and mesenteric, vascular, or lymphatic diseases.[9–11] Secretory diarrhea results when prosecretory stimulation overwhelms absorptive forces, such as that produced by cholinergic agents, gastrointestinal hormones, bacterial enterotoxins, deconjugated bile acids, hydroxy fatty acids, and neuropeptides.[9] Decreased intestinal absorption may occur because of loss of absorptive surface from surgery, cellular infiltration, or damage to the intestinal epithelial barrier (eg, parvovirus), with the latter also increasing intestinal permeability, which may predispose the patient to bacterial translocation and sepsis. An increase in osmolarity of the intestinal content may also lead to decreased absorption, owing to net water movement from plasma to the intestinal lumen. Diarrhea can occur via any or all of the above mechanisms. The presence of frank red blood (hematochezia) or black tarry stool (melena) should alert the clinician that there is a disruption to the integrity of the gastrointestinal epithelium and protein losses, and bacterial translocation should be anticipated. The fluid and electrolyte abnormalities associated with diarrhea include sodium derangements, hypokalemia, and a hyper-chloremic metabolic acidosis with a normal anion gap, and volume depletion.[12] It is imperative that these conditions and their sequelae are treated promptly and appropriately with fluid therapy to optimize a successful outcome.

INTRODUCTION TO FLUID THERAPY

Fluid therapy recommendations are constantly changing, and there is ongoing debate on the ideal fluid choice, dose, rate, and efficacy in different patient populations. This has given rise to empiric fluid therapy recommendations, based on extrapolations from human medicine. Fluid therapy can be the most lifesaving therapeutic measure when dealing with hypovolemia or dehydration from gastrointestinal losses. To properly administer fluid therapy to the vomiting or diarrhea patient, it is imperative to have a basic understanding of the fluid and electrolyte dynamic in this population of sick patients. The appropriate fluid and rate of administration should be based on history, signalment, physical examination, and laboratory findings (including electrolytes and acid-base status) and a careful assessment of interstitial and intravascular losses.

TOTAL BODY OF WATER AND COMPARTMENTALIZATION

Sixty percent of the adult mammal body weight (BW) is composed of fluid; this is referred to as the total body water (TBW). This percentage decreases with obesity and age. The TBW is categorized into 2 main compartments, the intracellular space, which constitutes 67% of this fluid, and the extracellular space (ECF), which makes up the remaining 33% (**Fig. 1**). The extracellular compartment is further divided into the interstitial space, which consist of 75% of the ECF, and the intravascular space, which creates the remaining 25%. The intravascular space is composed of 8% of BW in the canine and 6.5% of the BW in the feline. Loss of fluid in the intravascular compartment leads to hypovolemia. Dehydration occurs when there is a loss of water, from that which is deemed normal, in the intracellular and interstitial compartment.[13]

DEHYDRATION

There is no sensitive or specific marker available to assess dehydration. An estimate on dehydration can be achieved by means of the physical examination; however,

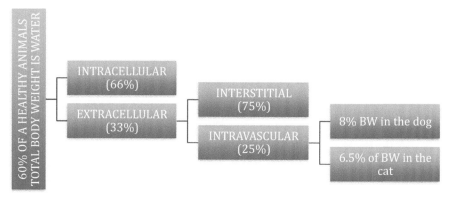

Fig. 1. Total body of water and fluid compartments within the body characterized by percentage of BW.

factors that influence accurate assessment exist, such as age and body condition. For example, the older and cachectic animal has less skin elasticity and fat compared with the obese patient that has extra lubrication between tissues. Because of these variables, it is best to assess the hydration status via a skin tent over the dorsum of the head or on the lateral thorax.[14] BW appears to be the most objective marker of hydration status. Having a recent past BW will be most useful in determining the degree of fluid loss. A loss of 1 mm of water is equivalent to 1 g; therefore, a loss of 1 kg suggests a loss of 1000 mm of body water.[9] A hyporexic and anorexic animal may lose ~0.1 to 0.3 kg/BW/d/1000 kcal of energy requirements.[12] An exception occurs in the case of third spacing when there is loss in the circulating volume and no appreciable loss in BW.

In addition to skin turgor and BW, other subjective parameters, such as mentation and mucous membrane moisture, can provide clues to detect the degree of dehydration (**Table 1**). Combining the history and laboratory measurements will aid the clinician in quantifying the extent of the dehydration most accurately. In the feline patient, a corneal response can be used to assess hydration because a delay in the nictating membranes sliding back into its normal anatomic position is a sign of dehydration.

In any disease process, the acute onset of fluid loss originates from the intravascular space. This results in a shift of water and electrolytes from the interstitial and intracellular compartment as a compensatory response. The tonicity and hydrostatic pressure of the remaining fluid in the ECF determine the extent of this shift. As a result, dehydration can occur to different degrees in various compartments and range from being not perceptible until approximately 5% of the BW has been lost in water to a loss of greater than 11% of BW (in water) being life threatening.

Table 1	
Subjective parameters used to assess the degree of dehydration	
Estimated Degree of Dehydration	**Clinical Signs**
<5% (subclinical)	Nonapparent on physical examination
5% (mild)	Tachy or dry mucous membrane (MM)
6%–8% (moderate)	Dry MM Decreased skin elasticity Tachycardia Normal pulse quality Normal arterial blood pressure
8%–10% (severe)	Dry MM Further decrease in skin elasticity Small increase in chemoreceptor trigger (CRT) Weak pulses
~12% (hypovolemia)	Dry MM Increased CRT Skin tent does not return to normal Tachycardia or bradycardia Weak to absent pulses Altered mentation Hypotension Cold extremities Hypothermia

ELECTROLYTES AND ACID-BASE DISORDERS

The loss of gastric and/or intestinal contents most commonly involves the loss of fluid that harbors chloride, potassium, sodium, and bicarbonate. The sequela of these losses can result in dehydration along with hyponatremia, hypochloremia, and hypokalemia. Large volumes of isotonic fluid are absorbed and secreted by the gastrointestinal tract. To place this in perspective, a 20-kg dog has approximately 2.7 L of fluid entering the duodenal lumen daily, and of this, greater than 98% is absorbed.[9] It is approximated that the jejunum absorbs 50% of fluid that passes through its lumen, the ileum 38%, and the colon 11%.[9] This makes it easy to understand why gastrointestinal pathologic condition can quickly lead to dehydration and hypovolemia. In the absence of endocrine and renal disease, the magnitude of gastrointestinal losses determines the extent of dehydration and acid-base disturbances.

In a retrospective study, 48% of dogs and 44% of cats with gastrointestinal disease presented with moderate to severe hypokalemia.[15] Emesis results in the loss of gastric secretions that contain potassium. It is calculated that the normal concentration of potassium in gastric secretions ranges between 10 and 20 mEq/L.[12] High potassium concentrations are found in fecal matter, and profound diarrhea can also result in hypokalemia. Furthermore, severe or chronic hypokalemia aggravates a patient's morbidity, leading to carbohydrate intolerance, anorexia, exacerbation of lethargy, and gastrointestinal hypomotility. When effective circulating volume is adequate, hypokalemia can cause persistent metabolic alkalosis by promoting renal acid excretion and bicarbonate reabsorption.[9]

Treatment of acute or severe hypokalemia requires intravenous (IV) intervention (**Table 2**). It is important to point out that the rate of potassium chloride IV is more important than the quantity, and it should at no time exceed a rate of 0.5 mEq/kg/h.[16]

The effect of gastrointestinal signs on acid-base balance is difficult to predict; hence, corrections should be based on blood gas analysis. The most prevalent acid-base disturbance seen in canines with gastrointestinal disease is metabolic acidosis, owing to hypovolemia and poor perfusion. This is typically corrected with the use of isotonic balanced crystalloids, such as PlasmaLyte or lactated Ringer solution, at a rate sufficient to correct hypovolemia, then provide for maintenance and ongoing losses.[14] It is worth mentioning that despite popular belief, there is no

Table 2			
Recommended amount of potassium chloride and rate of infusion			
Serum Potassium Concentration (mEq/L)	Potassium Chloride (mEq) to Add to Fluid (250 mL)	Potassium (mEq) to Add to Fluid (1 L)	Maximal Fluid Infusion Rate (mL/kg/h)
<2.0	20	80	6
2.1–2.5	15	60	8
2.6–3.0	10	40	12
3.1–3.5	7	28	18
3.6–5.0	5	20	25

So as not to exceed 0.5 mEq/kg/h.

Data from Schaer, M. Therapeutic Approach to Electrolyte Emergencies. Veterinary Clinics of North America: Small Animal Practice. 2008;38:516.; with permission.

significant association between electrolyte or acid-base abnormalities and the site of a gastrointestinal foreign body. However, the most common electrolyte and acid-base abnormalities regardless of the site or type of foreign body are hypochloremia, metabolic alkalosis, hypokalemia, and hyponatremia, with this last one being more prevalent in linear foreign bodies.[17] Metabolic alkalosis and hypochloremia usually respond to the correction of volume, chloride, and potassium deficits with 0.9% NaCl supplemented with KCl IV.

CRYSTALLOID FLUID

Isotonic crystalloids are the mainstay of treatment for most gastrointestinal disorders. This kind of fluid has an osmolality relative to that of plasma and the extracellular compartment. Sodium has the largest effect on fluid osmolality, as it has the highest concentration in the extracellular fluid compartment.[14,18] Water follows sodium; because of this intimate relationship, the sodium concentration of the fluid is important in selecting the appropriate fluid to treat a condition. The constitution of a fluid, with buffers and electrolytes, is also a consideration in making an adequate fluid choice. In general, vomiting and diarrhea result in isotonic dehydration. This is when the serum sodium concentration is within the normal reference range. A replacement fluid should be chosen that is nearly normal in serum sodium concentration and osmolality (**Table 3**). If there is a change in the sodium concentration from outside of the normal reference range, then an appropriate fluid should be chosen. If the derangement occurs acutely, the sodium can be corrected acutely; however, if it is chronic, it must be corrected slowly. If the serum sodium concentration is elevated, the patient has hypertonic dehydration and needs more free water than salt for replacement. Examples of hypotonic fluids are 5% dextrose and 0.45% NaCl in 2.5% dextrose. Correction of sodium derangements should not occur any faster than 0.5 mEq/L/h; lowering sodium too quickly in hypernatremia may produce cerebral edema, whereas increasing sodium in hyponatremia too quickly may lead to central pontine myelinolysis.[12] With hypotonic dehydration, the serum sodium concentration is low, and the patient needs more sodium relative to water.

ROUTE OF FLUID THERAPY

The route chosen for fluid administration depends on the severity, nature, and extent of the clinical disorder along with the fluid choice (**Table 4**). Oral fluid therapy should be reserved for the dehydrated patient that is not vomiting. Electrolyte solutions should be administered at frequent intervals to provide for adequate daily requirements. There has been promising preliminary data showing the benefit in the use of oral electrolyte solution for rehydration in patients with mild to moderate diarrhea as being safe, effective, and more cost- and time-effective, although further studies are lacking.[19] Subcutaneous fluid therapy can be used to treat the normovolemic patient with mild to no evidence of dehydration. A balanced isotonic polyionic crystalloid should be chosen, and the amount of fluid administered at each injection site should not exceed 20 mL/kg. The flow of the fluid is determined by the patient's comfort and is generally absorbed within 6 to 8 hours. If fluid pockets persist after this timeframe, intravenous fluid (IVF) administration should be implemented to reestablish peripheral perfusion. Avoid the use of subcutaneous acetated polyionic solutions like Normosol R and PlasmaLyte, as these have been described to cause patient discomfort. IVF therapy should always be chosen for the dehydrated patient because they allow rapid and accurate administration of volume resuscitation. Hypokalemia is a common finding in the vomiting patient, and thus, IVF allows for adequate and safe supplementation and

Table 3
Common fluids available, composition, indications, and contraindications

Fluid	Osm	Buffer	Na+	Cl-	K+	Ca++	Mg++	CHO-	Indications	Contraindication
Normosol R	296	Acetate 27 Gluconate 23	140	98	5	0	3	0	Replacement Metabolic acidosis Anorexia Vomiting Hypovolemic shock Diarrhea Renal failure	Metabolic alkalosis
PlasmaLyte-A	294	Acetate 27	140	98	5	0	3	0	Replacement Metabolic acidosis Anorexia Vomiting Hypovolemic shock Diarrhea Renal failure	Metabolic alkalosis
0.9% saline	308	0	154	154	0	0	0	0	Replacement Hypovolemic shock Anorexia Vomiting Diarrhea Metabolic alkalosis Hyperkalemia Hypercalcemia Renal failure Acute hyponatremia Chronic hypernatremia	Cardiac disease Metabolic acidosis
LRS	272	Lactate 28	130	109	4	3	0	0	Replacement Hypovolemic shock Vomiting Diarrhea Hypocalcemia Metabolic acidosis Renal failure	Hypercalcemia Lymphosarcoma Liver failure

delivery. Intraperitoneal and intraosseous routes are not commonly used and reserved for when access to IVF therapy is unsuccessful or not feasible.

FLUID REQUIREMENTS

1. Emergency phase: The IV administration rate should be based on parameters of hydration and perfusion with the end goal of achieving normovolemia. If the patient is hypovolemic, administer one-fourth of the total blood volume. Total blood volume is derived from the percent of body water that composes the intravascular compartment. In the dog, this is 80 to 90 mL/kg, and in the cat, this is 50 to 60 mL/kg. The choice of fluid is dependent on the acid-base status and sodium content of the patient. If the patient is acidotic, a balanced isotonic electrolyte solution is recommended; if the patient is alkalotic, 0.9% NaCl may be used instead. IV boluses should not be administered faster than over 15 minutes. This bolus can be repeated in aliquots as needed to correct volume loss, with a recommendation of boluses of 20 mL/kg in the dog and 10 mL/kg in the cat. In hypoproteinemic patients, fluid therapy should be administered cautiously to avoid overhydration and peripheral edema. It is rare that the total blood volume dose for each individual species is required to manage shock, and the patient should be reassessed for other derangements (vasodilation, hypocalcemia, hypoglycemia, hypoproteinemia, sepsis, and so forth) if this volume is about to be exceeded. Most patients are volume resuscitated with less than the maximum dose. If hypoproteinemia ensues, serum albumin and large volumes of fresh frozen plasma (FFP) may be needed depending on the nature and severity of the illness and is not addressed in this article. Fluid resuscitation should continue until there is an improvement in perfusion parameters: mentation, heart rate, pulse quality, mucous membrane color, capillary refill time, blood lactate, blood pressure, and urine output. In creating the appropriate fluid plan for a patient, the clinician must consider the fact that approximately 80% of IV isotonic crystalloid fluids is redistributed within an hour into the interstitial space.
2. Rehydration phase: If the patient is hypoperfused but not in hypovolemic shock, then fluids are calculated based on the hydration status. The rehydration phase is calculated based on percentage of dehydration (dehydration % × BW [kg] × 1000 = mL of fluid deficit), ongoing losses (vomiting and diarrhea), and the maintenance requirements. If the patient is febrile, 10% maintenance should be added for each degree Celsius above 39.5 C. The goal is to reestablish 80% to 100% of the fluid deficit within a 24-hour period.
3. Maintenance phase: The average figure chosen for total body of water in the adult mammal is 60%; hence, this is typically chosen in calculating maintenance fluid therapy. This figure is usually lower in feline patients and higher in pediatric and neonatal patients. The metabolic fluid requirement is estimated to approximate the metabolic energy requirement. One milliliter of water is required to metabolize 1 kilocalorie of energy; therefore, metabolic fluid requirements can be derived using the formula: (30 × kg) + 70 = mL of water required per day if the patient is greater than 2 kg and less than 100 kg.[20]
4. Monitoring: Frequent examination and reassessment are imperative to meet the unique fluid and protein losses of each individual patient. General guidelines for initial monitoring consist of weighing every 12 hours or more frequently, monitoring packed cell volume and total solids, blood glucose, electrolytes, and blood gas every 6 to 12 hours, and assessing perfusion parameters and ins/outs every 2 to 4 hours. A good rule of thumb to use in evaluating if the fluid requirements are

Table 4	
Routes of crystalloid fluid administration	
Route of Administration	Points to Consider
Oral (PO)	• Reserved for the euhydrated patient • Patients that are not vomiting • Offer ice cubes, small amounts of water, or an oral glucose and electrolyte solution • Give at frequent intervals to provide maintenance daily requirements
Subcutaneous (SQ)	• Use only to treat mild dehydration in absence of other systemic signs • Balance isotonic polyionic sterile fluids (eg, LRS) • Small dogs and cats without peripheral vasoconstriction • Do not exceed 10–20 mL/kg of fluid per injection site • Flow of fluids is based on patient's comfort • Fluid absorbed within 6–8 h • Do not use hypertonic crystalloids, colloids, or dextrose-supplemented fluid for this route
Intravenous (IV)	• Moderately to severely dehydrated • Use when accurate deliveries of fluid volume and pharmacotherapeutic agents are required • Benefit: Rapid and large administration of fluids, titration of fluids • Allows for potassium supplementation in IVF to replace that lost in vomitus
Intraperitoneal (IP)	• When IV catheter is not successful or possible as this provide a rapid access to the circulation • Most commonly needed in emergency situation when immediate IV access is not possible for the pediatric or neonatal patient
Intraosseous (IO)	• Severely anemic pediatric patient • Consider for rewarming hypothermic patients • Isotonic to mildly hypotonic fluid for rehydration • IV route preferred when possible • Medulla does not collapse during hypovolemia

met or need adjusting is remembering that 1 mL of fluid weighs 1 g. As the patient's clinical status progresses, these are tailored to fit the ongoing needs, response to the therapeutic regimen, and the course of the disease process.

FLUID OVERLOAD

Although widely recognized as a mainstay therapy for dehydration and hypovolemia in veterinary patients, fluid therapy is not always benign and can cause significant harm through fluid overload, which increases patient morbidity and mortality. Fluids exert physiologic effects when administered into the body and therefore should be considered "drugs." Clinically, fluid overload tends to manifest as either edema or cavity effusions (eg, pleural effusion and peritoneal effusion), or fluid deposition in peripheral tissues. Internal organ edema also occurs and may be difficult to identify on physical examination. Fluid overload can lead to decreased renal filtration (azotemia), decreased hepatic blood flow (liver enzyme elevations ± cholestasis), and decreased intestinal mobility (ileus, regurgitation or vomiting, and inappetence).[21] Preventing fluid overload is of extreme importance, because interventions to address it are limited to diuretics and fluid restriction. Fluid therapy is a constantly changing and dynamic process that should be continually reassessed in patients.[22]

MULTIMODAL THERAPY

Ongoing losses should be controlled as soon as possible to prevent exacerbation of fluid, electrolyte, and acid-base derangements. Maropitant and ondansetron can be used as an antiemetic, and the former may potentially provide adjunct visceral analgesia.[22–24] Gastro-protectants, such as proton-pump inhibitors and sucralfate, may be incorporated if there is suspicion or risk of gastric ulceration. If unobstructive ileus is present, a prokinetic agent can be added, such as metoclopramide. Antidiarrheal medications are not recommended, as these decrease peristalsis, which may result in bacterial translocation and severe intestinal bacterial overgrowth.[20] Antibiotics with broad-spectrum coverage of aerobes and anaerobes should be used if bacterial translocation or a bacterial cause is suspected, ensuring proper antibiotic stewardship to avoid bacterial resistance and gastrointestinal dysbiosis.

UPDATES IN TREATMENT

The diverse, complex, and dynamic microflora of pathogenic and nonpathogenic bacteria that inhabit the gastrointestinal tract of all mammals is an aspect of gastroenterology that has received a great deal of attention and research over the past few years. Much focus has been directed toward the microbiome of the dog and cat, and how alterations in its composition affect the patient. Prebiotics provide substrate to stimulate the growth of healthy gut bacteria. Probiotics are live organisms that when consumed may displace pathogenic microorganisms, may change motility and pain perception, improve the gastrointestinal tract epithelial barrier function, and modulate enteric and innate immune responses.[25,26] The clinical effect of treatment with probiotic strains continues to be researched to understand which strains are effective for each species and disease process.

Natural or synthetic colloids have historically been used to for oncotic support. A recent study in hypoalbuminemic dogs did not find any significant changes on plasma colloid osmotic pressure when hetastarch was administered as a constant rate of infusion, although additional studies are warranted to assess the impact of synthetic colloids in these patients.[27] It is important to note that the use of synthetic colloids is controversial and is an area under current scrutiny as new studies have revealed that colloids are not associated with improved survival.[28–31] This is due to the concern for it causing a proinflammatory state, fluid overload, acute renal injury, and hemodilution and coagulopathies (eg, decreased platelet adhesion, increased fibrinolysis, decreased circulating levels of von Willebrand factor, and decreased FVIII:C).[32–35] Research suggests that the weight-averaged molecular weight, degree of molar substitution, concentration, and administration technique may have an impact on the risk of toxicity of synthetic colloids. Tetrastarch has a lower molecular weight and molar substitution in comparison to hetastarch and hence may potentially have fewer side effects when compared with hetastarch; however, further studies are needed to assess appropriate dosage, administration method (bolus vs constant rate of infusion), indications, and safety profile.

The American College of Veterinary Internal Medicine consensus statement on pancreatitis in cats currently recommends considering supplementation of FFP for the treatment of cats with severe pancreatitis. FFP provides dose-dependent colloid

---

Box 3
Monitoring response to therapy

1. Underhydration
   a. Persistent tachycardia
   b Poor pulse quality
   c .Inadequate urine output
   d .Weight loss

2. Overhydration
   a .Chemosis
   b Serous nasal discharge
   c Weight gain exceeds that expected to accomplish rehydration
   d Excessive decrease in PCV/TS
   e Excessive urination
   f Sudden increase or persistently elevated central venous pressure
   g Increased respiratory rate and/or respiratory effort
   h Subcutaneous pitting edema
   i Pulmonary crackles (late indicator)

---

support by supplementing albumin and is therapeutic in inflamed patients for correction of coagulopathies secondary to disseminated intravascular coagulation.[36]

MONITORING

Monitoring weight is the most sensitive tool for assessment of dehydration and rehydration, as acute changes in weight reflect gain or loss of body water. The clinician must remember that a drastic gain or loss of 1 kg is approximately the equivalent of gaining or losing 1 L of fluid. Following PCV/TP serially during fluid therapy will also help evaluate the effectiveness of therapy, as a decrease in both suggests successful intravascular rehydration.

REASONS FOR TREATMENT FAILURE

Dehydration gives the clinician a preliminary assessment of the patient's clinical status; however, it must be remembered that this is purely an estimation and can result in a calculation error. Below are the most common reasons for calculation error:

- Inappropriate estimation of patient's dehydration status
- Larger losses than anticipated
- Diuresis from trying to correct fluid deficit too quickly
- Increased sensible losses (polyuria, panting, fever, and so forth)

Feline patients can also suffer from an inappropriate fluid plan, as they are less tolerant to aggressive fluid therapy owing to occult cardiac disease, a lower metabolic rate, and a smaller blood volume.[37] Overhydration can occur in both the feline and the canine patient from conditions like systemic inflammation, hypoproteinemia, kidney disease, and cardiac disease.[37] Therefore, the importance of reevaluating and reassessing the patient cannot be overemphasized; refer to **Box 3** for a complete list of clinical signs that should be used in assessing underhydration and overhydration.

SUMMARY

Adequate fluid therapy strongly relies on the astute clinician being able to detect and correct the underlying cause of fluid and electrolyte loss and/or sequestration.

Because gastrointestinal disease can be dynamic, fluid therapy should be tailored to the patient's needs, and fluid selection and volume requirements may change throughout the progression of therapy. Assessment of fluid loss is only an estimate, and therefore, it is most important to continually assess response to therapy to help guide the fluid plan. Developing an appropriate and evolving fluid therapy plan will be an important tool to decrease the length of hospitalization and improve care for the patient with gastrointestinal disease. Vomiting and diarrhea are common disorders encountered in veterinary medicine, and when treated appropriately, most often results in a positive outcome.

DISCLOSURE

The authors disclose no conflicts of interest.

REFERENCES

1. State of Pet Health™ 2016 Report, BARK group, Banfield Pet Hospital, 2016, Portland OR. Available at. www.stateofpethealth.com.
2. Washabau RJ, Holt DE. Pathophysiology of gastrointestinal disease. In: Slatter E, editor. Textbook Anim Surg3. Philadelphia: Saunders; 2003. p. 530–52.
3. Elwood C, Devauchelle P, Elliot J, et al. Emesis in dogs. J Small Anim Pract 2010; 51:4–22.
4. German A.J., Maddison J.E., Guilford G. Gastrointestinal drugs. In: Saunders small animal clinical Pharmacology. 2nd edition Philadelphia, Pennsylvania: Elsevier; Saunders:469-497
5. Washabau RJ. Vomiting. In: Washabau RJ, Day M, editors. Canine & feline gastroenterology. Saunders, Elsevier Inc.; 2013. p. p168–73.
6. Trepanier L. Acute vomiting in cats: rational treatment selection. J Feline Med Surg 2010;12(3):225–30.
7. Norsworthy GD, Estep JS, Kiupel M, et al. Diagnosis of chronic small bowel disease in cats: 100 cases: 2008-2012. JAVMA 2013;243(10):1455–61.
8. Ha YS, Hopper K, Epstein SE. Incidence, nature, and etiology of metabolic alkalosis in dogs and cats. J Vet Inten Med,27 2013;847–53.
9. DiBartola SP. Fluid and electrolyte disturbances in gastrointestinal and pancreatic disease. In: Fluid, electrolyte and acid-base disorders in small animal practice. 4th edition. St. Louis, Missouri: Elsevier; 2012. p. 436–55.
10. Marks SL. Diarrhea. In: Washabau RJ, Day M, editors. Canine & feline gastroenterology. Saunders, Elsevier Inc.; 2013. p. p99–108.
11. Hubbard K, Skelly BJ, McKelvie J, et al. Risk of vomiting and diarrhea in dogs. Vet Rec 2007;161:755–7.
12. Brown AJ, Otto CM. Fluid therapy in vomiting and diarrhea. Vet Clin North Am: Small Anim Pract 2008;38:653–75.
13. Rudloff ER, Kirby R. Fluid therapy. Vet Clin North America: Small Anim Pract 1998; 28:297–328.
14. Johnson S. Digestive system. In: Saunders Manual of small animal practice. St. Louis, Missouri: Elsevier; 2006. p. 664–739.
15. Hoehne SN, Hoppeer K, Epstein SE. Retrospective evaluation of the severity and prognosis associated with potassium abnormalities in dogs and cats presenting to an emergency room (January 2014-August 2015): 2441 cases. J Vet Emerg Crit Care 2019;653–61.
16. Schaer M. Therapeutic approach to electrolyte emergencies. Vet Clin North Am: Small Anim Pract 2008;38:513–33.

17. Boag AK, Coe RJ, Martinez TA, et al. Acid-base and electrolyte abnormalities in dogs with gastrointestinal foreign bodies. J Vet Intern Med 2005;19:816–21.
18. Mazzaferro E, Powell L. Fluid therapy for the emergent small animal patient. Vet Clin North Am: Small Anim Pract 2013;43:721–34.
19. Reineke EL, Walton K, Otto C. Evaluation of an oral electrolyte solution for treatment of mild to moderate dehydration in dogs with hemorrhagic diarrhea. J Am Vet Med Assoc 2014;243:851–7.
20. Hansen B. Fluid overload. Front Vet Sci 2021;8:668688.
21. Thomovsky E, Brooks A, Johnson P. Fluid overload in small animal patients. Top Companion Anim Med 2016;31(Issue 3):94–9.
22. Hickman MA, Cox SR, Mahabir S, et al. Safety, pharmacokinetics and use of the novel NK-1 receptor antagonist maropitant (Cerenia) for the prevention of emesis and motion sickness in cats. J Vet Pharmacolther 2008;31:220–9.
23. Boscan P, Monnet E, Mama K, et al. Effect of maropitant, a neurokinin-1 receptor antagonist, on anesthetic requirements during noxious visceral stimulation of the ovary in dogs. Am J Vet Res 2011;72:1576–9.
24. Encarnacion H, Parra J, Mears E, et al. Vomiting. Compendium 2009;31(3): 122–31. Available at: http://www.vetfolio.com/gastroenterology/vomiting-compendium. Accessed January 26.2016.
25. Jugan M.C., Rudinsky A.J., Parker V.J., Gilor C. Use of Probiotics in Small Animal Veterinary Medicine.
26. Rossi G, Pengo G, Caldin M, et al. Comparison of microbiological, histological, and immunomodulatory parameters in response to treatment with either combination therapy with prednisone and metronidazole or probiotics VSL#3 strains in dogs with idiopathic inflammatory bowel disease. PLoS One 2014;9(4):e94699.
27. Borrelli A, Maurella C, Lippi I, et al. Evaluation of the effects of hydroxyethyl starch (130/0.4) administration as a constant rate infusion on plasma colloid osmotic pressure in hypoabluminemic dogs. J Vet Emerg Crit Care 2020;30(5):550–7.
28. Hayes G, Beneddicenti L, Mathews K. Retrospective cohort study on the incidence of acute kidney injury and death following hydroxyethyl starch (HES 10% 250/0.5/5:1) administration in dogs (2007-2010). J Vet Emerg Crit Care 2016;26:35–40.
29. Morris BR, deLaforcade A, Lee J, et al. Effects of in vitro hemodilution with crystalloids, colloids and plasma on canine whole blood coagulation as determined by kaolin-activated thromboelastography. J Vet Emerg Crit Care 2016;26:58–63.
30. Adamik KN, Yozova ID, Regenscheit N. Controversies in the use of hydroxyethyl starch in small animal emergency and critical care. J Vet Emerg Crit Care 2015; 25(1):20–47.
31. Silverstain DC, Kleiner J, Drobatz KJ. Effectiveness of intravenous fluid resuscitation in the emergency room for treatment of hypotension in dogs: 35 cases (2000-2010). J Vet Emerg Crit Care 2012;22(6):666–73.
32. Glover P, Rudloff E, Kirby R. Hydroxyethyl starch: a review of pharmacokinetics, pharmacodynamics, current products, and potential clinical risks, benefits and use. J Vet Emerg Crit Care 2014;24(6):642–61.
33. Gauthier V, Holowaychuk CL, Kerr AM, et al. Effect of synthetic colloid administration on coagulation in healthy dogs and dogs with systemic inflammation. J Vet Intern Med 2015;29:276–85.
34. Helmbold K, Mellema M, Hopper K, et al. The effect of Hetastarch 670/0.75 administered in vivo as a constant rate infusion on platelet closure time in the dog. J Vet Emerg Crit Care 2014;24(4):381–7.

35. Wierenga JR, Jandrey KE, Haskins SC, et al. In vitro comparison of the effects of two forms of hydroxyethyl starch solutions on platelet function in dogs. Am J Vet Res 2007;68(6):605–9.

36. Forman MA, Steiner JM, Armstrong PJ, et al. ACVIM consensus statement on pancreatitis in cats. J Vet Intern Med 2021;35:703–23.

37. Mazzaferro E. Fluid therapy: the critical balance between life and death. NAVC Clinician's brief 2006;73–5.

Advanced Oxygen Therapy for the Small Animal Patient – High-Flow Oxygen Therapy and Mechanical Ventilation

Kate Hopper, BVSC, PhD[a], Lisa L. Powell, DVM[b],*

KEYWORDS

- Mechanical ventilation • Hypoxemia • Hypercapnia • Hypoventilation
- Intubation positive pressure ventilation • Respiratory
- High-flow nasal oxygen therapy

KEY POINTS

The indications for high-flow nasal oxygen therapy (HFNT) include:

- Failure to respond to traditional oxygen supplementation, including oxygen kennel or nasal cannula, as evidenced by increased work of breathing, hypoxemia, or low percent hemoglobin-oxygen saturation levels.
- The need for increased airway pressures to help support oxygenation.

The indications for mechanical ventilation include:

- Severe hypoxemia (defined as a $P_{aO_2} < 60$ mm Hg at sea level) that fails to respond to traditional or high-flow nasal oxygen therapy.
- Severe hypoventilation (defined as $P_{aCO_2} > 60$ mm Hg).
- Excessive work of breathing.

The prognosis of animals requiring high-flow nasal oxygen therapy or mechanical ventilation will depend on the underlying disease process, with many diseases having a good prognosis for recovery.

[a] Department of Veterinary Surgical and Radiologic Sciences, University of California, Davis, Room 2112, Tupper Hall, Davis, CA 95616, USA; [b] BluePearl Veterinary Partners MN, 7717 Flying Cloud Drive, Eden Prairie, MN 55344, USA
* Corresponding author.
E-mail address: ervet1@gmail.com

Vet Clin Small Anim 52 (2022) 689–705
https://doi.org/10.1016/j.cvsm.2022.01.006
0195-5616/22/© 2022 Elsevier Inc. All rights reserved.

INTRODUCTION

Animals with respiratory failure will need the support of oxygenation and/or ventilation as appropriate given their disease process. The common methods of respiratory support include traditional oxygen supplementation, high-flow nasal oxygen therapy (HFNT), and positive pressure ventilation (PPV). This discussion will review the indications and core principles of HFNT and PPV.

HIGH-FLOW NASAL OXYGEN THERAPY

High-flow nasal cannula oxygen therapy is a method of delivering heated, humidified oxygen at a high-flow rate to achieve higher inspired oxygen concentrations, with use in humans emerging within the past 2 decades (Ward 2013).[1] It has also been shown to increase pressure in the upper airway in human patients, further supporting respiration in hypoxemic patients (Groves 2007).[2] Traditional nasal cannula oxygen therapy can achieve a fraction of inspired oxygen (Fio_2) of 30% to 60%, depending on the oxygen flow rate and if unilateral or bilateral nasal cannulas are used.[3] However, flow rates above 4 to 6 L/min maybe difficult to achieve using this method, as higher flow rates can cause nasal mucosal damage and patient discomfort. HFNT is a noninvasion ventilation system that incorporates an oxygen concentrator, an air mixer, and a humidifier, delivering airflow from 2 to 60 L/min through heated tubing and nasal prongs. Through humidification at specific temperatures allowing increased airflow, higher Fio_2 concentrations can be achieved. Historically, patients that have failed traditional oxygen administration methods required mechanical ventilation. With the use of HFNT therapy, Fio_2 can be adjusted from 21% to 100%. The final concentration of oxygen the patient receives will depend on the Fio_2 selected and the flow rate applied. Flow rates that exceed the minute ventilation (product of tidal volume (TV) and respiratory rate) of the patient will mean the entire TV is provided by the machine. If HFNT is given with a Fio_2 of 100% at a flow rate that equals or exceeds the animal's minute ventilation, the animal will receive 100% oxygen. The ability to provide high levels of inspired oxygen benefits the severely hypoxemic patient as this can be delivered with little or no sedation, intubation, or mechanical ventilation. However, if the patient is unable to ventilate, or if they fail HFNT, mechanical ventilation would be indicated.

Veterinary Studies

Several veterinary studies have assessed the use of HFNT in dogs since 2016. The efficacy of HFNT of 100% oxygen at 20 L/min and 30 L/min was evaluated in 6 healthy dogs (17–36 kg). At both flow rates, arterial blood gases (ABGs) were consistent with the animals receiving a Fio_2 of 100% and there was no change in $Paco_2$ from baseline. No significant increase in end-expiratory pressure was evident in these dogs.[4] The first published clinical study retrospectively evaluated the use of HFNT in 6 dogs with hypoxemia that failed traditional oxygen therapy.[5] In this study, hypoxemia resolved in 4/6 patients. One dog developed pneumothorax, and one dog required sedation for nasal cannula discomfort. Carbon dioxide levels were increased in these patients but were not found to be significantly higher than when these dogs were receiving traditional oxygen therapy. Based on this small study, HFNT was found to be safe and effective, with minimal adverse effects. However, due to the higher flow rates that can cause increased airway pressures, patients should be monitored for the development of barotrauma.

In 2019, Jagodich and colleagues published an experimental study evaluating HFNT in healthy dogs.[6] The authors found that HFNT resulted in increased blood oxygen levels, mild increases in blood Pco_2 levels, and increases in measured airway pressures. This study also supported the use of flow rates of 1 to 2 L/kg/min based on target Fio_2 levels. At these flow rates, Fio_2 was measured at a mean of 95%; higher flow rates did not result in higher Fio_2 concentrations. These authors then published a prospective clinical study evaluating the use of HFNT in 22 hypoxemic dogs that failed traditional oxygen therapy.[7] This study showed that hemoglobin oxygen saturation levels (SpO_2) increase significantly within 30 minutes of starting HFNT, and 45% of the dogs survived to discharge. None were diagnosed with barotrauma.

A prospective, pilot study was published in 2020 evaluating the use of HFNT in dogs with hypoxemia that failed traditional oxygen administration therapy (the HOT-DOG study).[8] The 11 dogs evaluated in this study showed improved oxygenation and no adverse events, further supporting the use of HFNT in dogs with hypoxemia that fail traditional oxygen administration.

Guidelines for Clinical Use

High-flow nasal oxygen equipment uses purpose made, disposable circuits. These are generally useable for 30 days after initial use. The nasal cannulas are also purpose made and it is not recommended to use standard nasal oxygen therapy cannulas with a high-flow circuit. The nasal cannulas come in several sizes and the aim is for the cannula to be approximately (no larger than) 50% of the size of the nares. Once the circuit is connected, the machine is turned on and allowed to heat up. It is recommended to set the temperature to a value close to the patient (37° C is commonly used) to increase patient comfort. The initial flow rate selected is based on the size of the patient and is then titrated according to the patient's response and comfort. An initial flow rate of 0.5 to 1 L/kg/min is suggested and 1 to 2 L/min is a common range of flow rates used.

Summary

HFNT has been shown to be a viable and effective treatment of dogs that fail traditional oxygen administration modalities and can be used to escalate oxygen therapy without the intensiveness and increased morbidity associated with mechanical ventilation.

HFNT could be considered in cats; however, nasal prongs may be too large to facilitate high-flow support in this species. Flow should be adjusted to support blood oxygen levels and respiratory effort while avoiding excessively high flows, to minimize the risk of barotrauma and significant hypercarbia. Overall, there are minimal reports of adverse events. HFNT provides a noninvasive way to support dogs with significant hypoxemia which may avoid the need for PPV in many animals.

POSITIVE PRESSURE VENTILATION

Positive pressure ventilation (PPV) is becoming more common in veterinary medicine as a lifesaving intervention for animals with respiratory failure. This level of support can be provided by manual ventilation or a mechanical ventilator. Mechanical ventilators can be part of an anesthetic machine or be an independent piece of equipment that will be described as an intensive care unit (ICU) type ventilator for the purpose of this discussion. Anesthesia ventilators are effective and can be used for PPV of critically ill or injured patients although some are quite simple and may not have the ability to provide as much support as an ICU ventilator. In addition, ICU-type ventilators can vary the inspired oxygen concentration, which not all anesthetic ventilators are set up to do. In veterinary medicine, the role of long-term mechanical ventilation has been primarily assumed by specialists in emergency and critical care. However, patients that present with imminent respiratory failure must be managed quickly and assuredly by the primary attending veterinarian. First and foremost, an adequate and patent airway must be established. Following rapid induction of anesthesia, hand ventilation with an Ambu bag connected to an oxygen source can be administered. An anesthesia ventilator can be used for initial stabilization. If airway humidification is not available and/or the Fio_2 is fixed at 100% on the anesthesia ventilator, transition to an ICU ventilator as soon as possible is recommended (ideally within 8–10 hours).

INDICATIONS FOR VENTILATION

Mechanical ventilation is most commonly indicated when adequate gas exchange can no longer be maintained and there is a significant risk of patient death as a consequence. There are 5 main indications for mechanical ventilation. These are:[9–11]

1. Severe hypoxemia despite oxygen therapy (Pao_2 <60 mm Hg)
2. Severe hypoventilation (defined as Pco_2 >60 mm Hg)
3. Excessive work of breathing
4. Severe circulatory shock
5. Facilitate long-term endotracheal intubation

Severe Hypoxemia Despite Oxygen Therapy

The oxygenation status of a patient is ideally assessed by the measurement of the partial pressure of oxygen in an arterial blood sample (Pao_2). Hypoxemia is defined as a Pao_2 of less than 80 mm Hg at sea level, while a Pao_2 of less than 60 mm Hg is considered severe hypoxemia. The definition of hypoxemia will change with altitude. Severe hypoxemia is also known as hypoxemic respiratory failure.[9,10] The need for mechanical ventilation in the hypoxemic patient will depend on the underlying mechanism of hypoxemia and the patient's response to oxygen therapy. In animals with severe respiratory compromise, the collection of ABGs may not be feasible, especially in small patients. Venous blood gas (VBG) samples cannot be used to evaluate oxygenation but can be used to assess ventilation ($PvCO_2$) if the patient is hemodynamically stable. In the absence of ABG samples, pulse oximetry can provide a measure of oxygenation. Pulse oximetry is appealing, as it is noninvasive; however, it is prone to inaccuracies, especially in the awake patient.[12] A pulse oximeter reading of 95% is equivalent to a Pao_2 of ~80 mm Hg, while 90% is approximately 60 mm Hg (indicating severe hypoxemia).[9,13] Mechanical ventilation is a consideration for patients with severe hypoxemia identified as a Pao_2 of less than 60 mm Hg or a SpO_2 of less than 90% despite oxygen therapy. Given the lack of reliability of pulse oximetry, it may be necessary to decide to initiate PPV based on clinical judgment alone.

The role of PPV in the management of hypoxemia will depend on the underlying mechanism. General mechanisms of hypoxemia include:

1. Inadequate inspired oxygen
2. Hypoventilation
3. Venous admixture

Inadequate inspired oxygen is not likely to be relevant to the emergency room patient. It can occur in patients on a breathing circuit when the oxygen supply is disconnected, or the oxygen tank is empty. It is also the cause of hypoxemia when at high altitudes. This problem is readily resolved with oxygen administration.

Hypoventilation is defined by an elevation in the partial pressure of carbon dioxide (Pco_2) above the reference range. Elevations in Pco_2 will reduce the partial pressure of alveolar oxygen as defined by the alveolar air equation.[5] When patients are breathing room air, moderate-to-severe hypercapnia will be associated with hypoxemia. This cause of hypoxemia is readily resolved with oxygen administration and is not an indication for PPV.[9,10,13] Although, it is important to note that hypercapnia itself may be an indication for PPV.

Venous admixture describes any mechanism by which blood can pass from the right side of the heart to the left side of the heart without being fully oxygenated. This includes abnormalities such as ventilation-perfusion (V/Q) mismatch, right-to-left anatomic shunts, and diffusion defects.[13] Right-to-left anatomic shunts are associated with congenital cardiovascular defects (eg, right-to-left patent ductus arteriosus) and generally become clinically relevant in young animals. This cause of hypoxemia is not oxygen responsive and not considered an indication for PPV. Diffusion defects describe diseases that alter the alveolar-capillary interface, interfering in gas exchange. In small animal patients, potential causes include smoke inhalation, oxygen toxicity, and acute respiratory distress syndrome (ARDS). The alveolar changes typified by these diseases are the loss of type 1 alveolar pneumocytes and their replacement with the large, cuboidal type 2 pneumocytes. This process is slow, taking several days after the initial pulmonary insult to occur.[13] Hypoxemia subsequent to a diffusion defect improves with oxygen therapy and should not require PPV. But many causes of diffusion defects can also cause severe V/Q mismatch, necessitating mechanical ventilation. V/Q mismatch refers to pulmonary parenchymal disease that leads to alveoli receiving decreased ventilation for the degree of perfusion (low V/Q) or regions of no ventilation but ongoing perfusion (no V/Q or shunt). In small animal medicine, V/Q mismatch is associated with all forms of pulmonary parenchymal disease including pulmonary edema, hemorrhage, and pneumonia. When pulmonary parenchymal disease is associated with severe hypoxemia despite high levels of oxygen therapy, PPV is indicated. As a general guideline, lung disease resulting in a Pa_{O_2} of less than 60 mm Hg despite greater than 60% Fi_{O_2} is an indication for PPV unless the underlying cause for the hypoxemia can be readily resolved.[9-11] High V/Q describes alveoli that receive more ventilation than perfusion and this is not a mechanism of hypoxemia.

Severe Hypoventilation

Hypoventilation is marked by hypercapnia (P_{CO_2} >50 mm Hg). As arterial and venous carbon dioxide levels correlate well in hemodynamically stable patients, with Pv_{CO_2} running approximately 4 to 5 mm Hg higher than Pa_{CO_2}, VBGs can be used to evaluate ventilation (but not oxygenation) status in most patients.[13] In hemodynamically unstable animals, measurement of Pa_{CO_2} is ideal, as carbon dioxide can accumulate in venous blood in association with low flow states and is no longer representative of ventilation. Hypoventilation is defined as a P_{CO_2} greater than 50 mm Hg, while severe hypoventilation is a P_{CO_2} greater than 60 mm Hg (eg, hypercapnic respiratory failure).[9] Severe hypoventilation that cannot be readily resolved by treatment of the primary disease (eg, reversal agent for a sedative) may be an indication for PPV. The extreme of hypoventilation is apnea, a clear indication for PPV. As elevations of P_{CO_2} may be associated with increases in intracranial pressure, animals considered at risk of intracranial hypertension may require PPV to maintain a Pa_{CO_2} of 35 to 40 mm Hg.

The P_{CO_2} is directly proportional to the rate of carbon dioxide production and inversely proportional to alveolar minute ventilation.[13] In most clinical situations, alveolar minute ventilation is the primary determinant of P_{CO_2}. Alveolar minute ventilation is equal to the product of the respiratory rate and alveolar TV (total TV minus the volume of dead space). Consequently, causes of severe hypoventilation are diseases that impair the ability of patients to maintain an adequate respiratory rate and/or TV. Such diseases include brain disease, cervical spinal cord disease, peripheral neuropathies, diseases of the neuromuscular junction, and myopathies. Hypoventilation will cause hypoxemia when the patient is breathing room air, as it reduces (dilutes out) the partial pressure of oxygen in the alveolus.[13] The higher the Pco_2, the lower the alveolar oxygen partial pressure and hence the greater the severity of hypoxemia. This mechanism of hypoxemia should rapidly resolve with oxygen therapy, although the Pco_2 will be unchanged. For this reason, oxygen therapy should be provided as soon as hypoventilation is identified. Hypoventilation is associated with inadequate respiratory rate and/or TV, which can ultimately result in apnea and death. When hypoventilation is severe or the underlying disease is thought to be progressive in nature, PPV is indicated.[9]

Pulmonary parenchymal disease leading to low, or no V/Q regions will reduce the ability of the lung to remove carbon dioxide, but lung disease is not considered a direct cause of hypoventilation. This is because the respiratory center of the brain tightly controls Pco_2 and will stimulate an increase in respiratory rate and/or TV to target a normal Pco_2. When hypoventilation is evident in the patient with lung disease, it is most commonly secondary to muscle fatigue leading to inadequate ventilation.[14] Hypoventilation in the lung disease patient can be an indication of patient deterioration and PPV should be considered.

Excessive Work of Breathing

Animals that are breathing so hard that they are becoming exhausted or seem to be at risk of exhaustion (eg, orthopnea, inability to rest their head, inability to sleep) may require PPV to prevent imminent death. While some of these patients may be maintaining adequate blood gases, they are at risk for respiratory fatigue and arrest.[14] This indication for PPV is based on clinical judgment in patients that do not qualify for ventilation based on blood gases or no blood gas data is available.

Severe Circulatory Shock

In patients with severe circulatory shock that is persistent despite initial resuscitation efforts, PPV may be indicated. The main goal of PPV in these patients is to reduce oxygen consumption.[9] PPV also reduces afterload on the left ventricle and can have significant benefits for left-sided heart failure.[15] Circulatory shock is not a common indication for PPV in veterinary patients at this time but is well described in human patients, in particular for supportive management of cardiogenic shock.[16]

Facilitate Long-Term Endotracheal Intubation

It is not uncommon for mechanical ventilation to be used to support animals that require long-term endotracheal intubation. The anesthetic and sedative drugs required to maintain intubation often cause hypoventilation. In addition, prolonged recumbency can cause atelectasis and hypoxemia that can benefit from PPV.

PROGNOSIS

The prognosis of weaning from PPV is largely dependent on the underlying disease for which the animal requires ventilation. In general, patients that require PPV for hypoventilation (eg, cervical spinal cord disease) have a greater likelihood of weaning than those with pulmonary parenchymal disease (eg, ARDS, pulmonary contusions, pneumonia).[17–19] In a retrospective study of 111 dogs and 16 cats that received PPV, 22% of animals with pulmonary disease were successfully weaned and discharged from the hospital. In comparison 32% of animals with nonpulmonary disease were successfully weaned.[19] When only the animals ventilated for greater than 24 hours were considered in this study, 38% of animals with pulmonary disease were successfully weaned compared with 62% of animals with nonpulmonary disease.[19]

It is more helpful to consider the prognosis of weaning from PPV in terms of the primary disease process present. For example, cardiogenic pulmonary edema generally has a good prognosis with reported successful weaning rates of 33% to 69% and aspiration pneumonia has reported weaning rates of 50% to 72%.[17–21] In contrast, only 8% of dogs and cats with ARDS have been reported to wean from mechanical ventilation.[9,11] Other factors that have been reported to be associated with a poorer outcome from PPV include age, weight, and species. The weaning rates reported for feline patients are consistently lower than that of canine patients, in the range of 10% to 25%, overall.[17,19,21] Disease processes that can have a fair to good prognosis for weaning from PPV include:

- Congestive heart failure
- Pulmonary contusions
- Aspiration pneumonia
- Cervical spinal cord compression
- Polyradiculoneuritis
- Intoxications

Disease processes that may generally have a poor prognosis to be weaned from PPV include:

- Postcardiopulmonary arrest
- ARDS
- Pulmonary disease of unknown cause

OVERVIEW OF VENTILATION MODES

To understand how to appropriately manage a patient undergoing PPV, an understanding of the ventilation modes and ventilator settings is imperative.[9,10]

Pressure Versus Volume Control

Modern ICU ventilators have the capability to generate several different breath types. The more basic machines tend to be either volume control ventilators or pressure control ventilators. It can deliver a preset TV over a given inspiratory time (volume control, or VC), or the machine can maintain a preset airway pressure for a given inspiratory time (pressure control, or PC). In a volume-controlled breath, the peak-inspired airway pressure (PIP) generated will be dependent on the preset TV chosen by the operator and the compliance of the respiratory system. In a pressure-controlled breath, the TV will depend on the preset airway pressure chosen by the operator and the compliance of the respiratory system. There is no evidence that there is any clinical superiority of volume versus pressure control ventilation in the anesthetized, veterinary patient and at this time the choice is purely clinician preference.

Assist-Control Ventilation

In this mode of ventilation, a minimum respiratory rate is set by the operator. If the trigger sensitivity is set appropriately, the patient can increase the respiratory rate, but all breaths delivered will be full ventilator breaths, either pressure- or volume-controlled. Breaths triggered by the ventilator are controlled breaths, while breaths triggered by the patient are considered assisted breaths (eg, patient initiates the breath, but the ventilator generates the full breath). This mode of ventilation provides maximum support to the respiratory system and is used in patients with severe disease or patients with no respiratory drive.

Synchronized Intermittent Mandatory Ventilation

In this mode of ventilation, a set number of mandatory breaths is delivered. Between these breaths, the patient can breathe spontaneously, as often or as few times as desired. In modern ventilators, the machine tries to synchronize the mandatory breaths with the patient's inspiratory efforts, thus the term synchronized intermittent mandatory ventilation (SIMV). The operator can only control the minimum respiratory rate and minute ventilation; there is no control over the maximum rate or maximum minute ventilation. As this mode combines full ventilator breaths with spontaneous patient breaths, it is generally used for animals that do not require 100% assistance from the ventilator, such as neurologically inappropriate animals with an unreliable respiratory drive, or patients with lung disease that are improving and do not need as much support as assist-control provides.

Continuous Positive Airway Pressure

Continuous positive airway pressure (CPAP) is a completely spontaneous mode of ventilation; in other words, the patient determines both the respiratory rate and TV. The ventilator delivers no breaths; the operator can only control the baseline airway pressure, a form of positive end-expiratory pressure (PEEP). This mode of ventilation is only suited for patients with a strong respiratory drive and minimal pulmonary dysfunction. The ventilator will alarm if the animal does not generate adequate breaths or develops apnea, so it is a useful monitoring mode for weaning patients or for monitoring intubated patients.

Pressure Support Ventilation

Pressure support ventilation (PSV) allows the operator to augment the TV of spontaneous breaths. For example, a patient has a PSV of 6 cm H_2O. This patient will begin and end the breath, and the ventilator will maintain a pressure of 6 cm H_2O in the airway during inspiration; this effectively provides the patient with a greater TV for less patient effort. PSV is generally used in conjunction with CPAP or to support spontaneous breaths in SIMV. It can be particularly useful in animals with respiratory muscle weakness either due to their primary disease or secondary to a prolonged period of PPV.

OVERVIEW OF VENTILATOR SETTINGS

The parameters the operator will need to adjust on a ventilator will vary between machines. on advanced ICU ventilators, there tend to be more options for adjusting breath parameters compared with simpler, anesthesia-type machines. It is important to note that there is no consistency in the terminology for ventilator settings between companies; therefore, it may be necessary to read the manufacturer's instructions to fully understand how the settings on an individual machine operate.

Trigger Variable

This is the parameter that initiates a ventilator breath. In patients that are not making any respiratory effort, the trigger variable will be time (which is determined from the set respiratory rate). The patient trigger setting is usually a change in airway pressure or a change in flow within the circuit. Appropriate trigger sensitivity is an essential safety measure to ensure ventilator breaths are synchronized with genuine respiratory efforts made by the patient.[10,22] This increases patient comfort and allows the patient to increase its RR as required. The trigger variable can be too sensitive, such that nonrespiratory efforts such as patient handling may initiate breaths; this should also be avoided.

Respiratory Rate and Inspiration: Expiration Ratio

The respiratory rate can be set on all ventilators either directly or by the manipulation of variables such as minute ventilation, inspiratory time, or exhalation time. The ideal respiratory rate for an individual patient generally needs to be titrated according to patient comfort and Pco_2. Respiratory rates are commonly set in the range of 10 to 20 breaths per minute initially. The ratio of the duration of inspiration to expiration (called the I:E ratio) may be preset by the operator or may be a default setting within the machine. An I:E ratio of 1:2 is ideal to ensure the patient has fully exhaled before the onset of the next breath.[10] This is similar to a physiologic normal breath, whereby expiration lasts approximately twice as long as inspiration. As respiratory rates are increased, the expiratory time will have to be reduced accordingly. It is advised to prevent the I:E ratio from increasing more than 1:1 to avoid a situation known as breath stacking or intrinsic PEEP.[10,23]

Inspiratory Time and Flow Rate

Inspiratory time is commonly set at 0.8 to 1 second, with shorter inspiratory times for smaller patients and patients with high respiratory rates.[10,23] Many volume control ventilators have the option to set the flow rate instead of the inspiratory time. The faster the inspiratory flow rate, the more quickly the breath is delivered. Flow rates of 60 L/min are suggested as a good starting point.[10,23] The flow rate may be adjusted between 40 and 80 L/min as needed to provide an inspiratory time that suits the patient's needs.[23]

Tidal Volume

The normal TV reported for dogs and cats is in the range of 10 to 15 mL/kg. It is recommended to target lower TV (6–8 mL/kg) in animals with severe lung disease.[10,23] When using volume control ventilation, the operator presets the desired TV. Overdistension of the lung is to be avoided, as it is a major mechanism of ventilator-induced lung injury and can have severe, even fatal consequences. It is recommended to start with no more than 10 mL/kg as a preset TV. The TV can always be increased if it is determined to be insufficient once the patient is connected to the machine. If pressure control ventilation is used, then the operator presets the pressure used to generate inspiration; once the animal is connected to the machine, the TV achieved with the preset pressure is assessed. A TV of around 10 mL/kg would be a very acceptable result.

Positive End-Expiratory Pressure

Pulmonary parenchymal disease can lead to areas of poorly ventilated alveoli (eg, alveoli smaller than normal) and alveolar collapse; this is the primary cause of inefficient oxygenating ability of the diseased lung. PEEP will maintain pressure in the airway during exhalation. This prevents full exhalation from occurring, holding the lung in a semi-inflated state, which can help open collapsed alveoli to improve lung-oxygenating ability and potentially protect against some forms of ventilator-induced lung injury.[10,24] As lung disease tends to be heterogeneous, there is a risk that while increases in PEEP may recruit areas of diseased lung, it may also cause overdistension or volutrauma of healthier lung regions. Selection of optimum PEEP is a frequent challenge in the ventilator patient and careful monitoring is recommended following all changes in PEEP.

There are some potential dangers from the use of PEEP that must be considered. As PEEP increases peak airway pressure, it can contribute to ventilator-induced lung injury. PEEP also maintains elevated intrathoracic pressure during exhalation, as such, it may compromise venous return. Cardiovascular monitoring is recommended for all ventilator patients and is essential when high levels of PEEP and/or more aggressive ventilator settings are used. Ultimately, optimizing PEEP requires balancing the potential gain with the concern for adverse effects.[10,24]

Peak-Inspired Airway Pressure

Peak-inspired pressure (PIP) is dependent on the size of the TV and the compliance of the respiratory system. Animals with normal lungs, normal chest confirmation, and lean body condition are expected to have high compliance and should be able to be ventilated with PIP in the range of 8 to 15 cm H_2O, ideally not exceeding 20 cm H_2O. Pulmonary disease, abnormal chest confirmation, obesity, and abdominal distension are all factors that will reduce the compliance of the respiratory system and as a result, they will need a higher PIP to maintain an adequate TV. Generally, it is recommended to aim for a PIP no higher than 30 cm H_2O but higher pressures may be needed when compliance is extremely low.[10,23]

INITIAL STABILIZATION ON THE VENTILATOR

Initial stabilization on the ventilator requires an anesthetic plan, monitoring plan, and initial set up of the machine. The ventilator should be set up with the appropriate patient circuit attached and tested for leaks and the initial ventilator settings selected. It is essential to always have equipment for manual ventilation readily available. Mechanical ventilators can malfunction or there can be issues with set up or inappropriate settings that require time to troubleshoot. As such, the ability to manually ventilate patients is important. All patient monitoring equipment should be ready for immediate use and materials for airway suction set up. It takes time to be fully prepared to initiate ventilation and the unstable patient should be anesthetized, intubated, and manually ventilated in the interim.

Selection of Ventilator Settings

There is no way to accurately predict the ideal ventilator settings for a specific patient before the initiation of ventilation. The choice of initial settings is based on an understanding of the underlying disease process present and use of general guidelines.[10,23] Once the patient is attached to the ventilator, the settings are then titrated to target adequate blood gases with an accepza Fio_2. Before selecting settings, the operator must first decide what mode of ventilation they wish to use (see above). The settings required for machine operation will depend on the mode used.

Animals that do not have pulmonary disease are expected to have compliant, easy-to-ventilate lungs. As a result, low airway pressures, higher TV, and less PEEP are likely to be well tolerated (**Table 1**). When initially placing a patient on the ventilator, the use of 100% oxygen should be used as a safety measure. Reducing Fio_2 is a priority once appropriate ventilator settings are determined, and the patient stabilized.

Animals that require PPV for pulmonary disease are expected to have poor lung compliance and will require higher airway pressures than animals with healthy lungs (see **Table 1**). PEEP may improve the oxygenating efficiency of the diseased lung

Table 1		
Suggested initial ventilator settings		
Ventilator Parameter	**Normal Lungs**	**Lung Disease**
Fraction of inspired oxygen (%)	100	100
Tidal volume (mL/kg)	8–12	6–8
Respiratory rate (breaths per minute)	10–20	20–30
Inspiratory pressure above PEEP (cm H_2O)	8–12	10–15
PEEP (cm H_2O)	0–4	5–8
Inspiratory time (seconds)	0.8–1	0.8–1
Inspiratory: Expiratory (I:E) ratio	1:2	1:1
Inspiratory trigger (cm H_2O)	0.5–2	0.5–2
Inspiratory trigger (L/min)	0.5–2	0.5–2

and can be a very important aspect of the management of some ventilator patients. Studies in human patients have shown that limiting TV can improve outcomes in all patients, with an emphasis on the role of low TV in patients with lung disease.[25,26] As such, any opportunity to reduce TV should be taken. Part of ventilator set up also includes setting appropriate alarm parameters, given the size of the patient and the ventilator settings chosen.

Once the patient is attached to the ventilator, the patient's chest should be observed for appropriate movement. The thorax should then be auscultated bilaterally to ensure there is ventilation of all lung fields. All monitoring parameters need to be rapidly and continuously evaluated including blood pressure, electrocardiography (ECG), pulse oximeter, and end-tidal carbon dioxide ($ETCO_2$) monitoring. Any concerning changes should be addressed immediately.

Once the patient is considered adequately stabilized on the ventilator, the assessment of ABGs is ideally performed. The target of PPV is to maintain adequate gas exchange while minimizing the likelihood of ventilator-induced lung injury. Target values are commonly a Pao_2 between 80 and 120 mm Hg and a $Paco_2$ of 35 to 50 mm Hg. Lowering the target Pao_2 to 60 mm Hg (SpO_2 of ~90%) and increasing the tolerance for hypercapnia (eg, Pco_2 >50 mm Hg) may reduce the magnitude of the ventilator settings needed in animals with severe hypoxemic respiratory failure.

Pao_2

The first aim in the titration of ventilator settings is to lower the Fio_2 to 50% to 60% while maintaining an acceptable Pao_2. In the absence of ABGs, reductions in the Fio_2 will have to be based on SpO_2. If the Pao_2 is not high enough to allow adequate reductions in Fio_2, increases in PEEP may be of benefit.

$Paco_2$

The $Paco_2$ will be inversely proportional to alveolar minute ventilation. When titrating the initial ventilator settings, if $Paco_2$ is higher than desired, increases in TV and/or respiratory rate are made and vice versa if the $Paco_2$ is too low. If ABGs are not available, venous Pco_2 can be used to guide ventilator settings. Initially, Pco_2 should be measured on a blood gas machine to evaluate the correlation with $ETCO_2$. Once this relationship has been established, $ETCO_2$ can be used as a noninvasive measure to titrate ventilator settings further. If a significant change in the patient status occurs, the P_{CO_2} should be measured directly, as the relationship and accuracy with $ETCO_2$ can rapidly change.

Ventilator settings should be constantly adjusted as the patient status changes. For animals with lung disease, the magnitude of ventilator settings will be gradually reduced as the lung function improves. For animals with ventilatory failure, the level of machine support is reduced as the animal regains respiratory function.

Induction and Maintenance of Anesthesia

To successfully ventilate neurologically intact dogs and cats, appropriate anesthesia must be maintained. This is to allow maintenance of the endotracheal tube (ETT), to prevent patient movement, to provide patient comfort, and to stop animals from bucking or fighting the ventilator. In neurologically abnormal animals, anesthesia may not be necessary. Paralyzed animals may only need anesthesia to allow ETT intubation and may be ventilated without anesthesia via a temporary tracheostomy tube. Comatose patients may tolerate ETT intubation without drug administration and are another group of patients that often can be ventilated without anesthesia.

There are several options for the induction and maintenance of anesthesia in the ventilated patient. Induction of anesthesia should be performed using at least 1 fast-acting intravenous drug allowing rapid ETT placement. All animals should be pre-oxygenated before induction. Consideration of the patient's cardiovascular status when selecting induction drugs is important. Propofol or alfaxalone, administered slowly and to effect, are very effective induction drugs for hemodynamically stable patients. In hemodynamically unstable animals, the use of induction drugs such as ketamine or etomidate may be preferable. Severely compromised animals may only need minimal drug doses for induction. Lung disease generally increases vagal tone and is often associated with bradycardia. A dose of an anticholinergic drug such as atropine should be readily available during the induction and premedication of an anticholinergic drug should be considered if an opioid is to be included in the induction plan.

Maintenance anesthesia of the PPV patient is generally achieved by combinations of injectable drugs; however, if an anesthesia ventilator is used, low concentrations of inhalant anesthesia can also be used. The choice of anesthesia protocol for individual patients with PPV will be influenced by their cardiovascular stability, the duration of PPV anticipated, and in some situations, cost. A further consideration is recovery time. It is ideal to be able to recover animals as soon as they are ready to be weaned from PPV. This may require reducing drug doses ahead of time or changing the anesthetic protocol when weaning is thought to be imminent. Injectable anesthetics such as propofol and alfaxalone will provide an adequate plane of anesthesia when used as constant rate infusions (CRIs) and generally are the basis for most ventilator patient anesthetic protocols. It is ideal to provide balanced anesthesia by the addition of drugs such as benzodiazepines, dexmedetomidine, and/or opioids. This allows minimal dosing of any one drug to reduce the likelihood of adverse effects. See **Table 2** for suggested dosing regimens. Long-term administration of propofol in dogs can lead to lipemia, which can have adverse effects and should be avoided. By minimizing the dose of propofol with the addition of other drugs, lipemia can often be avoided. Animals on propofol infusions should be evaluated several times daily for lipemia. Cats cannot tolerate long-term (>36–48 hours) propofol administration, as it leads to Heinz body formation; therefore, other anesthetic regimes need to be considered for long-term PPV in this species.[27] Another concern for PPV in cats is the delayed recovery time they have after prolonged injectable anesthesia. After 24 hours of anesthesia, recovery time has been reported to be 18 to 35 hours in one study.[28] In the authors' experience, it can take many days for cats to recover from long-term anesthesia. As

Table 2	
Anesthetic/analgesic agents commonly used in ventilated patients	
Anesthetic/Analgesic Agent	**Suggested Dose**
Fentanyl	0.1–0.5 mcg/kg/min CRI Loading dose: 2–5 mcg/kg
Midazolam	0.1–0.5 mg/kg/h CRI Loading dose: 0.2–0.4 mg/kg
Diazepam	0.1–1.0 mg/kg/h CRI Loading dose: 0.5 mg/kg
Morphine-lidocaine-ketamine CRI	Morphine: 0.2 mg/kg/h; loading dose: 0.1–0.2 mg/kg slow intravenously Lidocaine: 3 mg/kg/h; loading dose 1–2 mg/kg Ketamine: 0.6 mg/kg/h; loading dose 0.5 mg/kg
Propofol	0.05–0.4 mg/kg/min CRI
Alfaxalone	0.05–0.4 mg/kg/min CRI
Dexmedetomidine	0.5–1.0 mg/kg/h

All doses indicate intravenous route.

they often require ventilator support during the prolonged recovery period, it adds significantly to the cost and challenge of management of cats needing PPV.

Patient Care and Monitoring

Mechanically ventilated patients require intense monitoring and supportive care. Multiple intravenous lines are usually needed, making a multilumen catheter ideal. In addition, an arterial catheter, a body temperature probe, and urinary catheterization are recommended in most cases. Monitoring should include continuous ECG, continuous pulse oximetry, continuous direct arterial blood pressure, intermittent blood gas analysis (via an arterial catheter), and continuous $ETCO_2$ measurements. Blood pressure monitoring is essential and in the absence of direct pressure monitoring, frequent indirect blood pressure measurement is required. Nursing care should include diligent catheter care protocols, oral cleaning and moisturizing, tracheal tube suction, passive range of motion of all limbs, ocular care, and intermittent change of body position. Readers are directed to other resources for more detail on the care of the ventilator patient.[29]

Airway humidification is essential for patients with an artificial airway for prolonged periods. The 2 main methods of humidification for the ventilator patient are either a heat moisture exchanger (HME) or an active heated water humidifier. The HME is a disposable airway adapter connected to the ETT that traps heat and moisture in the exhaled gas, transferring it to the inhaled gas on the next breath.[30] These are relatively inexpensive and very convenient and are as effective at humidification as the heated water devices. An HME does increase airway resistance and may not be tolerated by all patients. It adds dead space to the circuit so the appropriate size should be used for a given animal. It can easily become occluded by airway secretions and should be used with caution if obvious secretions are present. The heated water humidifiers are connected to the inspiratory limb of the breathing circuit and are ideally used in conjunction with heated wire circuits to avoid excessive moisture collecting in the circuit.[30] They do not have the issues of airway resistance, dead space, or occlusion associated with HMEs but they are a relatively expensive piece of equipment.

The ventilator itself requires management, including emptying water traps (if present) that collect condensation from the tubing and filling the humidifier with sterile water as needed. Ventilator patients need constant care by a dedicated veterinary nurse and an attentive veterinarian who can troubleshoot ventilator problems and adjust ventilator settings as needed. As such, placing and maintaining a patient on a mechanical ventilator is a significant commitment of both time and finances.

TROUBLESHOOTING

Hypoxemia is a common problem faced by patients undergoing PPV. The approach to the management of hypoxemia differs when it is an acute development versus a more gradual onset. If acute desaturation is detected on the pulse oximeter, repositioning of the pulse oximeter or confirmation with an ABG is ideal. Acute desaturation of a ventilator patient that was previously oxygenating adequately indicates a dramatic decrease in pulmonary function. Potential causes include pneumothorax, machine malfunction, circuit disconnection, and loss of oxygen supply. The Fio_2 should be immediately increased to 100%, the thorax auscultated, and the ventilator function reviewed. If a pneumothorax is suspected, thoracocentesis should be performed. A gradual decline in oxygenating efficiency of the lung is not uncommon in the ventilator patient and is more suggestive of progressive pulmonary disease such as pneumonia, ARDS, or ventilator-induced lung injury, rather than a pneumothorax or machine issue. This can be addressed in several ways. The Fio_2 can be increased as needed to keep the patient stable but efforts to improve oxygenation with the manipulation of ventilator settings are preferred. Increasing PEEP may improve the oxygenating ability of some lung diseases. In patients with low TV, consideration of increasing the TV may improve lung function if hypoxemia is severe.

Hypercapnia in the ventilator patient has many potential causes including pneumothorax, airway obstruction, malfunction of the ventilator or ventilator circuit, increased dead space, and inadequate ventilator settings. A sudden increase in $Paco_2$ in a previously stable patient is suggestive of an acute abnormality such as an ETT or tracheostomy tube obstruction or dislodgement, ventilator circuit leak, or pneumothorax. If the evaluation of the machine and patient rules out major complications, then it is to be assumed that there is insufficient alveolar minute ventilation, and appropriate changes in the ventilator settings should be made.

Hemodynamic compromise can be an adverse effect of PPV. Subatmospheric intrathoracic pressure generated during normal, spontaneous inspiration promotes venous return to the right side of the heart. When a patient is placed on PPV, it generates positive intrathoracic pressure during inspiration, which opposes venous return. As a result, venous return occurs primarily during exhalation during PPV and may be reduced compared with normal. With the addition of PEEP, which generates positive intrathoracic pressure during exhalation, venous return may be further compromised. Perfusion parameters and blood pressure should be closely monitored in the PPV patient, especially when high PEEP levels and high peak pressures are used. If hemodynamic compromise occurs, intravascular volume support to improve preload may be beneficial. In patients that are hypotensive despite fluid therapy, vasopressor therapy may be indicated.

When a patient fights or bucks the ventilator, it can prevent effective ventilation of the animal and may lead to desaturation and hypercapnia. In addition, it increases the work of breathing and can increase both patient discomfort and patient morbidity. Bucking the ventilator is one of the most common challenges for PPV patient management. It is ideal to have a thorough, systematic approach to this problem to avoid missing potential causes. Potential causes include hypoxemia, hypercapnia, pneumo-thorax, hyperthermia, patient-ventilator asynchrony, and/or inappropriate depth of anesthesia. Many anesthetic and sedative drugs lower the hypothalamic set point for temperature. As a result, mild increases in temperature may cause dogs to pant on the ventilator. This can make it very challenging to provide effective ventilation and active cooling is commonly required to control panting in patients with hyperther-mic ventilator. A common cause of hyperthermia is increased breathing efforts when patients fight the ventilator, making appropriate evaluation and resolution of active pa-tient breathing efforts important. Patient-ventilator asynchrony describes a mismatch between the nature of the ventilator breath (timing, flow rate, volume, etc.) and the pa-tient's respiratory demands. It is detected by evidence of active respiratory efforts dur-ing mandatory ventilation and interpretation of ventilator waveforms. Adjustment of ventilator settings is made in an effort to better meet the needs of the patient. An inad-equate depth of anesthesia may be the most common cause of animals fighting the ventilator, but care should be taken not to automatically increase the anesthetic drug dose when patients begin bucking the machine, without fully assessing the pa-tient or the ventilator settings.

SUMMARY

Mechanical ventilation can be a lifesaving tool for dogs and cats experiencing hypox-emic respiratory failure and those that develop ventilatory failure. Ventilation of pa-tients with ventilatory failure has been shown to have a better prognosis than the ventilation of those ventilated for hypoxemic respiratory failure.[19,27] An anesthesia ma-chine can be used to provide PPV to patients for short time periods. If longer-term ventilation is required, referral to a veterinary hospital with an ICU ventilator should be considered. Recognizing and treating dogs and cats with imminent respiratory fail-ure with anesthesia, intubation, and PPV can be practical and lifesaving.

CLINICS CARE POINTS

- Hypoxemic respiratory failure may be successfully managed with HFNT, avoiding the need for PPV
- Animals that fail HFNT or have ventilatory failure will require PPV
- Successful PPV requires an understanding of ventilator modes and key ventilator settings
- Long-term PPV (>12–24 hours) requires intensive nursing care and advanced patient monitoring
- There is an emphasis on minimizing TV, in particular in patients with pulmonary disease
- Clinicians need to constantly review and adjust ventilator settings in response to patient changes
- The duration of PPV and prognosis for weaning depends on the underlying disease process

DISCLOSURE

The authors have no financial or commercial conflict of interest to declare – K. Hopper and L. Powell.

REFERENCES

1. Ward JJ. High-flow oxygen administration by nasal cannula for adult and peri-natal patients. Respir Care 2013;58:98–122.
2. Groves N, Tobin A. High flow nasal oxygen generates positive airway pressure in adult volunteers. Aust Crit Care 2007;20(4):126–31.
3. Dunphy ED, Mann FA, Dodam JR, et al. Comparison of unilateral versus bilateral nasal oxygen catheters for oxygen administration in dogs. J Vet Emerg Crit Care 2002;12(4):245–51.
4. Daly J, Guenther CL, Haggerty J, et al. Evaluation of oxygen administration with a high-flow nasal cannula to clinically normal dogs. Am J Vet Res 2017;78:624–30.
5. Keir I, Daly J, Haggerty J, et al. Retrospective evaluation of the effect of high flow oxygen therapy delivered by nasal cannula on PaO2 in dogs with moderate-to-severe hypoxemia. J Vet Emerg Crit Care 2016;26(4):598–602.
6. Jagodich TA, Bersenas AME, Bateman SW, et al. Comparison of high flow nasal cannula oxygen administration to traditional nasal cannula oxygen therapy in healthy dogs. J Vet Emerg Crit Care 2019;29:246–55.
7. Jagodich TA, Bersenas AME, Bateman SW, et al. High-flow nasal cannula oxygen therapy in acute hypoxemic respiratory failure in 22 dogs requiring oxygen support escalation. J Vet Emerg Crit Care 2020;30:364–75.
8. Pouzot-Nevoret C, Hocine L, Nègre J, et al. Prospective pilot study for evaluation of high-flow oxygen therapy in dyspnoeic dogs: the HOT-DOG study. J Small Animal Pract 2019;60:656–62.
9. Laghi F, Tobin MJ. Indications for mechanical ventilation. In: Tobin MJ, editor. Indications for mechanical ventilation. 3rd edition. New York: McGraw-Hill; 2013. p. 101–36.
10. Hess DR, Kacmarek RM. Essentials of mechanical ventilation. 4th edition. New York: McGraw-Hill; 2018.
11. Cairo JM. Establishing the need for mechanical ventilation. In: Pilbeam's Mechanical ventilation: Physiology and clinical applications. 7th edition. St Louis (MO): Elsevier; 2019. p. 44–57.
12. Farrell KS, Hopper K, Cagle LA, et al. Evaluation of pulse oximetry as a surrogate for PaO$_2$ in awake dogs breathing room air and anesthetized dogs on mechanical ventilation. J Vet Emerg Crit Care 2019;29(6):622–9.
13. Lumb AB, Thomas CR. Nunn and Lumb's applied respiratory physiology. 9th edition. Elsevier; 2021.
14. Barton L. Respiratory muscle fatigue. Vet Clin North Am Small Anim Pract 2002; 32(5):1059–71.
15. Gomez H, Pinsky MR. Effect of mechanical ventilation on heart-lung interaction. In: Tobin MJ, editor. Indications for mechanical ventilation. 3rd edition. New York: McGraw-Hill; 2013. p. 821–50.
16. Alviar CL, Rico-Mesa JS, Morrow DA, et al. Positive pressure ventilation in cardiogenic shock: Review of the evidence and practical advice for patients with mechanical circulatory support. Can J Cardiol 2020;36(2):300–12.
17. Hopper K, Haskins SC, Kass PH, et al. Indications, management and outcome of long-term positive-pressure ventilation in dogs and cats: 148 cases (1990-2001). J Am Vet Med Assoc 2007;230:64–75.
18. Campbell VL, King LG. Pulmonary function, ventilator management, and outcome of dogs with thoracic trauma and pulmonary contusions: 10 cases (1994-1998). J Am Vet Med Assoc 2000;217:1505–9.

19. Cagle LA, Hopper K, Epstein SE. Indications and outcome associated with positive pressure ventilation in dogs and cats: 127 cases. J Vet Emerg Crit Care. In Print.

20. Edwards TH, Brainard BM, DeFrancesco TC, et al. Outcome of positive-pressure ventilation in dogs and cats with congestive heart failure: 16 cases (1992 – 2012). J Vet Emerg Crit Care 2014;24(5):586–93.

21. Lee JA, Drobatz KJ, Koch MW, et al. Indications for and outcome of positive-pressure ventilation in cats: 53 cases (1993-2002). J Am Vet Med Assoc 2005; 226:924–31.

22. Cairo JM. Final considerations in ventilator set up. In: Pilbeam's Mechanical ventilation: Physiological and clinical applications. 7th edition. St Louis (MO): Elsevier; 2019. p. 97–115.

23. Cairo JM. Initial ventilator settings. In: Pilbeam's Mechanical ventilation: Physiological and clinical applications. 7th edition. St Louis (MO): Elsevier; 2019. p. 80–96.

24. Cairo JM. Improving oxygenation and management of acute respiratory distress syndrome. In: Pilbeam's Mechanical ventilation: Physiological and clinical applications. 7th edition. St Louis (MO): Elsevier; 2019. p. 80–96.18.

25. Simonis FD, Juffermans NP, Schultz MJ. Mechanical ventilation of the healthy lungs: lessons learned from recent trials. Curr Opin Crit Care 2021;27(1):55–9.

26. Neto S, Simonis FD, Schultz MJ. How to ventilate patients without acute respiratory distress syndrome? Curr Opin Crit Care 2015;21(1):65–73.

27. Andress JL, Day TK, Day D. The effects of consecutive day propofol anesthesia on feline red blood cells. Vet Surg 1995;24(3):277–82.

28. Boudreau AE, Bersensas AM, Kerr CL, et al. A comparison of 3 anesthetic protocols for 24 hours of mechincal ventilation in cats. J Vet Emerg Crit Care 2012;22:239–52.

29. Epstein SE. Care of the ventilator patient. In: Silverstein DC, Hopper K, editors. Small animal critical care medicine. St Louis (MO): Elsevier-Saunders; 2009. p. P185–90.

30. Al Ashry HS, Modrykamien AM. Humidification during mechanical ventilation in the adult patient. Biomed Res Int 2014;2014:715434.

Fluid Therapy for Pediatric Patients

Leah A. Cohn, DVM, PhD[a], Amy J. Kaplan-Zattler, DVM[b],*, Justine A. Lee, DVM[b]

KEYWORDS

- Pediatric • Neonate • Fluid therapy • Crystalloids • Colloids • Blood transfusion
- Neonatal isoerythrolysis • Intraosseous

KEY POINTS

- Pediatric patients have a higher fluid requirement compared with adults because of increased extracellular fluid, decreased renal ability to conserve water, a larger surface area/body weight ratio, and larger fluid losses through the skin.
- In pediatric patients less than 6 weeks of age, hydration and volume status are difficult to assess.
- Fluids should be warmed to near body temperature (37°C/98.6°F) before administration to pediatric patients and should be kept warm, even in fluid lines.
- Multiple routes of fluid administration are used in the neonate or pediatric patient including oral, subcutaneous (SC), intraperitoneal (IP), intraosseous (IO), and intravenous (IV). Clinicians should be aware of the limitations and potential complications of each route of delivery.

INTRODUCTION

Although dogs and cats are often referred to as puppies and kittens until a year of age, the term pediatric generally refers to the first 6 months of life.[1] This terminology is further divided into the following: neonate aged 0 to 2 weeks, infant aged 2 to 6 weeks, and juvenile aged 6 to 12 weeks.[1–3] The term pediatric is used throughout this article, which focuses on the first 12 weeks of life. Medical treatment of pediatric patients presents challenges because of their small size and unique physiology, but understanding these challenges allows the veterinarian to provide life-saving supportive care to these young patients.

Sick pediatric patients can quickly become critically ill patients; any of several disease states, or even problems with basic animal husbandry or lack of maternal care, can result in a debilitated pup or kitten that requires critical care.[4] It is estimated that 12% to 15% of pups born at full-term will succumb by the time of weaning, with half of all deaths said to occur in the first 3 days of life.[5] Common causes of neonatal (ie, <2 weeks) illness are

[a] University of Missouri College of Veterinary Medicine, 900 East Campus Drive, Columbia, MO 65211, USA; [b] VETgirl, 2950 Busch Lake Boulevard, Tampa, FL 33614, USA
* Corresponding author.
E-mail address: ajzattler@gmail.com

Vet Clin Small Anim 52 (2022) 707–718
https://doi.org/10.1016/j.cvsm.2022.01.007
0195-5616/22/© 2022 Elsevier Inc. All rights reserved.

related to poor mothering, inadequate nutrition (eg, poor suckling, inadequate milk production), congenital defects, hypoxemia associated with dystocia, poor sanitation, neonatal isoerythrolysis (kittens only), or the poorly understood "fading" puppy or kitten syndrome.[4–6] These conditions are often manifested within the first week of life, but can also occur days or weeks after whelping if the mother herself becomes too ill to care for the puppies/kittens. During the infant period from 2 to 6 weeks of age, life-threatening diseases, such as juvenile hypoglycemia, parasitism (internal and external), trauma, or dehydration from diarrhea, are often seen.[2,4] Weakness, tremors, seizures, stupor, or coma can indicate severe hypoglycemia.[2,7] When hypoglycemia is suspected or confirmed, rapid treatment with intravenous (IV) or intraosseous (IO) glucose solution is imperative, along with monitoring and follow-up care. Infestation with fleas or parasitism with hookworms can result in severe anemia in these very small animals, seen clinically as listlessness, tachycardia, and pale mucous membranes. Dehydration often follows quickly from diarrhea of any cause, such as overfeeding, improper nutrition, parasites, or other infections (**Box 1**). During the juvenile period of 6 to 12 weeks, maternal antibodies are waning, resulting in increased susceptibility to infectious diseases.[4] Even pups vaccinated during this juvenile period may not be protected when there is just enough maternal antibodies to interfere with vaccine response or when only a single dose of vaccine has been recently administered. Among the most common juvenile infections of puppies and kittens are canine parvovirus and feline panleukopenia; these lead to diarrhea, vomiting, and anorexia, all of which predispose to severe dehydration and hypovolemia.

Dehydration and hypovolemia are 2 distinct conditions that can be seen either separately or together in critically ill juvenile patients. Dehydration refers to a water deficit in the interstitial and intracellular fluid compartments, whereas hypovolemia is a state of decreased intravascular volume. In the juvenile patient, severe dehydration can lead to hypovolemia as fluid is pulled from the intravascular space into the interstitial tissues and intracellular space. Because of their higher body water needs, this can happen quickly in young pups and kittens; hence, critically ill pediatric patients require appropriate fluid therapy to ensure survival.

Box 1
Infectious causes of diarrhea that can result in profound dehydration in the juvenile patient

1. Parasitism
   a. Coccidiosis
   b. Giardiasis
   c. Hookworms
   d. Roundworms

2. Viral infections
   a. Parvovirus
   b. Coronavirus
   c. Rotavirus

3. Bacterial infections
   a. *Salmonella*
   b. *Clostridia*
   c. *Campylobacter*
   d. *Escherichia coli*

4. Nutrition
   a. Overfeeding
   b. Inappropriate milk replacer (eg, cow's milk)
   c. Improper handling of the milk replacer diet
   d. Lactose intolerance

Unfortunately, the small size and physiologic differences between pediatric patients and mature animals can make clinical assessment of fluid status more difficult in these young patients.[8] For example, dehydration is typically graded as 5% to 7% in animals with "tacky" mucous membranes, but tiny mouths and frequent nursing can interfere with the assessment of oral mucous membranes. Skin tenting occurs at approximately 7% dehydration, but excess loose skin can affect this determination, and pups less than 6 weeks of age maintain skin turgor even when dehydrated.[8] Sunken globes are described at approximately 9% dehydration, and dull corneas at approximately 10% to 11%, but pups and kittens do not open their eyes until they are 1 to 2 weeks old. Clues to indicate hypovolemia usually include mucous membrane color and capillary refill time, pulse quality, and jugular venous distensibility. Each of these is far more difficult to gauge in very young animals. The other clue frequently used to assess volume status is heart rate, but heart rate in pediatric patients does not respond to volume change in a manner equivalent to mature animals. As difficult as it may be to gauge dehydration and hypovolemia, it is likewise difficult to judge overhydration. Signs of volume overload can include serous nasal discharge, chemosis (eg, particularly in the conjunctival region), tachypnea, altered breathing pattern, restlessness, cough, tachycardia, ascites, pulmonary crackles on auscultation, excessive weight gain, and polyuria. Careful monitoring of body weight, often several times per day, is absolutely crucial in neonates and helpful in all pediatric patients.

PEDIATRIC PHYSIOLOGY

Fluid requirements in pediatric patients are dramatically higher compared with adults.[1,2,5] As with humans and other species, neonatal dogs and cats have more extracellular fluid on a volume per kilogram body weight basis than older animals, and a higher water content (80% compared with 60% of body weight in adult animals).[9,10] Young pups and kittens use more water because of their higher metabolic rate. In addition, they have larger inherent fluid loss caused by a higher body surface area, a larger surface area/body weight ratio, and more permeable skin.[1,2] Their immature kidneys are not able to concentrate urine effectively to preserve water, and instead may contribute to their overall fluid loss.[1,11]

The unique cardiovascular physiology of pediatric patients contributes to their inability to adequately respond to hypovolemia.[12] Cardiac output is determined by heart rate multiplied by stroke volume. Adult animals compensate for hypovolemia through activation of the sympathetic nervous system thus increasing heart rate, activation of the renin–angiotensin system and release of antidiuretic hormone to retain fluid, and vasoconstriction, all in an attempt to maintain cardiac output. Pediatric patients lack the compensatory mechanisms to increase heart rate in an attempt to maintain cardiac output.[12,13] In the neonate, cardiac output cannot be increased by increasing cardiac contractility, because only 30% of fetal cardiac muscle is made up of contractile elements.[12] Puppies also seem to have fewer sympathetic nerve fibers supplying the myocardium than adults.[12,13] As a result, tachycardia in response to hypovolemia may not occur as it would in an older patient with hypovolemia.

Kidneys are not fully mature at birth, and renal physiology differs in pediatric patients compared with adults.[9,14,15] Even at 2 months of age, puppies have an increased glomerular filtration rate, higher daily urine volume, and greater fractional excretion of phosphorus than adult dogs.[16] There are conflicting data on the ability of young pups to concentrate urine. Traditionally, urine-specific gravity greater than 1.030 was not believed to occur before 8 weeks of age, but a study of healthy pups found that although neonates were unable to concentrate urine, pups 4 weeks and older generated urine comparable with that of adult dogs and could concentrate to specific gravity greater than or equal to 1.030.[17] Young puppies also have limited autoregulation of renal blood flow in response to changes in arterial blood pressure or hypovolemia, and may not be able to respond to rapid changes in sodium or water load.[9,11,15,18]

Importantly, pediatric patients are prone to hypoglycemia compared with adult animals and are perhaps more susceptible to the adverse effects of hypoglycemia than are adults.[10,12,19,20] Because of their limited glycogen stores, deficiency of gluconeogenic substrates, poor response to glucagon, and inefficient hepatic gluconeogenesis, pediatric patients are unable to maintain glucose homeostasis if deprived of food for even relatively short periods.[19,21] This tendency toward hypoglycemia is exaggerated by smaller size and younger age. Although the brain of all animals depends primarily on glucose as an energy source, lactate and ketones can be used as substitutes. However, the lack of fat and the time required to produce ketones prevents ketone bodies from being a substitute energy substrate in juveniles.[19] As a result, pediatric patients should have frequent blood glucose monitoring. Bolus administration of dextrose solution is often indicated during the acute presentation of weak pups and kittens (see fluid dosing). Routine ongoing dextrose supplementation in IV or IO fluid therapy should be considered for all pediatric patients that are not receiving complete and adequate enteral nutrition.

FLUID THERAPY

Crystalloid replacement solutions that resemble extracellular fluid in composition (eg, lactated Ringer solution, Normosol-R, Plasmalyte-A) can safely be administered to pediatric patients.[2] Some sources suggest avoiding lactate-containing fluids in animals less than 6 weeks of age because they do not effectively metabolize lactate into bicarbonate.[8] Other sources suggest that because lactate can be used as a substitute energy source by the neonatal brain, lactated Ringer solution may actually be preferred to other crystalloids.[10,22] At this time, there is no general consensus on what type of crystalloid solution should be used in the pediatric patient, only that it should be a balanced electrolyte solution. In the authors' opinion, the use of 0.9% NaCl as a replacement solution should be reserved for pediatric patients requiring higher sodium supplementation, as it is not a balanced, buffered solution. Supplementation with dextrose (2.5%-5% dextrose as a constant rate infusion [CRI]) and potassium (20–30 mEq potassium chloride per liter, or as guided by serum potassium concentration) is often necessary for critically ill pediatric patients.

Colloids are large-molecular-weight fluid solutions that stay within the intravascular space longer than do crystalloids, making them useful in the treatment of hypovolemia. Colloids are often used during volume resuscitation when crystalloids alone fail, or in patients with severe hypoalbuminemia. Examples include natural colloids (eg, plasma, whole blood, albumin) and synthetic colloids (eg, hydroxyethyl starch). The use of natural colloids such as fresh frozen plasma should be considered in coagulopathic pediatric patients (eg, anticoagulant rodenticide, congenital factor deficiency, inherited coagulopathy, disseminated intravascular coagulation) to replace deficient coaguloation factors. Likewise, with severe hypoproteinemia, natural colloids can supplement vital proteins in certain conditions, and both natural and synthetic colloids can provide oncotic support. Keep in mind that young animals have lower naturally occurring serum albumin and globulin concentrations compared with adults, and appropriate interpretation of total protein is warranted. As a result, life-threatening conditions such as inflammatory disease and blood loss can worsen the degree of hypoalbuminemia in pediatric patients. Plasma is not generally used in adult patients to replace albumin as such large volumes are needed (ie, approximately 22.5 mL/kg plasma is needed to increase albumin by 0.5 g/dL in a dog).[23] However, as pediatric patients tolerate high relative fluid volumes, the use of plasma as a source of colloidal support and fluid volume might be a viable consideration. Keep in mind that the use of plasma entails some risk of transfusion reaction (including future risk) or transmission of infectious disease, but naturally occurring antibodies in the administered plasma may offer limited benefit to neonatal patients deprived of colostrum.[24,25] Canine albumin, or less ideally human albumin, are other options for natural colloidal support. For anemic pediatric patients, transfusion of whole blood supplies oxygen-carrying support in addition to aiding with vascular volume (**Box 2** for more information on bolus dosing for volume resuscitation).

Any of several blood products may be necessary for the pediatric patient for a variety of reasons. Plasma can be useful when colostrum ingestion has not occurred.[24,25] The administration of plasma or serum from the mother or another healthy, well-vaccinated adult animal can provide protective antibodies. The recommended dose for this purpose is 16 mL for puppies and 15 mL for kittens, divided into 2 or 3 portions, administered subcutaneously (SC) every 6 to 8 hours.[3,24–26] Feline neonatal isoerythrolysis is another condition that often requires blood transfusion. Queens with type B blood have strong naturally occurring antibodies against type A blood. When these queens are bred to type A males, colostrum ingested by any resulting type A kittens may cause life-threatening hemolysis.[27] Clinical signs include tail tip necrosis, icterus, pale mucous membranes, listlessness, "fading," or sudden death. Ideally, kittens should be removed from the queen for the first 24 hours after birth to prevent colostrum ingestion, but if neonatal isoerythrolysis has already occurred, transfusion of washed red blood cells may be required. Initially, cells from the type B queen can be given at a dose of approximately 5 mL per kitten (IV, over several hours) because the circulating antibodies attack type A blood.[27] If further transfusions are required more than 3 days postpartum, the type A kitten may have formed antibodies to type B blood. At this point, washed cells from a type A donor should be used in place of the mother's cells.[27]

Pups and kittens have a lower red blood cell mass than adults even in health. Anemia from any cause, such as external or internal parasites or parvovirus, may warrant transfusion of red blood cells. Kittens should always be blood typed, and ideally crossmatched before transfusion. For pups, the same is ideal, but initial transfusions are often safe even from mismatched donors simply because dogs do not have preformed antibodies to other blood types.[28]

As for the use of synthetic colloids in pediatric patient, little evidence is available. Synthetic colloids are large molecular weight solutes carried in electrolyte and water

---

Box 2
Emergency fluid dosages for neonates

- Bolus isotonic crystalloid fluid for hypovolemia: 3 to 4 mL/100 g (pups); 2 to 3 mL/100 g (kittens)

- Bolus glucose for hypoglycemia: 1 mL to 3 mL of 12.5% dextrose (eg, 1:3 dilution of 50% dextrose with sterile water)

- Bolus colloid for hypovolemia that is nonresponsive to multiple crystalloid boluses: 2 mL/kg to 5 mL/kg, followed by 1 mL/kg/h as needed

- Whole blood for anemia: 10 mL/kg to 20 mL/kg

solutions. In the last decade, research in both human medicine and veterinary medicine have raised questions regarding the safety of their use in critically ill patients.[29–32] Based on current literature and recommendations, the use of synthetic colloids is considered contraindicated in patients with known kidney disease or potential for acute kidney injury (eg, nephrotoxicant, history of chronic kidney disease, and so forth); the use of synthetic colloids is also considered "under advisement" in septic patients.[29,33] Hyperoncotic synthetic colloids, such as HES 10%, have been suggested to cause renal damage in dogs with and without sepsis.[34] Lower oncotic solutions, such as HES 6%, appear safe at standard doses for conditions including hemorrhage, intraoperative hypotension, trauma, and others.[35–40] Keep in mind that the use of different sized synthetic colloids generally varies by country use, and the clinician must be aware of which type and size they are using when treating the critically ill patient. Currently, the exact mechanism for kidney injury secondary to synthetic colloid use is unknown; however, it is theorized to be due to osmotic injury resulting from the large molecular weight solutes lingering inside the renal epithelial cells.[31] There is also speculation that starch's carrier solution may play a role; specifically, the chloride found in the commonly used HES carrier solutions (0.9% NaCl) may act as a potent renal vasoconstrictor.[37,41] As there are no safety studies on the use of synthetic colloids in pediatric dogs and cats at this time, clinicians are limited to extrapolation from relevant emerging recommendations for use in human medicine and adult veterinary patients.

ROUTES OF ADMINISTRATION

Neonates and pediatric patients are unable to control their body temperature and are susceptible to chilling. As a result, it is advisable to warm the fluid—regardless of the route of administration—to approximate body temperature before administration. Remember that fluids that run through a length of administration tubing may cool rapidly, so temperature control of fluid in the tubing matters as much as warming of fluid in the bag or syringe. Warming the tubing close to the IV port can help lessen heat dissipation as fluids move through colder IV tubing. Fluid rates also affect heat dissipation through the IV line; faster rates will cool slower and can traverse longer distances, while slower rates will effectively cool the fluid within a shorter traveled distance.

Oral fluid replacement is generally recommended in the stable, normothermic, pediatric patient that does not have vomiting or nausea.[2,5,8,42] However, because oral replacement is the slowest means of replacing fluids, it should not be used in a dehydrated, hypovolemic, hypothermic, or hypoglycemic patient. An orogastric tube (eg, 5F or 8F premeasured red rubber catheter) is used for oral fluid administration. The tube should be measured from the tip of the nose to the last rib, and the tube marked accordingly. Although the gag reflex is not present until 10 days of age, the passage down the left side of the mouth allows for easy feeding of milk replacer, dextrose solution, or water. A small amount of water should be administered via the orogastric tube first, making sure that it does not come out through the nares. Once the orogastric tube is confirmed to be in the appropriate location, an appropriate amount of commercial milk replacer can be used. The exact amount depends on the labeled instructions and should be adjusted every several days for weight gain. Normal stomach volume is approximately 40 mL/kg to 50 mL/kg, and overfeeding must be avoided.[2,5,8,42] The fluid should be warmed to near body temperature and administered over a few minutes. In general, 10 mL can be fed to a puppy every 2 to 4 hours, whereas for kittens, 5 mL can be fed every 2 to 4 hours. The amount of feeding is increased by 1 mL per day in puppies and kittens.[2] After delivery of fluid, kink the tube before withdrawal to prevent aspiration pneumonia. Owners can be taught how to easily tube feed if the neonate has a weak suckle reflex or if nursing from the mother is discontinued or contraindicated (eg, rejection, eclampsia).

The use of SC fluids should be limited to stable patients with euvolemia and experiencing only mild dehydration. Advantages of the SC route include ease of administration and a low likelihood of overhydration, but disadvantages include slow fluid absorption, limitations in the types of fluid administered (ie, this route should be reserved for crystalloid fluids), and the potential for abscess formation. In general, fluids for SC administration should not contain dextrose, although 0.45% saline with 2.5% dextrose has been given by this route.[2] Ideally, only warm isotonic crystalloids, such as Norm-R, LRS, or 0.9% NaCl, should be given by the SC route.

Absorption of intraperitoneal (IP) fluids is slow, and therefore should not be used in hypovolemic or very dehydrated patients. Although it is sometimes used in very young neonates simply because of administration difficulties related to size, it is never preferred over the IV or IO route. Unlike the SC route, not only crystalloid fluids but also blood products (eg, whole blood, plasma, or red blood cells) can be given by the IP route.[2] However, hypertonic dextrose solutions should still be avoided because they can draw fluid from the interstitium and intravascular space into the abdominal cavity.[2] Absorption of blood cells by the IP route is very slow (up to 72 hours for most cells to be absorbed) and is therefore not acceptable for animals with hemorrhagic shock.[2,43] Although IP administration of a replacement crystalloid allows for large volume administration, it can cause patient discomfort, increased intraabdominal pressure that might interfere with respiration, and can result in peritonitis. Aseptic technique is of utmost importance with IP fluid administration, and fluids should be warmed to near body temperature before administration. Repeated IP fluid administration is not recommended because of the risk of septic peritonitis.

IV administration is the preferred route of fluid therapy in critically ill pediatric patients; however, depending on the size of the patient, it may be difficult to accomplish. Peripheral venous access with a 22- to 27-gauge catheter can be attempted. Provided there is no contraindication to doing so (eg, coagulopathy), a small cephalic catheter can often be placed in the jugular vein. The neck may be immobilized by a soft padded wrap when a jugular catheter is placed.If the animal is large enough to use a limb for the placement of a peripheral catheter, a tongue depressor and wrap can help prevent catheter dislodgement. Aseptic technique and catheter care are imperative. Although the placement of IV catheters is challenging, they offer instantaneous access to the vascular compartment for the administration of all fluid types. Heparin irrigation of IV catheters is not necessary,[44] and can easily lead to coagulopathy in very small patients. Normal saline should be used in place of heparinized saline during catheter placement and maintenance.

Although IV access is ideal, it is sometimes simply impossible in the smallest patients, and placement of an IO catheter for fluid administration may be life-saving. Access to the bone marrow sinusoids and medullary channels via IO catheter placement allows for the rapid administration of fluid therapy suitable for the treatment of hypovolemic shock.[8,45–47] In addition, such catheters allow for the administration of all fluid types including blood products, and for the administration of drugs typically meant for IV use.[45,46,48] The IO catheter must be placed and maintained in an aseptic fashion, even more so than for an IV catheter because not only sepsis but also osteomyelitis can result from infection at the site. Appropriate sites for pediatric IO catheterization include the greater tubercle of the humerus and trochanteric fossa of the femur; in larger patients, the tibial tuberosity and wing of the ilium can be used.[45–47] An 18-

to 22-gauge spinal needle or hypodermic needle is used for catheterization. Commercially available rotary devices for IO insertion are reserved for adult patients to avoid complications associated with the device's torque on immature bones. Although the placement of an IO catheter is fairly simple in even the smallest of patients, it is difficult to wrap and protect the catheter. Ideally, such a catheter is replaced with an IV catheter as soon as the animal has been stabilized. That said, IO catheters can remain in place for several days, provided they are protected and cared for. Rarely, IO catheterization can result in bone fracture, osteomyelitis, and pain.[8]

FLUID DOSAGE

As with mature animals, pediatric fluid dosage varies by goal, fluid type, and route of administration. In general, pediatric patients have higher fluid requirements than do mature animals but they are also more easily volume overloaded because of their small size and difficulties in monitoring volume and hydration status in very small patients. A syringe pump is ideal for the administration of very small fluid volumes by IV or IO CRI in neonatal patients, whereas larger pediatric patients may be treated using routine fluid pumps. If no syringe or fluid pump is available, intermittent bolus therapy is often a better option than relying on a drip set alone for CRI. Even microdrip sets are prone to error, and accidental fluid overdose is possible in very small patients. Alternatively, a newer, economic option is a spring-powered syringe pump with flow-control tubing, which allows more careful fluid bolusing when an electronic syringe pump is not available.[49]

The fluid volume required to replace a fluid deficit is calculated as for adults, but for reasons previously described, estimation of hydration is more difficult in the youngest patients. For pediatric patients with hypovolemia, an initial slow (eg, 10 minutes) bolus fluid administration by either the IV or IO route at a dosage of 3 to 4 mL per 100 g of body weight in neonatal pups or 2 to 3 mL per 100 g of body weight in neonatal kittens is a reasonable starting bolus dosage. Administration of additional bolus doses depends on serial examination, with the aim of normalizing volume and hydration. Over-aggressive crystalloid fluid administration can lead to pulmonary edema and death.[50]

Maintenance fluid requirements for pediatric patients are higher than for mature animals. A rate of 80 mL/kg to 120 mL/kg (8–12 mL/100 g) is reasonable for the youngest pups, whereas a slightly lower rate of 60 mL/kg to 80 mL/kg (6–8 mL/100 g) is reasonable for kittens. Some references suggest maintenance fluid rates of 200 mL/kg/d,[1,2,5] although this is likely overly aggressive once the animal is well hydrated if there are no ongoing fluid losses. Maintenance fluid rates decrease to those of adult animals by about 4 to 6 months of age. For euvolemic patients with mild dehydration, the total daily maintenance fluid requirement can be administered by the SC route. In the stable pediatric patients with normothermia and without gastrointestinal signs, maintenance fluids are ideally given in the form of milk replacer via the oral route to provide food and fluid requirements.[2,5,42]

Fluid losses caused by vomiting or diarrhea should be considered when calculating a parenteral fluid plan and the estimated volume of loss added to maintenance therapy. Appropriate electrolyte replacement is necessary for pediatric patients, especially when vomiting or diarrhea is present. After the initial fluid bolus is given, 20 mEq/L potassium supplementation is reasonable, or an amount guided by the measured serum potassium concentration.[8]

Many pediatric patients are hypoglycemic and weak when presented for care. A glucose bolus can be administered even before blood glucose concentration is measured, but additional bolus doses should only be given when necessary, based on measured blood glucose concentration. A 50% dextrose solution can be diluted 1:3 in sterile water to make a 12.5% dextrose solution, and 1 mL to 3 mL of this solution can be administered IV or IO. This should be further supplemented with crystalloid fluids given by IV or IO CRI, with dextrose supplementation to make a 2.5% to 5% solution. If a dextrose concentration greater than 5% is desired, such fluids should be administered only via a central (eg, jugular) catheter to avoid thrombophlebitis. Careful monitoring of blood glucose levels is warranted; if this is not available, or not practical given the patient's small size, it is generally considered safe to provide a 2.5% to 5% dextrose solution routinely until the pediatric patient is more stable and eating readily. Otherwise, keep in mind that over-supplementation of dextrose can result in osmotic diuresis and resultant worsening of dehydration.[12]

Although pups and kittens have lower colloid osmotic pressure (COP) than do adults, colloid dosages are similar in pediatric and adult animals. Hetastarch is typically administered at 20 mL/kg/d,[2] with a goal of maintaining COP in the range of 16 mm Hg to 25 mm Hg.[2] Tetrastarch is typically administered at 20 to 30 mL/kg/d and advised not to exceed 50 mL/kg/d.[51] For animals with anemia, red blood cells and plasma proteins are beneficial. Whole blood is collected at a ratio of 9:1 in citrate anticoagulant and given through a blood filter at a dosage of 20 mL/kg over 2 to 3 hours.[2]

DISCONTINUATION OF FLUID THERAPY

Fluid therapy can be discontinued when the pediatric patient is able to maintain hydration and blood glucose levels by eating and drinking. Usually, fluids are weaned slowly over 2 to 4 days to ensure the patient maintains adequate voluntary intake and remains hydrated.[8] In many cases, the pup or kitten may not yet be willing to take in enough food and water, but IV or IO fluid therapy can be replaced with forced oral fluid administration as long as the gastrointestinal tract is functional and there is no vomiting or nausea. As fluids are decreased, or when the route of fluid administration is changed, patients should be monitored carefully and frequently to ensure that rapid dehydration does not reoccur.

SUMMARY

Fluid therapy for neonate and pediatric patient can restore hydration and vascular fluid volume, and correct life-threatening electrolyte disturbances. Clinicians must be aware of the higher fluid requirement in pediatric patients compared with adults. Depending on the stability of the patient, the appropriate route of fluid administration (eg, oral, SC, IP, IO, IV) should be implemented for life-saving care. Appropriate dextrose supplementation is warranted in young patients in the face of hypoglycemia. Judicious use of transfusion products is warranted but may be life-saving in the pediatric patient. Clinicians should be aware of the limitations or potential complications of each route of delivery and appropriately monitor patients for improvement or overhydration.

DISCLOSURE

The authors have nothing to disclose.

REFERENCES

1. McMichael M, Dhupa N. Pediatric critical care medicine: physiologic considerations. Compend Contin Educ Pract Vet 2000;22(4):206–14.

2. Macintire DK. Pediatric fluid therapy. Vet Clin North Am Small Anim Pract 2008; 38(3):621–7.
3. Lee JA, Cohn LA. Pediatric critical care: part 2-monitoring and treatment. Clinician's Brief 2015;14:39–44.
4. Cohn LA, Lee JA. Pediatric critical care: part 1-diagnostic interventions. Clinician's Brief 2015;13:35–40.
5. Lawler DF. Neonatal and pediatric care of the puppy and kitten. Theriogenology 2008;70(3):384–92.
6. Bucheler J. Fading kitten syndrome and neonatal isoerythrolysis. Vet Clin North Am Small Anim Pract 1999;29(4):853–70.
7. Coates JR, Bergman RL. Seizures in young dogs and cats: pathophysiology and diagnosis. Compend Contin Educ Pract Vet 2005;27(6):447–60.
8. Hoskins JD. Fluid therapy in the puppy and kitten. In: Kirk RW, editor. Curr Vet Ther XIIvol. 1, 12th edition. Philadelphia (PA): W.B. Saunders; 1995. p. 34–7.
9. Kleinman LI, Reuter JH. Renal response of the new-born dog to a saline load: the role of intrarenal blood flow distribution. J Physiol 1974;239(2):225–36.
10. McMichael M. Pediatric emergencies. Vet Clin North Am Small Anim Pract 2005; 35(2):421–34.
11. Fettman M, Allen T. Developmental aspects of fluid and electrolyte metabolism and renal function in neonates. Compend Contin Educ Pract Vet 1991;13(3):392.
12. McMichael M, Dhupa N. Pediatric critical care medicine: specific syndromes. Compend Contin Educ Pract Vet 2000;22(4):353–9.
13. Mace SE, Levy MN. Neural control of heart rate: a comparison between puppies and adult animals. Pediatr Res 1983;17(6):491–5.
14. Horster M, Valtin H. Postnatal development of renal function: micropuncture and clearance studies in the dog. J Clin Invest 1971;50:779–95.
15. Kleinman LI, Lubbe RJ. Factors affecting the maturation of glomerular filtration rate and renal plasma flow in the new-born dog. J Physiol 1972;223:395–409.
16. Laroute V, Chetboul V, Roche L, et al. Quantitative evaluation of renal function in healthy beagle puppies and mature dogs. Res Vet Sci 2005;79(2):161–7.
17. Faulks RD, Lane IF. Qualitative urinalyses in puppies 0 to 24 weeks of age. J Am Anim Hosp Assoc 2003;39(4):369–78.
18. Jose PA, Slotkoff LM, Montgomery S, et al. Autoregulation of renal blood flow in the puppy. Am J Physiol 1975;229(4):983–8.
19. Atkins CE. Disorders of glucose homeostasis in neonatal and juvenile dogs: hypoglycemia. I. Compend Contin Educ Vet Pract 1984;6:197.
20. Atkins CE. Disorders of glucose homeostasis in neonatal and juvenile dogs: hypoglycemia (part II). Compend Contin Educ Pract Vet 1984;6:353–64.
21. Kornhauser D, Adam PA, Schwartz R. Glucose production and utilization in the newborn puppy. Pediatr Res 1970;4(2):120–8.
22. Hellmann J, Vannucci RC, Nardis EE. Blood-brain barrier permeability to lactic acid in the newborn dog: lactate as a cerebral metabolic fuel. Pediatr Res 1982;16(1):40–4.
23. Throop JL, Kerl ME, Cohn LA. Albumin in health and disease: causes and treatment of hypoalbuminemia. Compend Contin Educ Pract Vet 2004;26(12):940–9.
24. Levy JK, Crawford PC, Collante WR, et al. Use of adult cat serum to correct failure of passive transfer in kittens. J Am Vet Med Assoc 2001;219(10):1401–5.
25. Poffenbarger EM, Olson PN, Chandler ML, et al. Use of adult dog serum as a substitute for colostrum in the neonatal dog. Am J Vet Res 1991;52(8):1221–4.
26. Root-Kustritz MV. Small animal pediatrics and theriogenology. Washington (DC): Paper presented at Washington DC Veterinary Academy; 2011.

27. Silvestre-Ferreira AC, Pastor J. Feline neonatal isoerythrolysis and the importance of feline blood types. Vet Med Int 2010;2010:753726.
28. Kisielewicz C, Self IA. Canine and feline blood transfusions: controversies and recent advances in administration practices. Vet Anaesth Analg 2014;41(3): 233–42.
29. Perner A, Haase N, Guttormsen AB, et al. Hydroxyethyl starch 130/0.42 versus Ringer's acetate in severe sepsis. N Engl J Med 2012;367:124–34.
30. Schmid SM, Cianciolo RE, Drobatz KJ, et al. Postmortem evaluation of renal tubular vacuolization in critically ill dogs. J Vet Emerg Crit Care 2019;29(3): 279–87.
31. Adamik KN, Yozova ID, Regenscheit N. Controversies in the use of hydroxyethyl starch solutions in small animal emergency and critical care. J Vet Emerg Crit Care 2015;25(1):20–47.
32. Myburgh JA, Finfer S, Bellomo R, et al. Hydroxyethyl starch or saline for fluid resuscitation in intensive care. N Engl J Med 2012;367(20):1901–11.
33. Kampmeier TG, Arnemann PH, Hessler M, et al. Effects of resuscitation with human albumin 5%, hydroxyethyl starch 130/0.4 6%, or crystalloid on kidney damage in an ovine model of septic shock. Br J Anaesth 2018;121(3):581–7.
34. Hayes G, Benedicenti L, Mathews K. Retrospective cohort study on the incidence of acute kidney injury and death following hydroxyethyl starch (HES 10% 250/0.5/ 5:1) administration in dogs (2007-2010). J Vet Emerg Crit Care 2016;26(1):35–40.
35. Gillies MA, Habicher M, Jhanji S, et al. Incidence of postoperative death and acute kidney injury associated with i.v. 6% hydroxyethyl starch use: systematic review and meta-analysis. Br J Anaesth 2014;112(1):25–34.
36. Chappell D, van der Linden P, Ripollés-Melchor J, et al. Safety and efficacy of tetrastarches in surgery and trauma: a systematic review and meta-analysis of randomized controlled trials. Br J Anaesth 2021;127(4):556–68.
37. Boyd CJ, Sharp CR, Claus MA, et al. Prospective randomized controlled blinded clinical trial evaluating biomarkers of acute kidney injury following 6% hydroxyethyl starch 130/0.4 or Hartmann's solution in dogs. J Vet Emerg Crit Care 2021;31(3):306–14.
38. Zersen KM, Mama K, Mathis JC. Retrospective evaluation of paired plasma creatinine and chloride concentrations following hetastarch administration in anesthetized dogs (2002-2015): 244 cases. J Vet Emerg Crit Care 2019;29(3):309–13.
39. Boyd CJ, Claus MA, Raisis AL, et al. Evaluation of biomarkers of kidney injury following 4% succinylated gelatin and 6% hydroxyethyl starch 130/0.4 administration in a canine hemorrhagic shock model. J Vet Emerg Crit Care 2019; 29(2):132–42.
40. Yozova ID, Howard J, Adamik KN. Retrospective evaluation of the effects of administration of tetrastarch (hydroxyethyl starch 130/0.4) on plasma creatinine concentration in dogs (2010-2013): 201 dogs. J Vet Emerg Crit Care 2016; 26(4):568–77.
41. Suempelmann R, Witt L, Brutt M, et al. Changes in acid-base, electrolyte and hemoglobin concentration during infusion of hydroxyethyl starch 130/0.42/6:1 in normal saline or in balanced electrolyte solution in children. Paediatr Anaesth 2010;20(1):100–4.
42. Little S. Playing mum: successful management of orphaned kittens. J Feline Med Surg 2013;15(3):201–10.
43. Giger U. Transfusion therapy. In: Silverstein DC, Hopper K, editors. Small Anim Crit Care Medvol. 1. St Louis (MO): Elsevier; 2015. p. 327–32.

44. Ueda Y, Odunayo A, Mann FA. Comparison of heparinized saline and 0.9% sodium chloride for maintaining peripheral intravenous catheter patency in dogs. J Vet Emerg Crit Care 2013;23(5):517–22.
45. Beal MW, Hughes D. Vascular access: theory and techniques in the small animal emergency patient. Clin Tech Small Anim Pract 2000;15(2):101–9.
46. Hughes D, Beal MW. Emergency vascular access. Vet Clin North Am Small Anim Pract 2000;30(3):491–507.
47. Otto C, Kaufman G, Crowe D Jr. Intraosseous infusion of fluids and therapeutics. Compend Contin Educ Pract Vet 1989;11:421.
48. Goldstein R, Lavy E, Shem-Tov M, et al. Pharmacokinetics of ampicillin administered intravenously and intraosseously to kittens. Res Vet Sci 1995;59(2):186–7.
49. MILA syringe pump and flow control tube. Florence (KY). Available at: http://www.milainternational.com/index.php/spring-powered-syringe-pump-flow-control-tubes.html. Accessed September 9, 2016.
50. Strodel WE, Callahan M, Weintraub WH, et al. The effect of various resuscitative regimens on hemorrhagic shock in puppies. J Pediatr Surg 1977;12(6):809–19.
51. Brooks A, Thomovsky E, Johnson P. Natural and Synthetic Colloids in Veterinary Medicine. Top Companion Anim Med 2016;31(2):54–60.

Physical Rehabilitation for the Management of Canine Hip Dysplasia: 2021 Update

David L. Dycus, DVM, MS, CCRP, DACVS-SA[a],*,
David Levine, PT, PhD, DPT, CCRP, FAPTA[b],
Barbara Esteve Ratsch, DVM, PhD, CCRP[c],
Denis J. Marcellin-Little, DEDV, DACVS, DACVSMR[d]

KEYWORDS

- Canine rehabilitation • Canine physical therapy • Hip dysplasia • Hip laxity
- Osteoarthritis • Therapeutic exercises

KEY POINTS

- The goals of rehabilitation vary for various stages of canine hip dysplasia; initially, clinical signs most likely result from joint laxity. Later, signs result from chronic pain and loss of strength.
- Early surgical therapy focuses on improving femoral head coverage and reducing the development of osteoarthritis or removing the source of discomfort.
- Conservative management is centered on controlling pain control, while preserving or improving muscle mass and hip joint extension.
- Rehabilitation therapy for dogs with hip dysplasia needs to be multimodal and proportional to the level of disability and owners' objectives.

INTRODUCTION

Canine hip dysplasia (CHD) causes diffuse joint inflammation and subsequent coxofemoral osteoarthritis (OA).[1,2] Hip dysplasia was identified in more than 40% of Golden Retrievers and Rottweilers in one report.[3] Hip dysplasia was originally described more than 80 years ago. Its exact cause remains unknown; it is considered multifactorial with both genetic and environmental cues playing a role in its phenotypic expression.[3]

[a] Department of Orthopedic Surgery, Nexus Veterinary Bone & Joint Center, 3700 O'Donnell Street, Baltimore, MD 21224, USA; [b] Department of Physical Therapy, University of Tennessee at Chattanooga, 615 McCallie Avenue, Chattanooga, TN 37403, USA; [c] Evidensia Sørlandet Animal Hospital, Krittveien 2, Hamresanden 4656, Norway; [d] Department of Veterinary Surgical and Radiological Sciences, School of Veterinary Medicine, University of California, Davis, Davis, CA, USA
* Corresponding author.
E-mail address: dldycus@gmail.com

Vet Clin Small Anim 52 (2022) 719–747
https://doi.org/10.1016/j.cvsm.2022.01.012
0195-5616/22/© 2022 Elsevier Inc. All rights reserved.

vetsmall.theclinics.com

The central theme surrounding CHD is hip laxity, which is thought to play a major role in the development of OA. Hip laxity varies widely among dogs. Under a certain threshold, dogs are at a very low risk of CHD and greater than a certain threshold, dogs are at very high risk of developing CHD.[4]

Hip laxity leads to subluxation during growth, which can result in the abnormal development of the acetabulum and femoral head. Laxity results in lateralization of the femoral head during the swing phase of the gait and a rapid relocation ("reduction") of the femoral head into the acetabulum during foot strike. Subluxation leads to rapid focal cartilage wear of the femoral head and dorsal acetabular rim, leading to OA. Osteoarthritis and its clinical impact progress over time.[5] Management of CHD is centered around both conservative and surgical therapies as well as the age of the onset of clinical signs.[5–7] To date, there is only limited evidence that preventative measures in rehabilitation improve the long-term performance of dogs with hip dysplasia. However, a lean body condition decreases the rate of progression of OA.[7] Physical rehabilitation plays a role in the management of CHD by relieving pain through strengthening, maintaining hip range of motion (ROM), promoting optimal body condition, educating owners such as minimizing vigorous exercises that exacerbate the problem, and adapting living conditions. The purpose of this article is to present the rehabilitation steps that can be implemented to manage CHD at its various stages.

PHYSICAL REHABILITATION IN THE CONSERVATIVE MANAGEMENT OF CANINE HIP DYSPLASIA

Although CHD has been analyzed in several hundred scientific publications, few publications discuss the conservative management of CHD in skeletally immature and skeletally mature dogs, and fewer have assessed the long-term clinical signs and progression of OA as a secondary sequela of CHD.[8] The rehabilitation approach should be multimodal, with goals to improve function, reduce clinical signs of pain, improve hip ROM and strength, and thus potentially slow down or minimize the progression of OA. These goals are similar to management of OA. Loss of motion in patients with CHD results from the development of osteophytes and enthesophytes, thickening of the synovium, periarticular fibrosis, and from potential changes in muscle fiber elasticity. Motion should be assessed at regular intervals using goniometry as an objective assessment.[9,10] Loss of limb strength, core strength, and cardiovascular fitness result from a decrease in spontaneous activity, a decrease in owner-supervised exercise, and a reflex inhibition of muscle contractions secondary to joint pain.[11] Although hip OA in dogs with CHD is most often diagnosed using radiographs of affected joints, osteophyte size and severity of clinical signs correlate poorly. As a consequence, the management of CHD should not be based on radiographic appearance but rather on the specific physical limitations of the patient. Management goals are reached by weight optimization, by minimizing joint pain via medications, disease modifying osteoarthritic agents (DMOAs), manual therapy, therapeutic exercises, and physical modalities.

CONTROLLING PAIN

Nonpharmacologic, antiinflammatory options for peripheral pain management include cryotherapy (icing) and massage. Icing provides direct pain relief by decreasing nerve conduction velocity. It also provides secondary pain relief by decreasing acute edema (itself a source of pain) and decreasing the activity of catabolic enzymes in osteoarthritic cartilage.[12,13] Icing should be considered in osteoarthritic patients experiencing a flare-up, after a period of exercise, and before bedtime. Ice bags filled with ice chips or crushed ice or cold packs provide effective cold delivery. Ice cubes or frozen vegetables are not optimal because they have air pockets that decrease cold conduction. Most cold packs reach a therapeutic temperature after 2 hours in a freezer. For long-haired patients, cold packs are placed directly on the joint and can be held in place using a self-adhesive band or a neoprene sleeve. In patients with short or with clipped hair, a towel may be placed between the cold pack and the skin. Icing should last for 10 to 20 minutes to achieve effective cooling (**Fig. 1**).[12] Most dogs tolerate icing but patients should not be left unattended. The person applying the ice should make sure the patient is not uncomfortable and that the skin surface feels cold to the touch after icing.

Additional nonpharmacologic options for central pain management include low-level heating (thermotherapy) and possibly electrical stimulation, acupuncture, acupressure, or electroacupuncture. The short-term and long-term effects of massage in companion animals are not well known. Massage may decrease myofascial pain and muscle tension.[14] These methods primarily stimulate Aβ sensory fibers with rapid conduction velocities (30–70 m/s), sparing pain fibers with slower conduction velocities: Aδ (12–30 m/s) and C fibers (0.5–3 m/s). Heat is widely considered to positively affect patients with OA pain (**Fig. 2**).[13] The use of heat is 2-fold. Low-level heat (elevation of tissue temperature by 1–2°C) relieves pain through the stimulation of nonnociceptive Aβ sensory fibers and vasodilation leading to normalization of blood flow. This low-level tissue relaxation may be achieved by keeping osteoarthritic patients in relatively dry and warm temperatures throughout the day (eg, sleeping in heated indoor environments or providing a heated bed). Intense heating (tissue temperature elevation of 3–4°C) is used to increase the effectiveness of stretching while minimizing the risk of tissue damage during stretching. Vigorous heating is most often applied by a health care professional using a hot pack that is heated by a hydrocollator or a microwave oven. Four to six layers of dry towels are placed between the hot pack and skin, and heat is generally applied for 10 to 20 minutes.[15] Caution is used when placing a hot pack on a dog because of the risk of burn. Initially, a pack may not seem excessively hot to the touch, but it can induce thermal damage after several minutes of contact. Checking for excessive redness, skin swelling, or blistering every few minutes during vigorous heat therapy is important.

Therapeutic Exercises to Minimize Joint Pain, Maintain, or Increase Joint Motion

Active and passive ROM and stretching exercises help minimize hip pain and increase joint motion (**Fig. 3**). Hip joints with CHD seemingly lose extension but not flexion. In

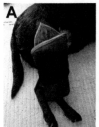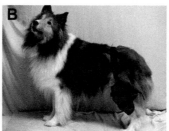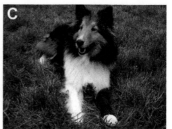

Fig. 1. Limb cryotherapy can be done using (*A*) a cold pack wrapped around the hind limb, (*B*) cryotherapy to the stifle, (*C*) cryotherapy to the carpus. (*Canine Rehabilitation and Physical Therapy 2ⁿᵈ edition* (Millis, Levine, eds.), Elsevier Saunders. Reproduced with permission.)

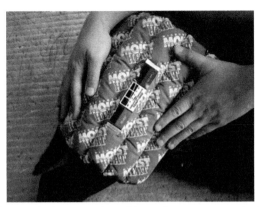

Fig. 2. A hot pack is applied over a dog's hip region. A tag on the hot pack indicates whether the pack should be reheated, whether its temperature is within therapeutic range, or whether it should not be used because it is excessively hot. (*Reproduced from* Canine Rehabilitation and Physical Therapy 2nd edition (Millis, Levine, eds.), Elsevier Saunders; with permission.)

one study, Labrador Retrievers with hip dysplasia had in average a decrease of 1° of hip extension for each year of life.[10] Minor (<20°) loss of joint motion is unlikely to affect limb function but severe loss of joint motion leads to a decrease or a loss of ability to gallop, trot, jump up, and climb steps or stairs. It seems beneficial, therefore, to assess joint motion in dogs with chronic CHD using a goniometer.[11] Because it is likely easier to maintain joint motion than to regain it once lost, it seems reasonable to recommend intermittent physical activity that leads to enhanced joint extension (compared with walking on a flat surface) without creating significant clinical signs. Passive ROM (pROM), active ROM (aROM) and stretching can be incorporated into the early phases of rehabilitation for CHD and continued as part of the daily exercise plan. These activities can help increase flexibility, prevent adhesions, help remodel periarticular fibrosis, and improve extensibility.[16] Passive ROM is completed without muscle contraction by moving the joint through its full ROM. Any additional force applied at the end of the ROM and held for at least a few seconds is defined as stretching. If

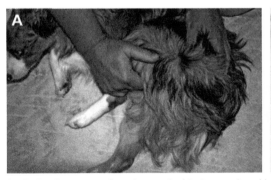
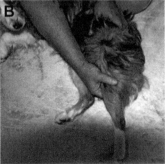

Fig. 3. Passive range of motion to the hip is completed by supporting the femur in one hand and the pelvis in the other. (*A*) Hip flexion; (*B*) hip extension. (*Reproduced from* Canine Rehabilitation and Physical Therapy 2nd edition (Millis, Levine, eds.), Elsevier Saunders; with permission.)

regaining joint motion is deemed important, a stretching program should be implemented. Stretching is more effective when tissues are heated immediately before and during the stretching session, and the tissues should be heated to a minimum of 2°C for effective stretching. pROM and aROM in patients with CHD can be beneficial in the early phases of rehabilitation to facilitate appropriate periarticular fibrosis that develops from laxity in younger patients or help realign fibrous tissue along lines of stress in older patients with clinical OA. In addition, ROM and stretching can be incorporated into part of the daily exercise program to maintain mobility between soft tissue layers, enhance blood and lymphatic flow, and improve synovial fluid production.[17,18] Ideally, ROM and stretching are applied to tissues that are warmed up; therefore, as part of a daily exercise program ROM and stretching can be completed after therapeutic exercises, as part of the cool down process. In the early phases of rehabilitation therapy, pROM and stretching can be performed 2 to 4 times daily for 10 to 20 repetitions. When used as part of the cool down process, ROM and stretching are performed at the end of the exercise program for 15 to 30 repetitions for ROM. For stretching, ten to fifteen 20- to 40-second-long sustained stretches are often recommended for each session. Sessions may be performed 2 to 3 times per day. With chronic loss of motion, a weekly gain of 3° to 5° of joint motion is anticipated. A more detailed explanation of how to perform ROM and stretching exercises is beyond the scope of this review and can be found elsewhere.[19,20] Joint mobilization may also be incorporated into a rehabilitation program to help increase ROM. Joint mobilization differs from stretching in that when a stretch is applied, a low load is placed on the tissues for a specified amount of time (often 10–30 seconds) to help elongate them. In joint mobilization, the force is applied in an oscillatory manner rather than a sustained manner (**Fig. 4**). A more thorough explanation of how to perform point mobilizations can be found elsewhere.[20]

Proprioception can be negatively affected in patients with OA from chronic CHD. Although little is known about the negative impact of naturally occurring OA on proprioception in dogs, there is clear evidence that OA progresses rapidly in patients with joint injuries that have sensory deficits. In older humans with decreased proprioception, balance exercises readily improve proprioception.[21] In dogs with OA, it is logical to dedicate a small portion of the exercise program to focus on proprioception and balance. In the early phases, this may include weight-shifting exercises (**Fig. 5**)

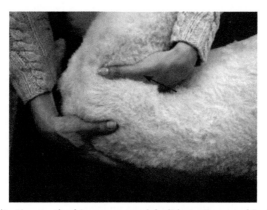

Fig. 4. Joint mobilization to the hip uses a caudal glide to increase hip flexion. The black arrow indicates the direction of the mobilization. (*Reproduced from* Canine Rehabilitation and Physical Therapy 2nd edition (Millis, Levine, eds.), Elsevier Saunders; with permission.)

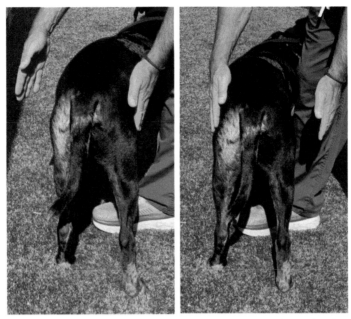

Fig. 5. Weight shifting being applied to the pelvic limbs. This is accomplished by the therapist standing beside the patient with hands on either side of the pelvis. Pressure is gently applied to one side, then applied to the other side in slow, rhythmic fashion.

requiring rapid and unpredictable side-to-side weight shifts and, to a lesser extent, front-to-back and back-to-front weight shifts; this is completed by supporting the animal on either side and gently pushing on one side, followed by pushing back the other way. The weight-shifting exercises can be done in slow, rhythmic fashion for 15 to 25 repetitions, 2 to 4 times daily. As balance and proprioception improve, perturbation exercises can be added to weight shifting to disturb the patient's balance and allow recovery, without risking a fall. Perturbation exercises are performed by gently pushing the hip region without supporting the other side. More complex weight shifting exercises can be incorporated while the patient is walking to improve dynamic stability; this is accomplished by gently bumping or pushing the dog to one side as it is walking, to challenge the dog's balance. Additional proprioception and balancing exercises include balance boards, wobble boards, and exercise balls and rolls. A balance board uses a board placed over a fulcrum to rock the dog side to side or forward to back (**Fig. 6**). A more challenging aspect to balance and proprioception improvement is using a wobble board (**Fig. 7**). Exercise balls and rolls for human exercises can be used to improve balance, coordination, and strength in dogs. For example, the front limbs can be placed on the ball requiring the dog to maintain static balance of the pelvic limbs (**Fig. 8**). For dynamic challenges, the ball can be rolled forward, back, and side to side; this challenges the limbs to maintain balance as movement is occurring. The most challenging use of the exercise balls and rolls is having the patient stand on a therapy ball or roll. This exercise will challenge and engage core stabilizing muscles; therefore, this exercise is limited to dog with strength and balance, and sessions are kept short to minimize fatigue and avoid an injury.

Other exercises that promote balance and proprioception include standing or walking on foam rubber (**Fig. 9**), mattress, air mattress, or a trampoline. Patients

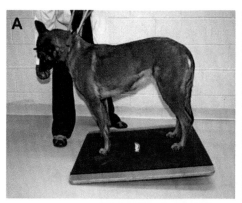
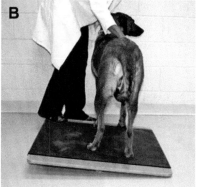

Fig. 6. A balance board is used to provide balance and proprioceptive training (*A*) from the front limbs to the hind limbs (*B*) from side to side. (*Reproduced from* Canine Rehabilitation and Physical Therapy 2nd edition (Millis, Levine, eds.), Elsevier Saunders; with permission.)

can walk on surfaces such as grass, concrete, sand, or mulched paths. Altering the texture and evenness of the surface challenges patients' proprioception. To facilitate improving balance and proprioception for daily activities, animals should be encouraged to walk over or around obstacles such as low rails, pole weaving, walking on a teeter-totter, and negotiating stairs.

Additional therapeutic exercises are incorporated into formal rehabilitation therapy, and a home exercise program is geared toward continued improvement in ROM, specifically in extension of the hip, improving comfortable weight bearing, building muscle mass and endurance. An understanding of basic biomechanics of exercise modification is helpful to select exercises. Information of the biomechanics and kinematics of exercise can be found elsewhere.[21]

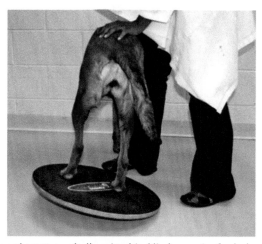

Fig. 7. A wobble board creates a challenging hind limb exercise for balance and proprioceptive training. (*Reproduced from* Canine Rehabilitation and Physical Therapy 2nd edition (Millis, Levine, eds.), Elsevier Saunders; with permission.)

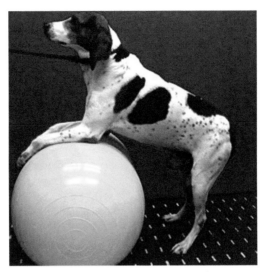

Fig. 8. An exercise ball can improve hind limb balance, coordination, and strength. (*Reproduced from* Canine Rehabilitation and Physical Therapy 2nd edition (Millis, Levine, eds.), Elsevier Saunders; with permission.)

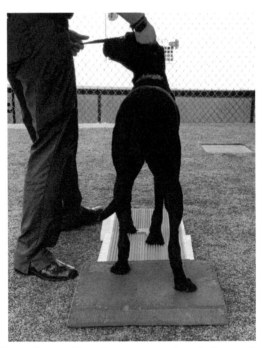

Fig. 9. When walking on foam rubber, the uneven surface challenges the dog's proprioception and balance.

The patient can warm up for 5 to 10 minutes before therapeutic exercises. The simplest of the therapeutic exercises consist of slow controlled leash walking. Walking can be instituted in the early phases of rehabilitation and continued throughout. In regard to the hind limbs, walking will generate approximately 35° of motion in the hip and 40° and 35° of motion in the stifle and hock, respectively.[22,23] Treadmill walking (≤10° incline) has been shown to result in the same joint motions as land walking; however, 3° of additional hip extension are obtained while walking on a treadmill inclined 10°, compared with walking on land.[21] Although trotting is ideal to increase the speed of muscle contractions and the forces on the limb, it does little to improve hip ROM compared with walking.[24] Walking up and down stairs or a ramp can facilitate additional flexion and extension to particular joints; however, some consideration has to be placed on the particular exercise for CHD management. For example, incline ramp walking can increase hip flexion by 11% but does not contribute to improvement in hip extension, which is more commonly targeted in patients with CHD.[25] Walking up stairs is helpful to improve hind limb ROM: hip extension is increased by up to 10° compared with walking on level ground (**Fig. 10**).[26] Stair descent results in greater ROM in the hip (27°) compared with ramp descent (23°).[27]

With knowledge of the kinematics of exercises, one can create a plan to improve hip ROM and improve muscle mass and comfort. For example, in the beginning stages, one may use slow controlled leash walking on level ground beginning at 15- to 20-minute intervals 2 to 3 times daily. Once the animal has developed the ability to perform this comfortably, 5 minutes can be added weekly to reach 30 to 45 minutes of exercise. Inclined walking along with stair ascent and decent can be added after several weeks of flat land walking to further improve hip ROM and muscle mass. It is also beneficial to add walking down a declined slope and walking over uneven terrain such as a trail, high grass, or sand to force the patient to increase flexion and extension of various joints. Walking exercises should only become more challenging once the dog successfully completes simpler walks.

Depending on existing comorbidities, additional therapeutic exercises such as dancing, Cavaletti rail walking, and sit-to-stand exercises can help improve hip ROM. These exercises are performed during rehabilitation therapy or are incorporated in a home exercise program. Dancing exercises (**Fig. 11**) are designed to increase weight bearing on the rear limbs by raising the forelimbs off the ground and walking the patient either forward or back. The kinematics of walking forward or backward

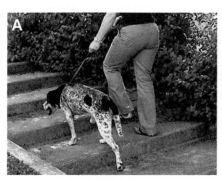
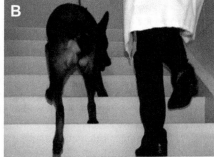

Fig. 10. Walking up stairs to improve hip extension more so than walking on level ground. (A) Stairs with a gradual rise; (B) steeper stairs can be used as the patient progresses. (*Reproduced from* Canine Rehabilitation and Physical Therapy 2nd edition (Millis, Levine, eds.), Elsevier Saunders; with permission.)

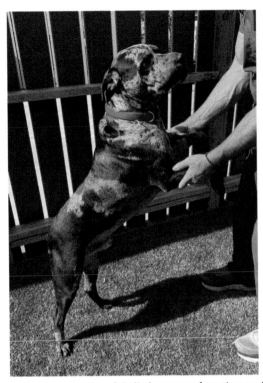

Fig. 11. Dancing exercise encourages pelvic limb range of motion and strength. Initially, dancing the patient forward is less painful and helps to improve quadriceps strength. As a patient becomes stronger, dancing the patient backwards is more challenging and exercises the hamstrings.

differ: dancing forward results in less hip flexion and ROM (22°) compared with walking on level ground (ROM, 33°). Dancing backward, however, increases hip extension more than walking on level ground. That difference influences the direction of dancing exercises. During the early phases of rehabilitation when hip extension is painful, it may be more comfortable to improve gluteal muscle strengthening by walking the patient forward rather than back. Depending on pain level and degree of hip extension, forward dancing exercises can begin with the patients front limbs lower to the ground (such as on a low chair). The chair can slide as the patient is moving forward. As comfort increases, the height the patient is off the ground can increase. In the later phases when hip extension is improved, walking the patient backwards will be more challenging and will help improve hip extension.[28] ROM is increased by using Cavaletti rail walking (**Fig. 12**). That increase is proportional to the height of the rails. Compared with walking (36° hip ROM), ROM is improved by 2° with a Cavaletti rail in the low position (level of the carpus), 4° in a medium position, and 7° in a high position (mid-antebrachium). Cavaletti rail waking does not improve joint extension but helps in the overall reeducation of the joint motion pattern.[29] Sit-to-stand exercises are beneficial in improving both quadriceps and hamstring muscle mass as well as improving aROM. Hip extension with sit-to-stand exercises is less compared with walking; however, aROM is larger (66°) than when walking (36°)[30]; this is beneficial in the early rehabilitation, while hip extension is painful, to allow a comfortable exercise that improves hip aROM.

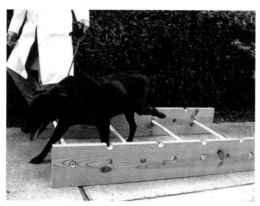

Fig. 12. Example of Cavaletti rail walking to help improve active range of motion (flexion). (*Reproduced from* Canine Rehabilitation and Physical Therapy 2nd edition (Millis, Levine, eds.), Elsevier Saunders; with permission.)

Aquatic therapy has become more widely used in veterinary rehabilitation. It allows active muscle contractions with decreased weight bearing on joints and bones. In patients with CHD, aquatic therapy can help with muscle spasm, muscle weakness, and pain associated with OA. The most significant benefit of aquatic therapy is likely buoyancy, which allows the patient to exercise in an upright position and may decrease pain by minimizing the amount of weight bearing on joints. The higher the water level, the more stress that is taken off of the joints. With water at the level of the lateral malleolus of the fibula, dogs support about 91% of their body weight. With water to the lateral condyle of the femur, dogs support 85% of their body weight. With water to the greater trochanter, dogs are supporting only 38% of their body weight (**Fig. 13**).[31] Another feature of aquatic therapy is hydrostatic pressure and its ability to reduce edema and decrease pain during exercise; this is thought to decrease

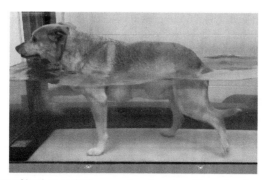

Fig. 13. The amount of body weight borne when immersed in water changes with the water level. For the dog in the picture, with water at the level of the greater trochanter, forces resisted by limbs are reduced to 38% of the body weight. At the stifle, forces are reduced to 85% of the body weight and at the lateral malleolus, forces are reduced to 91% of the body weight.[31] (*From* Levine D, Marcellin-Little DJ, Millis DL, et al. Effects of partial immersion in water on vertical ground reaction forces and weight distribution in dogs. Am J Vet Res 2010;71:1413-1416; with permission.)

pain perception, which allows the patient to exercise longer and with less pain.[32] An additional feature of aquatic therapy is the resistance needed to move through the water versus air. This resistance can help to strengthen weak muscles and improve endurance. In patients with OA from associated CHD, underwater treadmill therapy improves comfort, while increasing muscular work and building endurance while unloading painful joints. Initially, many dogs only tolerate 2 to 5 minutes of aquatic therapy once or twice weekly. The goal is to increase to 10 to 20 minutes with as few breaks as necessary. Because of the different kinematics of underwater treadmill versus swimming and walking on dry land, in patients with CHD, underwater treadmill therapy is likely more beneficial than swimming. Compared with walking on ground, joint flexion is increased in both underwater treadmill walking and swimming; however, almost near normal joint extension is noted in underwater treadmill therapy compared with swimming, where hip joint extension is limited.[33] Furthermore, walking or trotting in the underwater treadmill encourages a more normal gait pattern than swimming. For a more in-depth discussion on the indications, contraindications, parameters, settings, and usages for various physical modalities the reader is encouraged to refer to additional resources.[34–38]

In summary, dancing backwards maximally increases hip extension, whereas sit-to-stand, ramp descent, ramp ascent, and stair descent minimize hip extension. Hip ROM is maximized with sit-to-stand exercises and minimized when dancing forward. Aquatic therapy can further be added to improve muscular strength and endurance and decrease weight bearing on painful bones and joints. Potential therapeutic exercises used to manage canine CHD are listed in **Table 1**. For more in-depth therapeutic exercises to improve joint motion, strengthen, and improve endurance and speed, the reader is encouraged to read additional sources.[39]

PHYSICAL MODALITIES TO IMPROVE RANGE OF MOTION, COMFORT, AND FUNCTION

Physical modalities can be used in rehabilitation therapy to decrease pain, augment therapeutic exercises, and promote tissue healing. Modalities such as therapeutic ultrasound, electrical stimulation, laser therapy, and extracorporeal shockwave therapy can be used to manage CHD. Therapeutic ultrasound can be beneficial to patients with OA associated with CHD by improving ROM and decreasing pain and muscle spasm. It allows heating of deeper tissues that cannot be reached using superficial moist heat. Therapeutic ultrasound depth penetration changes based on frequency:

Table 1
Therapeutic exercises potentially included in the management of canine hip dysplasia

Purpose	Possible Therapeutic Exercises
Increasing limb strength	Daily walk or trot longer than 10 minutes; tunnel-walk, sit-to-stand, and stand-to-sit repetitions, swimming
Increasing core strength	Daily walk or trot longer than 10 minutes; swimming
Increasing cardiovascular fitness	Daily walk or trot longer than 10 minutes
Stretching pelvic limbs	Climbing up slopes, hills, and stairs; low jumps
Increasing proprioception	Daily walk or trot longer than 10 minutes; walk on soft surfaces: sand, mulch, gravel, leaves, grass; teeter-totter or pole weaving

1.0 MHz heats to a depth ranging from 2 to 5 cm, whereas 3.3 MHz heats from 0.5 to 3 cm.[40] Hot packing can heat tissue up to 2 cm; however, the greatest temperature change is noted from the skin surface to approximately 1 cm in depth. The thermal effect of therapeutic ultrasound may increase collagen extensibility, blood flow, pain threshold, and enzyme activity. Therapeutic ultrasound can be incorporated into a rehabilitation protocol in the management of CHD to heat the tissues to further improve stretching and ROM for maximal benefit. An intensity of 1.0 to 2.0 W/cm^2 is used at a frequency of 1.0 or 3.3 MHz, depending on depth of target tissue. Treatment typically lasts 8 to 12 minutes, based on the sizes of the area treated and the sound heard. The thermal effects of therapeutic ultrasound are short-lived. Therefore, ROM and stretching exercises should occur while the tissue is being heated whenever possible or should occur immediately afterward.

Electrical stimulation increases muscle strength and ROM, improves muscle tone, improves pain control, and decreases edema and muscle spasm.[41] Neuromuscular electrical stimulation (NMES) is used for muscle reeducation, prevention of muscle atrophy, and enhanced joint movement, whereas transcutaneous electrical nerve stimulation (TENS) is commonly used for pain control. In patients with CHD, electrical stimulation can be incorporated into a rehabilitation program to manage long-term muscle atrophy or selectively strengthen muscle groups (hamstrings, gluteal muscles, or quadriceps) by using NMES twice weekly for 10 to 20 minutes. In patients with chronic OA pain associated with CHD, TENS can be used for relief of pain. Treatment frequency and duration can be 2 to 3 times weekly for 30 minutes.

Laser therapy can be used to relieve pain, reduce inflammation, and increase microcirculation through the concept of photobiomodulation. The antiinflammatory and analgesic benefit of laser therapy for patients with OA has been described.[42–44] For patients with OA from CHD, 8 to 20 J/cm^2 are used and the entire hip area is treated. Therapy starts at the greater trochanter followed by the cranial, medial, and caudal surfaces of the hip in a circumferential pattern. Laser dosage can be difficult to calculate and compare between devices due to the number of diodes and terminology used. The wavelength is chosen to minimize absorption in the melanin of the skin and oxygenated and deoxygenated hemoglobin. Because of possible compensatory changes, referred pain from the lumbosacral and epaxial areas can be treated as well. Treatment protocols vary, but initially 6 treatments are applied over a 3-week period, followed by maintenance treatments every 3 to 4 weeks.

The usage of extracorporeal shockwave therapy (ESWT) is centered around the pain-relieving response in patients with OA from chronic CHD. Shock waves are acoustic waves with various frequencies that are delivered and travel through soft tissues to the target area. Once the shockwave reaches the target, energy is then released, which creates a biological response promoting analgesia and decreasing inflammatory mediators. The analgesic effect following ESWT is poorly understood but thought to be due to release of cytokines and growth factors centered around decreasing inflammation and swelling. In dogs with hip OA, ESWT improved ground reaction forces following 4 weeks of treatment and benefits lasted up to 3 months.[45] In a human study of arthritic chondrocytes, inflammatory factors (tumor necrosis factor alpha and interleukin-10) were found to be decreased in patients treated with ESWT when compared with the pretreated chondrocytes.[46] The effects of ESWT on articular cartilage is an area of concern that warrants additional investigation because preliminary research suggests that high-energy ESWT applied directly to cartilage may cause degenerative changes.[47,48] Patients may or may not need to be sedated before ESWT. The number of shocks applied vary by manufacturer but may be as high as 1000 shocks per treatment.

SELECTING A TREATMENT PROGRAM FOR A CONSERVATIVE APPROACH TO CANINE CANINE HIP DYSPLASIA

Arthritic dogs with minor locomotion problems will have a treatment program focused on decreasing pain, maintaining optimal weight, maintaining limb and core strength, stretching affected joints, and stimulating proprioception. Pain management is generally achieved with simple pharmacologic steps, rest, and exercise supervision and customization. Pharmacologic and other forms of pain relief may be intermittent, as long as dogs adhere to a long-term exercise program. Because OA screening is not done routinely in dogs, OA is most often discovered in its later stages. Losing mobility because of severe hip OA is common in large-breed dogs. For patients with severe OA, it is important to implement all possible support strategies to decrease the impact of the disease on the dogs' well-being and mobility. These may include multimodal pharmacologic management, ice, heat, massage, acupuncture, acupressure, electro-acupuncture, transcutaneous electrical nerve stimulation, and avoiding activities such as high impact exercise. Once pain is managed, it is important to initiate an initially conservative and subsequently progressive exercise program. Patients with severe OA may need temporary or permanent ambulation assistance. Slings are the most common and cost-effective ambulation assistance devices. Severely impaired dogs may benefit from an ambulation cart. Underwater treadmills significantly reduce pelvic limb peak vertical force[32] and are useful in building muscle in a weight-minimized environment. Overall, a management program for companion animals with OA should be simple and logical. Managing pain is the first priority for all patients. The program must then address the most critical aspects of each patient's unique situation and, over time, improve the patient's mobility, strength, proprioception and, above all, quality of life.

HOME MANAGEMENT (HOME EXERCISE PROGRAMS AND ERGONOMICS)

The home exercise program of dogs with CHD is individually designed depending of the dog profile, disease severity, and owners objectives.[49] Attentive dog owners provide valuable information about the general health of their pets.[50] It is important not to overwhelm the pet owner at the time of diagnosis with an extensive array of home treatment possibilities. A basic home exercise plan in patients with CHD is described in **Table 2**. All companion animals with CHD benefit from trained owners capable to

Table 2
Home exercise plan for dog with hip dysplasia

5–10 min warm-up period	
Controlled leash walking (2–3x daily)	Begin on level flat ground and work up to 20 min Once at 20 min add inclined/declined walking Comfort with inclined/declined walking adds stair ascent/descent Add uneven terrain
Return from walking	Sit-to-stand exercises (10–20 reps) Dancing (10–20 reps) Cavaletti walking
5–10 min cool-down period	pROM (10–20 reps Stretching (20–30 s hold at end range) Massage Cryotherapy (10–20 min)

evaluate chronic pain.[51] The owner's documented observations and monitoring skills are critical to the overall success in managing chronic conditions.[50] Accordingly, it is important that the owner learns to recognize when their companion animal is in pain or when a flare-up may be occurring. Having owners keep a daily journal can be helpful for them to track trends that could indicate a flare up or progression of the problem. Alternatively, the owners can use the "popsicle method"; this can be achieved by having the owner use green, yellow, or red popsicle sticks or other objects to indicate a good day, an okay day, or a bad day. Once the yellow or red popsicles outnumber green popsicles, the presence of a flare up or chronic pain is suspected.

The home exercise programs have several components: (1) pain management: home exercise should start after the implementation of a tailored effective pain management program. Owners assist in monitoring pain and alert their veterinarian about a flare ups. Questionnaires such as the Canine Brief Pain Inventory should be filled at regular intervals to monitor pain[52]; (2) weight loss and conditioning: weight loss and nutritional management are needed in overweight dogs with CHD (**Table 2**). Weight loss improve gait in dogs with CHD.[53] Conditioning improves proprioception and balance and is likely to decrease the frequency of falls; (3) ergonomics.

Ergonomics includes strategies that make living conditions safe and comfortable. The home life and home exercise program of dogs with CHD should be ergonomic. If a dog is falling, throw rugs or yoga mats can improve traction and stability. If stairs are challenging, dogs should only negotiate them under supervision, and exercises aimed at increasing the ability to climb stairs are incorporated into the home exercise program. As the disease progress or as dogs respond to treatment, gradual ergonomic changes are made and new exercises or modalities are introduced.

PHYSICAL REHABILITATION AFTER SURGICAL MANAGEMENT OF HIP DYSPLASIA

Surgical intervention is used in young patients with CHD and in older patients that failed medical, conservative, and rehabilitative therapies to positively improve quality of life. The surgical intervention is dictated by the clinical signs, age, and the presumptive source of clinical signs: joint laxity in young dogs and severe OA in older dogs. Rehabilitation therapy is standard after surgery for CHD to decrease pain, promote healing, maintain or improve ROM, and promote early use of the operated limb.

Rehabilitation Therapy Following Juvenile Pubic Symphysiodesis

The fusion of the medial growth plates of the pubis, referred to as juvenile pubic symphysiodesis (JPS) is sometimes performed in dogs around the age of 16 weeks with the intent to alter pelvic growth to increase dorsal coverage of the femoral head. Dogs undergo JPS to control hip subluxation.[54] Subluxation persists after surgery but altered growth of the pubis increases the dorsal coverage of the femoral head by the dorsal acetabular rim. Tissue trauma after a JPS is relatively minor and does not warrant specific rehabilitation strategies to accelerate the resorption of edema or decrease focal pain. Also, pelvic strength is not compromised after a JPS, unlike the double or triple pelvic osteotomy where the ilium is osteotomized and stabilized with a bone plate. The focus of rehabilitation after JPS is to minimize the impact of hip subluxation during skeletal development. Dogs with hip subluxation will benefit from having strong muscles in hip region (gluteal muscles, pectineus, adductor, rectus femoris, and so forth). Growth optimization is also important. Large breed puppies should not be eating *ad libitum* (as much as they want to eat). They should not overeat carbohydrates[55,56] or receive calcium or phosphorus supplementation.[57] The primary focus of rehabilitation is to promote muscular development of the hind limbs with low-impact exercises. Growing dogs with hip laxity that exercise off leash have fewer clinical signs of hip dysplasia than growing dogs that do not exercise off leash.[58]

Rehabilitation Therapy Following Triple or Double Pelvic Osteotomy

Triple or double pelvic osteotomies (TPO or DPO) are performed on dogs that have early clinical signs of CHD but do not have radiographic evidence of OA. Most dogs that fit these criteria are between 4 and 10 months of age.[6] The TPO or DPO also improves dorsal femoral head coverage by the dorsal acetabular rim. The technique involves making 2 or 3 osteotomies: one in the pubis and the ilium and one in the ischium in the TPO but not the DPO. The caudal ilial segment is commonly rotated by 20°. A bone plate is applied to stabilize the ilial osteotomy.[6] Rehabilitation includes specific activity supervision for approximately 6 weeks until bone healing is confirmed on radiographs. During that time, nonsteroidal antiinflammatory drugs (NSAIDs), cryotherapy, and pROM are used to maintain and normalize hip motion. Controlled, low-impact therapeutic exercises, such as sit-to-stand exercises, and aquatic walking may be useful to attenuate muscle atrophy while avoiding excessive stress on the repair. Strengthening is achieved using controlled walking, aquatic walking, and low-impact exercises. The duration of these activities increases gradually during the first 3 months. Dogs are restricted to leash walking, with no running or jumping for the first 3 months to reduce the chances of implant loosening or hip joint luxation.

Rehabilitation Therapy Following Femoral Head and Neck Ostectomy

Rehabilitation after femoral head and neck ostectomy (FHO) emphasizes gaining hip extension, muscle mass, and increasing use of the operated limb. Rehabilitation must begin within 48 hours of FHO and continue until normal weight bearing is achieved on the surgical limb. A sample rehabilitation protocol after FHO is included in Appendix 1. After surgery, NSAIDs, cryotherapy, and hip pROM (especially hip extension) should be performed daily to enhance scar development of the pseudoarticulation. Ambulation on land, a ground treadmill, or an underwater treadmill promotes limb use and active hip extension. Walking up inclines will emphasize strengthening of the hip extensor muscle groups. Dancing exercises may encourage muscle strengthening and improve hip ROM, especially in extension. Most dogs toe touch consistently within 1 to 2 weeks, partially weight-bear within 3 weeks, and be actively using the operated limb within 4 weeks. In patients lacking hip extension, deep heating (up to 5 cm) may be accomplished using of therapeutic ultrasound[59] and may be performed before stretching. The dog should regain near-normal walking and trotting gaits, but full hip extension is rarely achieved and a pain response to maximal extension is likely to persist. After FHO, the prognosis for return to daily function is good but is influenced by the chronicity of the preexisting lameness and the presence of comorbid conditions, including body condition and OA in other joints. Overall athletic ability is likely to be decreased. Recovery is less predictable in large dogs compared with small dogs and in unfit or overweight dogs compared with fit or athletic dogs.

Rehabilitation Therapy Following Total Hip Replacement

Total hip replacement is most often delayed until CHD can no longer be managed by the use of medical therapy and exercise. Rehabilitation after total hip replacement can be divided into conventional rehabilitation, performed in uncomplicated patients, and targeted rehabilitation, performed to address specific situations relating to total hip replacement. The goal of rehabilitation after total hip replacement is to restore long-term, pain-free use of the operated limb.[60] In retrospective or prospective studies of canine total hip replacement,[61–64] information regarding postoperative rehabilitation is generally limited to initial supportive care and progressively longer leash walks. In a long-term prospective clinical trial, physical rehabilitation was limited to walking dogs on a leash to void during the first 8 weeks after surgery and increasing the length of leash walks 9 to 12 weeks after surgery. Hip pROM was normal in 29 of 31 dogs (94%) that were free of complications 5 years after surgery.[63] Hip extension was decreased in 3 dogs with long-term implant luxation and in 1 dog with a femoral osteosarcoma. In the same study, thigh girth was equal or larger to the opposite thigh in all complication-free dogs. To the authors' knowledge, there are no published reports describing dogs that did not achieve proper limb function after total hip replacement, provided that the hips were free of complication (implant malposition, failure of implant fixation, infection, or fracture). Functionally, dogs undergoing routine total hip replacement have normal limb use 3 months after surgery.[62] This suggests that specific rehabilitation programs or long hospitalization periods are probably not necessary in uncomplicated total hip replacements but may be considered in patients with limited hip joint motion because of tissue tightness. For example, some patients with dorsal femoral displacement for extended periods of time before surgery have tight periarticular muscles and other soft tissues after joint replacement. Rehabilitation includes acute, subacute, and chronic phases. Acutely, the rehabilitation after total hip replacement is focused on providing pain relief and avoiding catastrophic complications, including implant luxation or femoral fracture. Subacute rehabilitation after total hip replacement is focused on completing the recovery of joint motion and strengthening of the operated and contralateral limbs. Because healing is still progressing, exercises that place stress on the joint capsule and bone-implant interfaces are avoided. Excessive stress on the joint capsule could result from external rotation, excessive adduction, or excessive abduction of the operated limb. Walking exercises are generally performed in a straight line. Slippery and unsteady surfaces are avoided. Chronic rehabilitation after total hip replacement is focused on strengthening the operated and contralateral limbs. A wider range of therapeutic exercises is introduced, and the intensity of these exercises increases over time (**Fig. 14**).

Targeted Rehabilitation After Total Hip Replacement

Tissue tightness
Dogs with tissue tightness and limited hip extension benefit from a stretching program. Manual stretching is not critical when the loss of hip extension is modest (<20°) and the patient's limb use is acceptable. When the loss of hip extension is severe, moist heat and manual stretching techniques are used. Extension tightens the cranial aspect of the joint capsule and can be safely performed after surgery. Some patients are not receptive to stretching techniques, and owners may not be able to safely perform stretching at home Active hip extension exercises also increase ROM. Targeted therapeutic exercises are to gain hip extension for a more normal gait pattern and better function. Walking up a gentle incline, stepping up a single step or a series of steps with adequate traction, and stepping over objects all place the trailing limb in increased hip extension.

Sciatic neurapraxia
Patients with sciatic neurapraxia after total hip replacement scuff and show signs of weakness of the muscles innervated by the sciatic nerve, including the hamstrings and crus musculature. Rehabilitation is needed for days to months, depending on the severity of the deficits.[64] Rehabilitation focuses on minimizing hip complications due to decreased active muscular stabilization and protection (such as luxation), avoiding skin abrasions resulting from scuffing or knuckling, decreasing the loss of

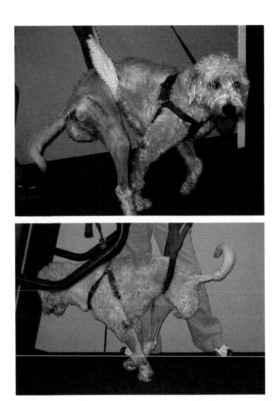

Fig. 14. Example of a patient walking on a land treadmill following a THR for severe CHD; this patient had previously had a contralateral midfemoral amputation, note the sling being used to support the pelvic limb so the patient cannot slip or fall during the exercise session. (*Reproduced from* Marcellin-Little DJ, Doyle ND, Pyke JF. Physical Rehabilitation after Total Joint Arthroplasty in Companion Animals. Elsevier. Vet Clin Small Animal 45, 2015; with permission.)

muscle mass in muscles innervated by branches of the sciatic nerve, and strengthening the affected muscle groups. Neuromuscular electrical stimulation can be used to elicit muscle contractions of the affected muscles and attenuate atrophy[35] but is not universally accepted by patients. If active hock extension is absent for weight bearing, the hock can be stabilized by an orthosis during therapeutic exercises (**Fig. 15**). Once hock flexion improves, the dog can exercise without an orthosis.[65] To avoid abrasions, affected dogs should avoid walking on abrasive surfaces and metacarpals and toes should be protected by a thin bootie or bandage. If the patient frequently knuckles, bootie systems with support straps that pull the hock into flexion and the digits into extension (TheraPaw, Lebanon, NJ, USA or Kruuse, Langeskov, Denmark) can be used during ambulation and therapeutic exercise sessions to create more normal posture for functional limb use while simultaneously protecting the skin from abrasions. In dogs with weak hock flexion, an exercise band or rubber traction band (Anti-Knuckling Device; Canine Mobility, Seattle, WA, USA or Biko Mobility, Raleigh, NC, USA) can be used to facilitate more normal flexion ROM during exercises. Exercises to strengthen hock flexion include stepping over progressively taller objects, such as segments of PVC pipe, walking in water at the height of the hock, and elicitation of a flexor withdraw reflex by pinching the digits. Most dogs fully recover from sciatic neurapraxia.[64]

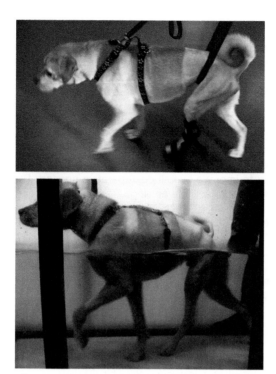

Fig. 15. A patient with sciatic neurapraxia following a THR. In the upper image the patient is wearing a tarsal orthotic, which will allow the patient to exercise without scuffing or knuckling while walking. Utilization of underwater treadmill therapy allows the patient to exercise without scuffing or knuckling. (*Reproduced from* Marcellin-Little DJ, Doyle ND, Pyke JF. Physical rehabilitation after total joint arthroplasty in companion animals. Vet Clin North Am Small Anim Pract 2015;45:145-165; with permission.)

Implant luxation following a total hip replacement (dorsal/ventral)

Following the acute management of a luxation, either traumatic or following a total hip replacement (with reduction/hobbles and/or surgical revision), targeted strengthening of the appropriate muscle groups provides improved dynamic joint support to help prevent a recurrence. Dogs that experienced a dorsal luxation need additional strengthening of the muscles lying on the dorsal aspect of the hip. Suggested exercises include 3-legged standing (lifting the unaffected pelvic limb and cuing the dog to shift weight onto the operative limb while maintaining a level pelvis), balancing on a soft or unsteady surface (commercial balance discs or an air mattress), walking perpendicular to an incline with the operative limb "downhill," and the previously mentioned hip extension exercises. Dogs experiencing a ventral luxation require strengthening of adductor muscles. Suggested exercises include resisted TheraBand exercises (TheraBand, Akron, OH, USA) while walking on a treadmill or alongside the handler (pull the hip into abduction with the band wrapped around the thigh to stimulate a contraction of the adductors), walking sideways, or walking perpendicular to an incline with the operative limb uphill. Underwater treadmill walking also can effectively and safely target the desired muscle group in both situations, particularly in the earlier phases of recovery. Proprioceptive retraining should also be used to improve body awareness and coordination for decreased risk of future falls.

SUMMARY

The goals of rehabilitation therapy at various stages of CHD vary. Initially, clinical signs and discomfort seem related to the underlying joint laxity. Rehabilitation therapy as part of conservative management in patients with laxity or in older patients with OA focuses on pain control and comfort while improving hip ROM in extension and maintenance of muscle mass. This is accomplished with weight reduction and fitness, minimizing joint pain, medications, DMOAs, manual therapy, physical modalities, and therapeutic exercise.[49] Surgical therapy for patients with CHD is focused at improving femoral head coverage and reducing the development OA (JPS, TPO, or DPO) or decreasing the source of pain (FHO or total hip replacement). Initially, rehabilitation therapy is designed to improve overall postoperative comfort, ROM, early usage of the postoperative limb, and facilitate healing.

CLINICS CARE POINTS

- An orthopedic examination is necessary to identify comorbid and premorbid conditions and simultaneously manage all conditions.
- Ensure that pain control is being adequately addressed when managing canine hip dysplasia through physical rehabilitation.
- Factors critical to maintaining optimal function in dogs with hip dysplasia include a regular exercise program and the optimization of body condition to eliminate excess body weight.
- The home environment and adequate physical activity is often overlooked but needs to be considered and discussed when managing canine hip dysplasia.

DISCLOSURE

The authors report no conflict of interest.

REFERENCES

1. Johnson JA, Austin C, Breur GJ. Incidence of canine appendicular musculoskeletal disorders in 16 veterinary teaching hospitals from 1980-1989. Vet Comp Orthop Traumatol 1994;7:56–69.
2. Riser WH. The dog as a model for the study of hip dysplasia. Growth, form, and development of the normal and dysplastic hip joint. Vet Pathol 1975;12:234–334.
3. Paster ER, LaFond E, Biery DN, et al. Estimates of prevalence of hip dysplasia in Golden Retrievers and Rottweilers and the influence of bias on published prevalence figures. J Am Vet Med Assoc 2005;226:387–92.
4. Smith GK, Mayhew PD, Kapatkin AS, et al. Evaluation of risk factors for degenerative joint disease associated with hip dysplasia in German Shepherd Dogs, Golden Retrievers, Labrador Retrievers, and Rottweilers. J Am Vet Med Assoc 2001;219:1719–24.
5. Smith GK, Karbe GT, Agnello KA, et al. Pathogenesis, diagnosis, and control of canine hip dysplasia. In: Tobias KM, Johnston SA, editors. Veterinary surgery, small animal. 1st edition. St. Louis (MO): Elsevier Saunders; 2012. p. 824–48.
6. Roush JK. Surgical therapy of canine hip dysplasia. In: Tobias KM, Johnston SA, editors. Veterinary surgery, small animal. 1st edition. St. Louis (MO): Elsevier Saunders; 2012. p. 849–64.

7. Davidson JR, Kerwin S. Common orthopedic conditions and their physical reha-bilitation. In: Millis DL, Levine D, editors. Canine rehabilitation and physical ther-apy. 2nd edition. Philadelphia (PA): Elsevier Saunders; 2014. p. 543–81.
8. Smith GK, Paster ER, Powers MY, et al. Lifelong diet restriction and radiographic evidence of osteoarthritis of the hip joint in dogs. J Am Vet Med Assoc 2006;229: 690–3.
9. Jaegger G, Marcellin-Little DJ, Levine D. Reliability of goniometry in Labrador Re-trievers. Am J Vet Res 2002;63:979–86.
10. Greene LM, Marcellin-Little DJ, Lascelles BD. Associations among exercise dura-tion, lameness severity, and hip joint range of motion in Labrador Retrievers with hip dysplasia. J Am Vet Med Assoc 2013;242:1528–33.
11. Millis DL, Levine D. The role of exercise and physical modalities in the treatment of osteoarthritis. Vet Clin North Am Small Anim Pract 1997;27:913–30.
12. Millard RP, Towle-Millard HA, Rankin DC, et al. Effect of cold compress applica-tion on tissue temperature in healthy dogs. Am J Vet Res 2013;74:443–7.
13. Oosterveld FG, Rasker JJ. Treating arthritis with locally applied heat or cold. Semin Arthritis Rheum 1994;24:82–90.
14. Danneskiold-Samsoe B, Bartels EM. Massage-is it really a reliable method of treatment? Eur J Pain 1999;3:244–5.
15. Millard RP, Towle-Millard HA, Rankin DC, et al. Effect of warm compress applica-tion on tissue temperature in healthy dogs. Am J Vet Res 2013;74:448–51.
16. Millis DL, Levine D. Range-of-motion and stretching exercises. In: Millis DL, Levine D, editors. Canine rehabilitation and physical therapy. 2nd edition. Phila-delphia (PA): Elsevier Saunders; 2014. p. 431–46.
17. Brody LT. Mobility impairment. In: Hall CM, Brody LT, editors. Therapeutic exer-cise: moving toward function. Philadelphia (PA): Lippincott Williams & Wilkins; 1999. p. 87–111.
18. Marcellin-Little DJ, Levine D. Principles and application of range of motion and stretching in companion animals. Vet Clin North Am Small Anim Pract 2015;45: 57–72.
19. Westlake KP, Wu Y, Culham EG. Sensory-specific balance training in older adults: effect on position, movement, and velocity sense at the ankle. Phys Ther 2007;87: 560–8.
20. Saunders DG, Walker JR, Levine D. Joint mobilization. Vet Clin North Am Small Anim Pract 2005;35:1287–316.
21. Weigel JP, Arnold G, Hicks DA, et al. Biomechanics of rehabilitation. Vet Clin North Am Small Anim Pract 2005;35:1255–85.
22. Hottinger HA, DeCamp CE, Olivier NB, et al. Noninvasive kinematic analysis of the walk in healthy large-breed dogs. Am J Vet Res 1996;57:381–8.
23. DeCamp CE, Riggs CM, Olivier NB, et al. Kinematic evaluation of gait in dogs with cranial cruciate ligament rupture. Am J Vet Res 1996;57:120–6.
24. DeCamp CE, Soutas-Little RW, Hauptman J, et al. Kinematic gait analysis of the trot in healthy greyhounds. Am J Vet Res 1993;54:627–34.
25. Holler PJ, Brazda V, Dal-Bianco B, et al. Kinematic motion analysis of the joints of the forelimbs and hind limbs of dogs during walking exercise regimens. Am J Vet Res 2010;71:734–40.
26. Durant AM, Millis DL, Headrick JF. Kinematics of stair ascent in healthy dogs. Vet Comp Orthop Traumatol 2011;24:99–105.
27. Richards J, Holler P, Bockstahler B, et al. A comparison of human and canine ki-nematics during level walking, stair ascent, and stair descent. Wien Tierärzt Mschr 2010;97:92–100.

28. Millis DL, Schwartz P, Hicks DA, et al. Kinematic assessment of selected thera-peutic exercises in dogs. 3rd International Symposium on Physical Therapy and Rehabilitation in Veterinary Medicine. Research Park (NC), August 7-11, 2004.

29. Headrick JH, Hicks DA, McEachern GL. Kinematics of walking over cavaletti rails compared to over ground walking in dogs. 2nd World Veterinary Orthopedic Congress Veterinary Orthopedic Society 2006.

30. Feeney LC, Lin CF, Marcellin-Little DJ, et al. Validation of two-dimensional kinematic analysis of walk and sit-to-stand motions in dogs. Am J Vet Res 2007;68:277–82.

31. Levine D, Marcellin-Little DJ, Millis DL, et al. Effects of partial immersion in water on vertical ground reaction forces and weight distribution in dogs. Am J Vet Res 2010;71:1413–6.

32. Johns KM. Aquatic therapy: therapeutic treatment for today's patient. Phys Ther Prod 1993;24–5.

33. Marsolais GS, McLean S, Derrick T, et al. Kinematic analysis of the hind limb dur-ing swimming and walking in healthy dogs and dogs with surgically corrected cranial cruciate ligament rupture. J Am Vet Med Assoc 2003;222:739–43.

34. Levine D, Watson T. Therapeutic ultrasound. In: Millis DL, Levine D, editors. Canine rehabilitation and physical therapy. Philadelphia (PA): Elsevier Saunders; 2014. p. 328–41.

35. Levine D, Bockstahler B. Electrical stimulation. In: Millis DL, Levine D, editors. Canine rehabilitation and physical therapy. Philadelphia (PA): Elsevier Saunders; 2014. p. 342–58.

36. Pryor B, Millis DL. Therapeutic laser in veterinary medicine. The Vet Clin North America Small Anim Pract 2015;45:45–56.

37. Durant A, Millis DL. Applications of extracorporeal shockwave in small animal rehabilitation. In: Millis DL, Levine D, editors. Canine rehabilitation and physical therapy. 2nd edition. Philadelphia (PA): Elsevier Saunders; 2014. p. 381–92.

38. Levine D, Millis DL, Flocker J, et al. Aquatic therapy. In: Millis DL, Levine D, ed-itors. Canine rehabilitation and physical therapy. 2nd edition. Philadelphia (PA): Elsevier Saunders; 2014. p. 526–42.

39. Millis DL, Drum M, Levine D. Therapeutic exercises: joint motion, strengthening, endurance, and speed exercises. In: Millis DL, Levine D, editors. Canine rehabil-itation and physical therapy. 2nd edition. Philadelphia (PA): Elsevier Saunders; 2014. p. 506–25.

40. Shulthies SS. Interview with Dr. David O Draper. Sports phys ther sect newslett, Am Phys Ther Assoc; 1995. p. 12–3.

41. Nelson RM, Hayes KW, Currier DP. Clinical electrotherapy. 3rd edition. Norwalk (CT): Appleton & Lange; 1999.

42. de Morais NC, Barbosa AM, Vale ML, et al. Anti-inflammatory effect of low-level laser and light-emitting diode in zymosan-induced arthritis. Photomed Laser Surg 2010;28:227–32.

43. Rubio CR, Cremonezzi D, Moya M, et al. Helium-neon laser reduces the inflam-matory process of arthritis. Photomed Laser Surg 2010;28:125–9.

44. Brosseau L, Robinson V, Wells G, et al. Low level laser therapy (Classes I, II and III) for treating rheumatoid arthritis. Cochrane Database Syst Rev 2005;CD002049.

45. Mueller M, Bockstahler B, Skalicky M, et al. Effects of radial shockwave therapy on the limb function of dogs with hip osteoarthritis. The Vet Rec 2007;160:762–5.

46. Moretti B, Iannone F, Notarnicola A, et al. Extracorporeal shock waves down-regulate the expression of interleukin-10 and tumor necrosis factor-alpha in osteoarthritic chondrocytes. BMC Musculoskelet Disord 2008;9:16.

47. Dorotka R, Kubista B, Schatz KD, et al. Effects of extracorporeal shock waves on human articular chondrocytes and ovine bone marrow stromal cells in vitro. Arch Orthop Trauma Surg 2003;123:345–8.

48. Mayer-Wagner S, Ernst J, Maier M, et al. The effect of high-energy extracorporeal shock waves on hyaline cartilage of adult rats in vivo. J Orthop Res 2010;28:1050–6.

49. Marcellin-Little DJ, Levine D, Millis DL. Multifactorial rehabilitation planning in companion animals. Adv Sm Anim Care 2021;2:1–10.

50. Fortney WD. Implementing a successful senior/geriatric health care program for veterinarians, veterinary technicians, and office managers. Vet Clin North Am Small Anim Pract 2012;42:823–34, viii.

51. Hielm-Bjorkman AK, Kuusela E, Liman A, et al. Evaluation of methods for assessment of pain associated with chronic osteoarthritis in dogs. J Am Vet Med Assoc 2003;222:1552–8.

52. Alves JC, Santos AM, Jorge PI. Effect of an oral joint supplement when compared to carprofen in the management of hip osteoarthritis in working dogs. Top companion Anim Med 2017;32:126–9.

53. Marshall WG, Hazewinkel HA, Mullen D, et al. The effect of weight loss on lameness in obese dogs with osteoarthritis. Vet Res Commun 2010;34:241–53.

54. Dueland RT, Adams WM, Fialkowski JP, et al. Effects of pubic symphysiodesis in dysplastic puppies. Vet Surg 2001;30:201–17.

55. Hedhammar A, Krook L, Whalen JP, et al. Overnutrition and skeletal disease. An experimental study in growing Great Dane dogs. IV. Clinical observations. Cornell Vet 1974;64(Suppl 5):32–45.

56. Kasström H. Nutrition, weight gain and development of hip dysplasia. An experimental investigation in growing dogs with special reference to the effect of feeding intensity. Acta Radiol Suppl 1975;344:135–79.

57. Hazewinkel HAWG, Poulos SA, Wolvekamp PW, et al. Influences of chronic calcium excess on the skeletal development of growing Great Danes. J Am Anim Hosp Assoc 1985;21:377–91.

58. Krontveit RI, Trangerud C, Saevik BK, et al. Risk factors for hip-related clinical signs in a prospective cohort study of four large dog breeds in Norway. Prev Vet Med 2012;103:219–27.

59. Levine D, Millis DL, Mynatt T. Effects of 3.3-MHz ultrasound on caudal thigh muscle temperature in dogs. Vet Surg 2001;30:170–4.

60. Marcellin-Little DJ, Doyle ND, Pyke JF. Physical rehabilitation after total joint arthroplasty in companion animals. Vet Clin North Am Small Anim Pract 2015;45:145–65.

61. Peck J, Liska W, DeYoung D, et al. Clinical application of total hip replacement. In: Peck J, Marcellin-Little D, editors. Advances in small animal total joint replacement. 1st edition. Ames (IA): Wiley-Blackwell; 2013. p. 69–108.

62. Lascelles BD, Freire M, Roe SC, et al. Evaluation of functional outcome after BFX total hip replacement using a pressure sensitive walkway. Vet Surg 2010;39:71–7.

63. Marcellin-Little DJ, DeYoung BA, Doyens DH, et al. Canine uncemented porous-coated anatomic total hip arthroplasty: results of a long-term prospective evaluation of 50 consecutive cases. Vet Surg 1999;28:10–20.

64. Andrews CM, Liska WD, Roberts DJ. Sciatic neurapraxia as a complication in 1000 consecutive canine total hip replacements. Vet Surg 2008;37:254–62.

65. Levine JM, Fitch RB. Use of an ankle-foot orthosis in a dog with traumatic sciatic neuropathy. J Small Anim Pract 2003;44:236–8.

APPENDIX 1: SAMPLE PROTOCOL FOR FEMORAL HEAD AND NECK OSTECTOMY

Phase	Expected Time Frame[a]	Rehabilitation Clinic Program	Home Program	Outcome Assessment Measures	Criteria for Movement to Next Phase
Non–weight-bearing to toe-touching	Immediate to 48–72 h postoperative	Therapeutic exercises • Slow, gentle hip PROM for operated limb focusing on extension (10 reps TID-QID beginning immediately postoperative while recovering from anesthesia) • Slow leash walking with sling support available, only to go outside (up to 5 min, TID-QID) • Balance exercises on a soft foam pad or bidirectional balance board for weight-bearing Modalities • Gentle massage around the surgery site, thigh, and lumbosacral regions • Transcutaneous electrical stimulation for pain relief (15–20 min SID-TID) • Cryotherapy (15–20 min TID after activities)—first	Inpatient status preferred during this phase If Home: Therapeutic Exercises • Slow, gentle hip PROM for operated limb focusing on extension (10 reps TID-QID beginning immediately postoperative) • Slow leash walking with sling support available, only to go outside (up to 5 min, TID-QID) • Balance exercises on a semi-firm surface for weight-bearing Modalities • Gentle massage around the surgery site, thigh and lumbosacral regions • Cryotherapy (15–20 min TID after activities) – first session immediately post-operative	• Postoperative bilateral "hip" PROM and other joints as applicable via goniometry • Postoperative bilateral thigh circumference • Response to activity and subjective pain level • Lameness score at a stance and walk • Weight	• Early toe-touching • Adequate resting analgesia • Decreased perioperative swelling and lack of incisional drainage.

Phase	Interventions	Outcome measures	Goals
	session immediately postoperative in combination with slow PROM while recovering from anesthesia • Therapeutic laser therapy SID		
Early weight-bearing 72 h to 2 wk postoperative	Therapeutic exercises • PROM and flexion/ extension hip stretches of operated limb (10–15 reps BID-TID). Bicycling and flexor reflex exercises • Slow, controlled walking on a land treadmill, 5–10 min including mild incline settings to encourage hip extension and target gluteal muscles • Balance exercises on a soft foam pad or bidirectional balance board for weight-bearing BID-TID Modalities • Heat therapy before activity (10–15 min BID-TID, NOT within 72 h after surgery or if S/S of acute inflammation are still present) Therapeutic exercises • PROM and flexion/ extension hip stretches of operated limb (10–15 reps BID-TID). • Slow, controlled leash walking, 5–20 min including mild inclines to encourage hip extension and target gluteal muscles • Balance exercises on a soft foam pad for weight-bearing BID-TID Modalities • Heat therapy (10–15 min BID-TID, prior to exercises, NOT within 72 h after surgery or if CS of acute inflammation are still present) • Cryotherapy (15–20 min BID) following exercises	• Goniometry - hip ROM and other joints if applicable • Response to activity and subjective pain level • Lameness score at a stance and walk • Weight	• Consistent partial weight-bearing on operated limb on all strides at a walk • Minimal pain with light activities • Incisional healing without complications

(continued on next page)

(continued)

Phase	Expected Time Frame[a]	Rehabilitation Clinic Program	Home Program	Outcome Assessment Measures	Criteria for Movement to Next Phase
		• Therapeutic ultrasound SID • Massage • Therapeutic laser therapy PRN • Cryotherapy (15–20 min BID) following exercises			
Consistent weight-bearing at a walk	2–4 wk postoperative	• Therapeutic exercises • PROM and flexion/extension hip stretches of operated limb (10–15 reps SID-BID • Controlled walking on a land treadmill, 10–15 min with increased incline angle and speed SID • Balance exercises on an inflatable disk or 360° wobble board for weight-bearing 5 min BID-TID • Encourage increased weight-bearing on operated limb (eg, initiating dancing exercises as tolerated 5 min BID-TID, applying weight on operated limb at 3%–5% body weight	• Therapeutic exercises • PROM and flexion/extension hip stretches of operated limb (10–15 reps BID-TID) • Leash walks 15–20 min including 5–10 min of inclines • Balance exercises on an inflatable disk for weight-bearing BID-TID • Sit-to-stand exercises 5–10 reps BID • Light jogging 3–5 min per day • Stairs: 1 flight SID-BID Modalities • Heat therapy (10 min) before activity • Cryotherapy (15–20 min) following exercises	• Goniometry - hip ROM and other joints if applicable • Reevaluate thigh muscle girth at 3–4 wk postoperative • Response to activity and subjective pain level • Lameness score at a stance, walk, and trot • Weight	• Consistent weight-bearing on operated limb on all strides at a walk, consistent partial weight-bearing at a trot • Minimal pain with light activities

or syringe cap under contralateral foot)
- Sit-to-stand exercises 5–10 reps BID
- Aquatic therapy: UWTM walking 5–10 min once incision is sealed SID-BID
- Swimming 3–5 d per wk
- Cavaletti Rails 5–10 reps BID

Modalities
- Heat therapy before activity
- Therapeutic ultrasound PRN
- Massage PRN
- Therapeutic laser therapy PRN
- Cryotherapy (15–20 min BID) following exercises

| Consistent weight-bearing at a Trot | 5–8 wk postoperative | Therapeutic exercises
• PROM and flexion/extension hip stretches of operated limb PRN
• Controlled walking or light jogging on a land treadmill, 15–20 min with increased incline angle and speed SID
• Balance exercises on an inflatable disk or 360° wobble board for | Therapeutic exercises
• PROM and flexion/extension hip stretches of operated limb PRN
• Leash walks 20–30 min including up to 10–15 min of inclines, may use weights on affected limb or pulled with a harness as tolerated/required
• Incorporate challenging surfaces to walks that is, | • Goniometry - hip ROM and other joints if applicable
• Reevaluate thigh muscle girth at 7–8 wk postoperative
• Response to activity and subjective pain level
• Lameness score at a stance, walk and trot
• Weight | • Consistent weight-bearing on operated limb at a trot
• Minimal to no pain with moderate to extensive activities |

(continued on next page)

(continued)

Phase	Expected Time Frame[a]	Rehabilitation Clinic Program	Home Program	Outcome Assessment Measures	Criteria for Movement to Next Phase
		weight-bearing 10 min BID-TID • Sit-to-stand exercises 10–20 reps BID • Aquatic therapy: UWTM walking 15–30 min SID-BID • Swimming 2–5 d per week Modalities • Heat therapy PRN before activity • Cryotherapy PRN after exercises	snow, sand, when possible • Controlled ball-playing with gradually increasing times and distances • Sit-to-stand exercises 10–20 reps BID • Light jogging 3–5 min per day • Stairs: 2–4 flights SID-BID Modalities • Heat therapy PRN before activity • Cryotherapy PRN after exercises		
Trotting at speed with minimal to no lameness	9 wk postoperative and beyond	Aquatic therapy as desired; otherwise exercises may be continued as part of a home exercise program.	Therapeutic exercises • PROM for operated limb PRN • Leash walks at times and distances tolerated, including fast walks up inclined surfaces • Sit-to-stand exercises 20–30 reps as needed • Jogging: working up from 10-15 min per day • Stairs: walking and trotting, increasing number of flights as tolerated	• Goniometry every 3–4 wk if needed • Reevaluate thigh muscle girth every 3–4 wk PRN • Response to activity and subjective pain level • Lameness score at a stance, walk, and trot • Weight	• Consistent weight-bearing on operated limb at a trot; permanent mild gait deficits may persist • Minimal to no pain with extensive activities

- Swimming or walking in mid-to-upper-thigh-level water
- Ball-playing with gradually increasing times and distances, becoming more vigorous over time

[a] This protocol is for use by licensed veterinary professionals. It is intended as a guideline and may be influenced by many factors affecting individualized patient care.

Brachycephalic Obstructive Airway Syndrome

Dorothee Krainer, Dr Med Vet, MBA*, Gilles Dupré, Dr Med Vet, Dr Hc

KEYWORDS

- Brachycephalic obstructive airway syndrome • Soft palate
- Nasopharyngeal collapse • Laryngeal collapse • Surgery

KEY POINTS

- Skull conformation anomalies in brachycephalic breeds lead to shortening and compression of nasal and nasopharyngeal passages.
- Additional mucosal hyperplasia and secondary collapse of the upper airway contribute to a multilevel obstruction and the genesis of the so-called brachycephalic obstructive airway syndrome.
- Surgical treatments usually include widening of stenotic nares and various palatoplasty techniques to improve airflow through the nasopharynx and rima glottidis.
- The overall prognosis for a significant improvement is excellent.

 Video content accompanies this article at http://www.vetsmall.theclinics.com.

INTRODUCTION

Brachycephalic obstructive airway syndrome (BOAS) is an established cause of respiratory distress in brachycephalic breeds.[1–3] Breeds most commonly affected are English and French bulldogs, pugs, and Boston terriers; however, Pekingese, Shih tzu, Lhasa apsos, Cavalier King Charles spaniels, Boxers, Dogue de Bordeaux, Brussels griffon, and Bullmastiffs are also categorized as brachycephalic dogs.[4]Most owners report heat, stress, and exercise intolerance, snoring, inspiratory dyspnea, and, in severe cases, cyanosis and even syncopal episodes. Sleep apneas can be observed,[5] and occasionally gastrointestinal signs such as vomiting and regurgitation.

With the diagnostic advancements of the recent years, the problem list of brachycephalic breeds has expanded from an upper airway syndrome to a much wider scope. Further organ systems that are described to be affected by brachycephaly are:

Department for Small Animal and Equine, Clinic for Small Animal Surgery, University of Veterinary Medicine Vienna, Veterinärplatz 1, A- 1210 Vienna, Austria
* Corresponding author.
E-mail address: dorotheeheidenreich@hotmail.com

Vet Clin Small Anim 52 (2022) 749–780
https://doi.org/10.1016/j.cvsm.2022.01.013   vetsmall.theclinics.com

- Brachycephalic ocular syndrome.[6]
- Dental and oral health problems.[7]
- Vertebral malformation and spinal disease.[8–12]
- Brain disorders.[13]
- Middle ear effusion and inflammation.[14–17]
- Patella luxation.[18]

This article focuses on the BOAS, including its effects and new aspects. The discussion on ethics or genetic aspects is beyond the scope of this article and the reader is asked to view the appropriate literature elsewhere.

ANATOMIC AND PATHOPHYSIOLOGIC CHANGES OF THE RESPIRATORY SYSTEM OBSERVED IN BRACHYCEPHALIC DOG BREEDS
Primary Static Anomalies: Bony Tissue Changes

Skull conformation anomalies
Brachycephalic breeds have a shorter and wider skull compared with mesaticephalic and dolichocephalic breeds,[19,20] which leads to a compressed nasal passage[21] and altered nasopharyngeal anatomy.[22–24] In addition, pugs are reported to have a dorsal rotation of the maxillary bone, miniscule or absent frontal sinuses,[25,26] a ventral orientation of the olfactorial bulb,[27] and, altogether, shorter craniofacial skull dimensions than French and English bulldogs.[25,27–30] This dorsal rotation has been discussed as a potential cause for aberrant nasopharyngeal turbinates, which are also more commonly reported in pugs (**Figs. 1 and 2**).[3,25,31–33]

Aberrant conchae, and nasopharyngeal turbinates
Abnormal conchal growth obstructing the intranasal airways and the nasaopharyngeal meatus are common findings (43%) in the extreme brachycephalic breeds, such as pugs, French bulldogs, and English bulldogs.[25] However, their impact on airway obstruction is difficult to assess and remains unclear. Vilaplana and colleagues[34] (2015) reported aberrant caudal turbinates in 100% of English bulldogs with no or mild clinical signs of brachycephalic airway syndrome. Other studies evaluating the intranasal airway obstruction with computed tomography (CT) and rhinoscopy state that the presence of aberrant conchae contribute to the heat and exercise intolerance of brachycephalic breeds.[21] Pugs seem to be most affected by rostral aberrant turbinates (90.9%) and nasal septum deviation compared with French bulldogs (56.4%) and English bulldogs (36.4%), which might be due to the dorsorotation of their skull.[31,32,35] These abnormal turbinates are thought to be more present in these

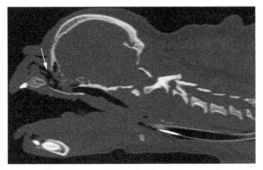

Fig. 1. Dorsal rotation maxillary bone. Midsagittal CT image of a 4-year-old pug depicting dorsal rotation (*arrow*) of the maxillary bone.

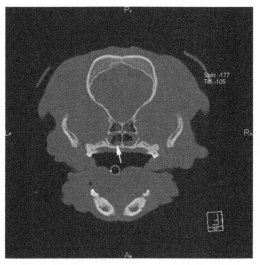

Fig. 2. Aberrant turbinates. Transverse CT image of a French bulldog depicting aberrant nasopharyngeal turbinates (*arrow*).

breeds, because their growth fails to stop.[3] Interconchal and intrachonal contact points were found in 91.7% of brachycephalic and 24% of normocephalic dogs. Regrowth of aberrant turbinates is reported as a common complication after laser-assisted turbinectomy (LATE) and revision surgery was required in 20% of French bulldogs and pugs.[36]

Primary Static Anomalies: Soft Tissue Changes

Stenotic Nares

BOAS-affected dogs have stenotic nares, which decrease each nostril often to a vertical slit (**Fig. 3**). Liu and colleagues[37] (2017) described stenotic nares in English bulldogs, French bulldogs, and pugs with the following grading system:

- 0 = open = wide open
- 1 = mild = slightly narrowed, lateral nostril wall not in contact with septum

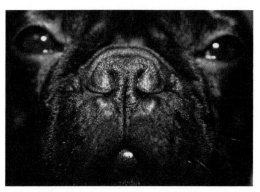

Fig. 3. Stenotic nares. Stenotic nares in a 2-year-old French bulldog.

- 2 = moderate = lateral nostril wall in contact with septum dorsally but nostrils open ventrally
- 3 = severe = nostrils almost closed

This typical and easily recognized primary anatomic component of brachycephalic syndrome is widely accepted as a major cause of upper airway obstruction in these breeds.[38]

Soft Palate Hyperplasia

Although the literature originally describes an elongated soft palate fluttering, and obstructing the rima glottidis as a primary component of BOAS,[2,31,39] it is now commonly agreed that an additional pathologic thickening of the soft palate plays a major role in the nasopharyngeal obstruction.[3,26,40–45] Radiographic, CT, fluoroscopic, and histologic examinations demonstrated a hypertrophy of the soft palate.[3,26,40–45] Grand and Bureau[40] (2011) found a positive correlation between the thickness of the soft palate and the severity of the clinical signs. A CT study evaluating the upper airway dimension in pugs and French bulldogs showed that French bulldogs have a significantly thicker soft palate compared with pugs. Pugs, however, have a smaller nasopharyngeal airway space with a complete airway obstruction dorsal to the soft palate in 81%.[26]

In addition to soft palate hyperplasia, CT and endoscopic studies reported hyperplasia of the nasopharyngeal mucosa,[46,47] hypertrophy and eversion of the tonsils,[48] and an overlong and thickened tongue (macroglossia), which further displaces the soft palate dorsally.[49]

Macroglossia and Hyoid Malformation

Macroglossia has already been identified as part of BOAS by Fox in 1963[49] and is described in many textbooks. Recent anatomic CT-aided measurements of the tongue size and its extent within the oropharynx and nasopharynx quantify the potential contribution of macroglossia to upper airway obstruction. Jones and colleagues[50] (2020) describe a relative macroglossia and an associated decrease of upper airway space in extreme brachycephalic breeds (ie, pugs, French bulldogs, English bulldogs, and Boston terriers) compared with mesaticephalic dogs. The tongues of brachycephalic dogs were denser than those of mesaticephalic dogs.[50] The other study comparing the size of the tongue, soft palate and airway space in the oropharynx and nasopharynx revealed smaller tongues in pugs compared with French and English bulldogs. However, pugs were still the breed of these 3 that had the smallest air volume in the oropharynx at the base of the tongue.[51]

The effect of tongue size on the air volume in the upper airway is difficult to assess because its position and the dynamic changes of the oropharynx space during a breathing circle can vary significantly.

A hyoid malformation was reported in a French bulldog.[52] A comparison of the hyoid conformation of French bulldogs compared with mesaticephalic dogs showed more acute curvature and greater ventrodorsal thickness of the basihyoid bone in French bulldogs, which might be an additional distorted anatomic component of brachycephalic skull morphology.[52]

Glottis and Cricoid Cartilage Narrowing

There are few data available on the laryngeal and cricoid anatomy of brachycephalic dogs. A laryngeal morphometric study comparing English and French bulldogs, and pugs found that pugs have a more oval-shaped and narrower glottis than English and French bulldogs. The glottis was reported to be round in English Bulldogs and elliptical in pugs.[53]

The cricoid cartilage was also found to be more oval-shaped in pugs and French bulldogs compared with mesaticephalic dogs. However, the dimensions of the cricoid were similar for BOAS- affected and BOAS nonaffected brachycephalic dogs. The smallest diameter of the tracheal and cricoid airway was found to be located in the trachea.[54]

A recent report of a Pekinese and a French bulldog with BOAS found difficulties during tracheal intubation owing to narrowing of the cricoid cartilage and a thickened mucous membrane. The rostral level of cricoid cartilage was markedly narrower than the ring level of the cricoid cartilage in both dogs. The shape of the rostral part of the cricoid cartilage was vertically ovoid in the Pekinese and gourd-shaped in the French bulldog.[55]

Tracheal Hypoplasia
Tracheal hypoplasia,[2,31,56] defined as a tracheal diameter to the thoracic inlet ratio of less than 0.20 in nonbrachycephalic and less than 0.16 in brachycephalic dogs,[57] has been described in 13% of BOAS-affected dogs.[23,58] The English bulldog has the highest incidence of tracheal hypoplasia among brachycephalic breeds, and tracheal hypoplasia in this breed has been defined as a tracheal diameter to the thoracic inlet ratio of less than 0.12. Tracheal hypoplasia was found to occur more often in screw-tailed brachycephalic dogs compared with non–screw-tailed brachycephalics.[59] A comparison of tracheal dimensions assessed with radiography, CT scans, and thoracoscopy showed that the latter was the most reliable technique to identify tracheal hypoplasia and did not correlate with the 2 other imaging techniques. CT measurements were 19% greater than those assessed was radiographs.[60] Although tracheal hypoplasia increases airway resistance, its contribution to the syndrome is likely minimal,[3] and tracheal hypoplasia was found not to improve after surgical correction for BOAS.[61]

Middle Ear Effusion and Inflammation
Incidental middle ear effusion is common in brachycephalic dogs,[62] with a prevalence of up to 41%.[16,17,63] French bulldogs and Cavalier King Charles spaniels seem to be the most affected.[14,15] The middle ears of brachycephalic dogs have a smaller luminal size than normal dogs,[16,17,64] and French bulldogs and English bulldogs have an increased thickness of the ventral tympanic wall.[15,16] Obstruction or dysfunction of the eustachian tube is thought to cause this middle ear effusion.[62] Potential reasons are a smaller opening of the eustachian tube secondary to an abnormal shape and rostral position of the tympanic bulla.[17] A decreased pharyngeal aperture was found to be related to middle ear effusion in Cavalier King Charles spaniels,[14] but not in French bulldogs or pugs.[15] However, a correlation of soft palate hyperplasia and middle ear effusion was found in bulldogs, French bulldogs, and pugs.[16] French bulldogs were reported to be more commonly affected with middle ear effusion and inflammation (41.6%) compared with pugs (5.0%). These dogs also showed an increased incidence of regurgitation, which might contribute to middle ear effusion and inflammation.[15]

Secondary Dynamic Changes of the Airway

Nasopharyngeal Obstruction and Collapse
The nasopharyngeal airway space is decreased in brachycephalic dogs owing to a thickened soft palate, enlarged and everted tonsils, redundant mucosal folds,[65] and relative macroglossia. Static CT measurements of this region showed that its smallest

airway space is located dorsal to the caudal end of the soft palate and was smaller in pugs compared with French bulldogs, who have a significantly thicker soft palate.[26] The increased thickness of the soft palate was also identified as the most relevant pharyngeal CT parameter in dogs severely affected by BOAS.[40] Kim and colleagues[66] (2019) found that body weight and maximum soft palate thickness are the key factors associated with decreased nasopharyngeal airway dimensions. The maximal naso-pharyngeal occlusion was found to be located about 1 cm caudal to the hamuli pter-ygoidei. but this distance varied in the individual dogs.[67] The tongue and palatal tissues were reported to decrease the nasopharyngeal airway dimension by 60% in brachycephalic dogs when compared with mesaticephalic ones.[50]

Dynamic nasopharyngeal collapse assessed with fluoroscopy was significantly more common in brachycephalic dogs compared with mesaticephalic dogs.[68] Another fluoroscopy assessment of pharyngeal collapse found that it is likely second-ary to a long-term negative pressure of the upper airway. It was most seen in dogs with bronchial or tracheal collapse, but also in dogs with brachycephalic syndrome.[69] These fluoroscopic studies did not quantify the airway dimensions of the collapsed pharynx, but differentiated its degree as complete or partial if more than 50% of the airway was collapsed. Interobserver and intraobserver agreement of the nasopharyn-geal dimensions in pugs and French bulldogs by means of fluoroscopic examination is currently under investigation.[70]

More recent studies applied dynamic CT to assess nasopharyngeal collapsibility: Hara and colleagues[71] (2020) identified the order of the pharyngeal motion during inspiration as pharyngeal collapse followed by pharyngeal contraction and laryngo-spasm. The second dynamic CT study quantified the nasopharyngeal collapsibility in normal dogs and found that the caudal end of the soft palate and the level of the foramen lacerum are useful locations for its assessment. Factors that might influence nasopharyngeal collapsibility are thickening of the soft palate, weight gain, or epiglottis location.[72]

Tonsillar Eversion and Hypertrophy

Palatine tonsillar enlargement and eversion have been reported in 9% and 56% of dogs with BOAS, respectively.[48,73] It is thought that the hypertrophy and associated eversion from the tonsillar crypts occur secondary to an increased negative pressure during inspiration. Histopathology of excised tonsils in BOAS- affected dogs showed mild to marked inflammation and edema.[74] Inflammation of the tonsils was also diag-nosed in 15 of 73 dogs (20.5%), predominately French Bulldogs, with BOAS.[75] This finding was thought to be secondary to chronic inflammation of the pharyngeal area caused by gastroesophageal reflux. Enlarged tonsils can contribute to the upper airway obstruction in these dogs. Tonsillectomy as part of multilevel surgical approach is performed routinely by some surgeons,[74,76] whereas other surgeons prefer not to because they expect the tonsillar inflammation to resolve after treating the primary anomalies of these dogs.

Laryngeal Collapse

Laryngeal diseases associated with BOAS are thought to be mainly secondary to the turbulent airflow and chronic high negative pressures in the pharynx.[2,39,41,77,78] They are characterized by a relatively high-pitch sound when air flows through the narrowed rima glottidis. They include.

- Mucosal edema
- Everted laryngeal saccules (ELS)
- Laryngeal collapse

In an early classification, ELS were considered the first stage of laryngeal collapse[79] (**Fig. 4**). Stage 2 was characterized by a medial displacement of the cuneiform processes of the arytenoid cartilages, and stage 3 by a collapse of the corniculate processes with loss of the dorsal arch of the rima glottidis. Altogether, the incidence of laryngeal collapse varies from 50%[80,81] to as many as 95%[82] in BOAS-affected dogs. Studies report that the size of the rima glottidis is smaller in pugs[53] and that they are also significantly more often affected by severe laryngeal collapse than French bulldogs.[83] In this breed, the arytenoid cartilages can even invert into the laryngeal lumen as a consequence of lack of rigidity (chondromalacia), which makes the larynx incapable to withstand high negative pharyngeal pressures[41] (Video 1). Altogether, an evaluation of the movements of the larynx remains critical to objectivate the laryngeal collapse. Unfortunately, endoscopic examination under anesthesia may not reflect the actual situation of the laryngeal cartilages during inspiration under increased negative pressure situation such as exercises, heat, or excitement. Ultrasound examination has been evaluated as an alternative way to objectivate laryngeal collapse.[84]

Although some authors describe laryngeal collapse as a negative prognostic indicator for the surgical outcome,[76] other authors found no correlation between the severity of laryngeal collapse and overall respiratory signs or prognosis.[83] Other reported abnormalities of the larynx associated with BOAS are epiglottic cysts, and laryngeal granulomas.[85]

Tracheal Collapse and Bronchial Collapse

Tracheal collapse and bronchial collapse were found to be significantly correlated with the severity of the laryngeal collapse ($P = .45$), and pugs were found to be most severely affected. Left-sided bronchi were generally more affected by bronchial collapse (52.1%) than the right, with the cranial left bronchus most commonly collapsed.[82] Whether the etiology is loss of rigidity (chondromalacia), increased negative pressure, or compression within the chest remains to be investigated (Video 2). Rubin and colleagues[69] (2015) also found an association of bronchial and tracheal collapse with dynamic pharyngeal collapse, which is likely secondary to increased negative gradients during inspiration.

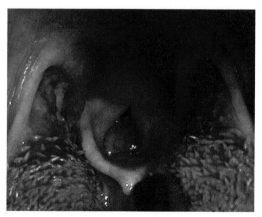

Fig. 4. ELS. Laryngoscopic view of the rima glottides of a dog a French bulldog with stage 1 laryngeal collapse with ELS.

GASTROINTESTINAL DISEASE ASSOCIATED WITH BRACHYCEPHALIC OBSTRUCTIVE AIRWAY SYNDROME

Dysphagia, vomiting, and regurgitation are common clinical signs in brachycephalic breeds.[77] The prevalence of gastrointestinal disease in BOAS-affected dogs has been reported to be as high as 97%,[4,48,75] and investigations of these dogs showed concurrent esophageal, gastric, or duodenal anomalies.[47,75,86] Brachycephaly was found to be significantly associated with esophageal dysmotility, prolonged esophageal transit time, and gastroesophageal reflux.[87] The negative intrathoracic pressures generated by increased inspiratory effort[88–92] is believed to be a major cause of gastroesophageal reflux. The associated regurgitation and vomiting can contribute to upper esophageal, pharyngeal, and laryngeal and middle ear inflammation.[93] French bulldogs exhibit significantly more often and more severe digestive signs than pugs.[75,83,94,95] A recent comparison of 3 brachycephalic dog breeds showed an overall prevalence of gastrointestinal signs in 56%, with 93% of the French bulldogs, 58% of the English bulldogs, and 16% of pugs affected.[95] Gastrointestinal signs, gastritis, and regurgitation significantly improved after surgical treatment of stenotic nares and soft palate hyperplasia,[47,83,95] especially in French bulldogs, whereas pugs and English bulldogs showed little alleviation, most likely owing to the small number of pugs affected with gastrointestinal disease.[95]

Possible explanations for the persistent gastrointestinal problems in these unresponsive dogs might be that their origin is not related to upper airway obstruction. Another explanation might be that staphylectomy alters the airway pressures with different efficiency in brachycephalic breeds that were reported to have breed-specific anatomic variations: French bulldogs are reported to have a significantly thicker soft palate compared with pugs and English bulldogs,[26,40,51] which might explain why staphylectomy leads to a greater improvement in these dogs. Pugs are reported to have a smaller nasopharyngeal and laryngeal space compared with French bulldogs.[26,53,69] These airway obstructions were not addressed during the surgical treatment, which might explain why these dogs continue to have residual upper airway resistance with concurrent gastrointestinal signs. English bulldogs can have a hypoplastic trachea, which will also not be addressed with the standard BOAS surgical treatment.

Gastroesophageal Reflux and Hiatal Hernia

Brachycephalic dogs are predisposed to hiatal hernia and accompanied gastroesophageal reflux,[96] which is thought to be secondary to increased negative intrathoracic pressure and increased inspiratory effort.[89,92,97] The increased inspiratory effort leads to a decrease in the intraesophageal and intrapleural pressures, with subsequent axial displacement of the distal esophagus and stomach into the thoracic cavity during inspiration.[89] In a recent esophageal imaging study, 8 of 8 dogs diagnosed with hiatal hernia were brachycephalic,[87] and the prevalence of sliding hiatal hernia in French bulldogs with BOAS was found to be 44%[98] Transient manual obstruction of the endotracheal tube to increase the transdiaphragmatic pressure gradient was found helpful to identify gastroesophageal junction abnormalities in BOAS-affected dogs.[98–100]

Aspiration pneumonia is a common complication of reflux and regurgitation, which should be investigated before anesthesia (see Preoperative and Perioperative Treatment).

DIAGNOSIS

Diagnosis is usually based on owners' reports, clinical examination, and diagnostic imaging. Additional respiratory function testing and scoring to document the severity of BOAS can be performed.

Clinical Diagnosis

Snoring, inspiratory dyspnea, exercise intolerance, sleep disturbances, cyanosis, and, in the most severe cases, syncopal episodes are most often reported by owners.[2,4,83,85,94,101–103] On inspection, stenotic nares and inspiratory efforts with even abdominal breathing can be observed. A particular attention shall be paid to respiratory sounds. These sounds can be more apparent during exercise tests.

Whereas snoring is most likely caused by air turbulences in the oropharyngeal region, the high-pitched sound associated with extreme inspiratory effort is related to more severe airway compromise when turbulent air is passing through the collapsed larynx or nasopharynx.

Risk Factors

Conformational risk factors for BOAS that were identified are stenotic nostrils, high body condition score, and large neck girth compared with the chest girth (neck girth ratio).[37] Packer and colleagues[101] (2015) also showed that obesity and a thicker neck girth are BOAS risk factors but also showed that a relative short muzzle length (less than one-half the cranial lengths) is an additional conformation risk factor for BOAS.

GRADING SYSTEMS, CLINICAL SCORES, AND RESPIRATORY FUNCTION TESTING

To classify the severity of BOAS, several grading systems and function testing including exercise tolerance tests and whole-body barometric plethysmography have been introduced. The Poncet-Dupré score is a grading system based on the frequency of the respiratory and digestive clinical signs.[75] Bernaerts and colleagues[85] (2010) also introduced a respiratory scoring system, which is a combination of a symptom score (noisy breathing and exercise intolerance) and lesion score based on anatomic abnormalities of the nose, soft palate, ventricle, larynx, trachea and lower airways. Similar grading systems assess the upper airway dimensions and obstruction at the different anatomic levels such as the

- Nares
- Nasopharyngeal turbinate protrusion
- Soft palate elongation
- Narrowed pharyngeal dimensions (dorsoventral flattening, thickness of base of tongue, tonsillar protrusion, diffuse pharyngeal edema)
- Narrowed laryngeal dimensions (laryngeal hypoplasia, laryngeal collapse)[34,104–106]

Most of these systems describe the severity as mild, moderate, or severe.

A functional grading system based on respiratory signs (respiratory noise, inspiratory effort, dyspnea/cyanosis/syncope) combined with an exercise tolerance test was established by Liu and colleagues (2015).[103] A slow trot test provides more effective grading of upper airway obstruction than a walk test based on results from whole-body plethysmography in 44 dogs.[107] A 3-minute slow trot tests should be included in the clinical examination to identify dogs that display respiratory noise only when stressed or exercised.[107] Other suggested exercise test assess how far dogs can walk and if they can walk 1000 m in 6 minutes[108] or the time taken to walk 1000 m.[109]

Whole-body barometric plethysmography can be used for respiratory function testing. A dog is placed in a sealed chamber with biased airflow moving across it. Changes in the air pressure within the chamber that result from the humidification and expansion of air on breathing are detected by a pressure transducer. These whole-body barometric plethysmography flow traces are 93% specific and 90% sensitive to identify respiratory obstruction and has been validated to discriminate BOAS-affected versus nonaffected brachycephalic dogs. With whole-body barometric plethysmography, a BOAS index can be calculated, which allows an objective evaluation of BOAS severity, risk for BOAS, and effectiveness of surgical treatment.[103,104]

DIAGNOSTIC IMAGING

Radiographic, fluoroscopic, CT, and endoscopic studies all contribute to the evaluation of the static and dynamic obstruction of the respiratory tract.[21,25,26,40,41,69] In a clinical practice setting, a proper evaluation of BOAS patients should include at least neck and thoracic radiographs, and endoscopic examination of the upper airways.

- Thoracic radiographs are performed to document secondary heart or lung diseases and to rule out aspiration pneumonia. Also, on occasion a sliding hiatal hernia can incidentally be found on a lateral radiograph.
- Lateral radiographs of the neck (when a CT scan is not available) can help to assess the soft palate thickness as defined by the soft tissue density present between the nasopharynx and oropharynx.[1]
- A CT evaluation of the head and neck allows a detailed assessment of the nostrils, vestibule, nasal cavity, nasopharynx and oropharynx, and cricoid and tracheal size (**Fig. 5**).[25,26,40,54]
- Endoscopic examination provides more information on the dynamic changes within the upper airways:
  - With the dog intubated, retrograde rhinoscopy performed with a 120° rigid scope or a flexible endoscope allows for good evaluation of nasopharyngeal tissue hyperplasia and collapse as well as for the presence of caudal aberrant turbinates (**Fig. 6**, Videos 3 and 4). Rhinoscopy is a complementary method to assess cranial aberrant turbinates in the nasal cavity.[21]
  - With the dog extubated, a laryngoscopic examination can expose ELS and also help to evaluate laryngeal dynamics. With laryngeal collapse, a lack of

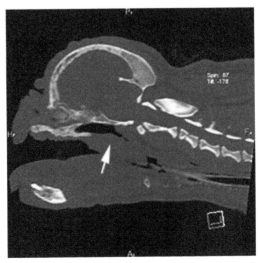

Fig. 5. Soft palate thickening. Midsagittal CT image of 2-year-old French bulldog with thickening of the soft palate (arrow).

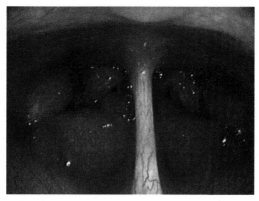

Fig. 6. Nasopharyngeal turbinates. Images of a retrograde rhinoscopy displaying aberrant nasopharyngeal turbinates.

abduction during inspiration or even paradoxic movements of the arytenoid cartilages can occur. In pugs and other dogs affected by laryngeal chondromalacia, the dorsal border of the cuneiform process of the arytenoid cartilages can even invert into the laryngeal lumen (Video 5). Tracheoscopy was reported to be more accurate for diagnosing tracheal hypoplasia compared with radiography and CT.[60]

CONTROVERSY REGARDING THE GENESIS OF BRACHYCEPHALIC SYNDROME

The genesis of BOAS is thought to be due to anatomic changes, which lead to increased inspiratory resistance.[58,77,79,110] With significant negative pressure, the soft tissues are drawn into the lumen, resulting in the collapse of the upper airway.[41,77] Eversion of the laryngeal saccules and tonsils, nasopharyngeal collapse, and laryngeal collapse are suspected to contribute to the clinical signs and further deterioration of BOAS, which might ultimately cause syncopal episodes and death from suffocation.[48,58,110]

Although, in the past, an overlong soft palate fluttering in the rima glottidis has been considered as the main cause of BOAS, it remains difficult to estimate the greatest contributor to the clinical signs. The nose is known to be the greatest source of flow resistance in the total airway system,[111,112] and rhinomanometric studies confirm that intranasal resistance is significantly higher in brachycephalic dogs compared with normal dogs.[113,114] The major upper airway obstruction was postulated to be intranasal secondary to aberrant turbinates[25] or located in the compressed nasopharynx.[40] CT studies comparing pugs and French bulldogs found that the smallest airway space is located dorsal to the soft palate, even in dogs with aberrant nasopharyngeal turbinates.[26] The maximal nasopharyngeal occlusion was found to be located about 1 cm caudal to the hamuli pterygoidei.[67] Aberrant turbinates were also described in clinically normal English bulldogs,[34] which suggests that the contribution of the aberrant turbinates to BOAS needs to be further investigated.

Although laryngeal collapse has usually been considered to be associated with progression of the disease, a significant correlation between age and the severity of laryngeal collapse was demonstrated only recently.[83] In another study including pugs and English and French bulldogs with stage 1 laryngeal collapse, no correlation between the glottic index and age or weight could be demonstrated.[53] Whereas some authors describe laryngeal collapse as a negative prognostic indicator for the surgical outcome,[76] other authors found that the overall postoperative prognosis was not affected by the grade of laryngeal collapse.[39,83]

Overall, although it is clear that air cannot flow through the nose as long as the nostrils are obstructed, it remains uncertain which part of the obstructed airway—nasal cavity, nasopharynx, or rima glottis—is most responsible for the clinical signs associated with BOAS. In that regard, the effect of soft palate resection might be due to the opening of the nasopharyngeal space and not to the relief of the rima glottidis obstruction.

TREATMENT OF BRACHYCEPHALIC SYNDROME
Medical Therapy

Patients presented with acute signs of respiratory distress should be treated accordingly with cooling, tranquilizers, oxygen therapy, and anti-inflammatory drugs. Whenever digestive signs are observed in dogs with BOAS, medical treatment, including inhibition of hydrogen ion secretion and gastric prokinetic drugs, is recommended before and immediately after surgery.

Surgical Therapy

Timing
According to the pathophysiology of the syndrome, relief of the proximally located obstruction should be attempted early to prevent deterioration or possibly reverse tissue collapse.[23,38,58] However, the optimal time to correct upper airway obstruction has not yet been determined and was recommended to be performed after the age of 6 months. Recent studies suggest that improvement in clinical signs is still obtained when surgery is performed on mature and middle-aged dogs.[83]

Preoperative and Perioperative Treatment

To decrease the risk of perioperative aspiration pneumonia and reflux esophagitis, medical treatment to decrease the incidence of gastroesophageal reflux should be administered. Younger dogs and those with a history of regurgitation seem to be especially predisposed to postoperative regurgitation and should receive preventive treatment.[115] At least dogs with gastrointestinal signs should receive omeprazole (1 mg/kg twice daily per os) and metoclopramide (0.2–0.5 mg/kg 3 times daily per os) for 1 to 2 weeks before surgery. Preoperative and postoperative antacid treatment was found to positively influence the digestive clinical signs and was recommended to be administered to all dogs scheduled for BOAS surgery, even those without digestive clinical signs.[100] Other combinations of perioperative prokinetics (metoclopramide, cisapride), gastroprotectants (famotidine, omeprazole, sucralfate), and antiemetics (maropitant, ondansetron) can also be given to decrease postoperative regurgitation.[47,75,86,116,117] However, adverse reactions after administrating of histamine-2 blockers (famotidine) to French and English bulldogs have been reported anecdotally.

General Considerations of Anesthesia

Brachycephalic dogs have a 1.57 higher risk for complications[118] during anesthesia and need to be monitored closely during the recovery phase to address any potential postanesthetic complications, such as acute airway blockage, regurgitation, vomiting, aspiration pneumonia, prolonged recovery, and stertorous breathing. Brachycephalic dogs are also 4.33 times more likely to have postanesthetic complications, with aspiration pneumonia being the most common complication.[118] To minimize the critical recovery phase, the airway assessment and corrective surgery should be performed under the same anesthetic. A light meal of wet food 3 to 4 hours before anesthesia was found to decrease the incidence of gastroesophageal reflux in dogs.[119] Intravenous lidocaine (2 mg/kg IV 2%) was found to reduce coughing during endotracheal intubation compared with locally applied lidocaine. This practice may also aid in decreasing the risk of regurgitation during induction and intubation.[120]

In-depth descriptions of anesthesia in brachycephalic dogs can be found elsewhere,[121] but important aspects to consider are:

- No emetic opioids.
- Add prokinetics, gastroprotectants, and/or antiemetics (discussed elsewhere in this article).
- Patient preoxygenation for 3 minutes.[122]
- Addition lidocaine 2% intravenously during induction.
- Range of endotracheal tube sizes available.
- Rapid induction and intubation.[77]
- Potential need of anticholinergic drugs to combat the bradycardic effects of vagal stimulation secondary to glottic handling.[23,58]
- Placement of a nasotracheal oxygen tube.[83]
- Delayed extubation.[65]
- Supplemental oxygen.

Although dogs used to be monitored at least 12 to 24 hours after BOAS surgery in an intensive care unit, a newer less stressful practice is to have the dogs recover with the owner present and to discharge them the same day. The complication rate of a subsequent anesthetic after corrective BOAS surgery was found to be decreased by 79%.[123]

CONTROVERSY OF WHICH SURGICAL TECHNIQUES TO APPLY

Surgical treatment options to address upper airway obstruction are manifold and there is a discrepancy whether to perform multilevel surgery or to focus on the 2 most relevant primary obstructions—the nares and the elongated, hypertrophic soft palate. Traditionally, BOAS surgery consisted of alarplasty, staphylectomy, and sacculectomy if the laryngeal saccules were everted. Nowadays, there is an ongoing debate regarding the additional improvement in airflow achieved by sacculectomy, particularly when balanced against concerns regarding the increased risk of complications, such as laryngeal webbing or regrowth.[124,125] A higher complication rate was found in patients undergoing additional sacculectomy compared with patients undergoing nares resection and staphylectomy alone.[126] However, the theory that the saccules return to their original position ones the negative inspiratory pressure has resolved was also found unrealistic.[127] A recent study evaluation the short-term outcome of 2-level BOAS surgery found that 70.7% of dogs improved after alarplasty and staphylectomy. This improvement was associated with the severity of inspiratory effort, but not with any other clinical sign or anatomic abnormality. This study also found an association between snoring and pharyngeal dimensions, but not with soft palate length.[105] This finding strengthens the argument that the thickness of the soft palate needs to be corrected-either by a palatoplasty reducing its thickness or by a rostrally extending staphylectomy.

A comparison of 2 types of multilevel surgery—a traditional one consisting of vertical wedge resection alaplasty, staphylectomy, sacculectomy, and partial tonsillectomy—and a modified one that included a modified rhinoplasty technique combining a Trader's alaplasty and nasal vestibuloplasty, folded flap palatoplasty, bilateral sacculectomy, partial cuneiformectomy, and partial tonsillectomy was in favor for the modified version. Treated dogs showed improvement of their BOAS index by 10%, but were not clinically normal.[76] LATE was added to the treatment for severely affected dogs and those that did not improve enough after the multilevel surgery.[128]

Stenotic Nares

Several surgical options have been described for the correction of stenotic nares: amputation of the ala nasi,[129,130] various alaplasty techniques, alapexy,[131] and vestibuloplasty.

Alaplasty is the most used procedure and consists of the excision of a wedge of the ala nasi with primary closure of the defect. This wedge excision can be made vertically, horizontally,[38,65] or laterally.[23,58,132] Incisions are made with a No. 11 or 15 scalpel blade or alternatively with a punch.[133] Two to 4 simple interrupted sutures, using absorbable monofilament material, are placed to appose the wedge margins. Hemorrhage resolves quickly when the wound is sutured (Video 6).

Vestibuloplasty has been advocated instead of alaplasty to further improve airflow.[134] It involves the dorsomedial and caudal portion of the ala and results in a wide and open vestibule.

Turbinectomy

Turbinectomy[135] and its laser-assisted variation (LATE)[136,137] are aimed at removal of malformed obstructive parts of the ventral and medial nasal turbinates. The LATE, combined with vestibuloplasty and staphylectomy, resulted in a decrease of 55% of intranasal resistance 3 to 6 months after surgery compared with preoperative values.[113] When LATE was performed 2 to 6 months after modified multilevel surgery, an additional improvement of the BOAS index by 25% was observed.[128] Complications were reverse sneezing, nasal noise, and hemorrhage. Partial regrowth of the removed turbinates, but with fewer mucosal contact points, is also being reported.[138] The long-term positive effects of turbinectomy on intranasal resistance and adverse effects on thermoregulation require further investigation.

Elongated–Hyperplastic Soft Palate

Common surgical techniques for the correction of an elongated soft palate are aimed at shortening the soft palate by simple resection of its caudal portion (staphylectomy) to prevent it from obstructing the rima glottidis on inspiration. Different landmarks have been recommended, varying from the tip of epiglottis[65,77,139–142] or the middle to the caudal aspect of the palatine tonsils.[23,78,139,141,142] A more recent trend is to extend the staphylectomy rostrally to the level of the rostral end of the tonsils.[105,143,144] The hamuli pterygoidei was found useful as a landmark to identify the maximal nasopharyngeal occlusion intraoperatively.[67]

During staphylectomy, the caudal border of the soft palate is grasped and held with Allis forceps or stay sutures,[140,143] and resection of excessive length of soft palate can be performed with a scalpel blade,[5,38,140] scissors,[58,65,77,145] monopolar electrocoagulation,[38,139,144] carbon dioxide laser,[2,141,144,146,147] diode laser,[144] or bipolar sealing device (Ligasure, Valleylab, Covidien, Boulder, CO).[143,147,148]

Because these palate-trimming techniques may not address the soft palate hyperplasia, techniques designed to more extensively shorten and thin the soft palate have been described.[42,143,144,149,150] The folded flap palatoplasty has been developed to correct both the excessive length and excessive thickness of the soft palate, thus relieving also nasopharyngeal obstruction.[42,149,150] In this technique, the soft palate is made thinner by excision of a portion of its oropharyngeal mucosa and underlying soft tissues. In addition, the palate is made shorter by being folded onto itself until the caudal nasopharyngeal opening is readily visible transorally (**Box 1, Figs. 7–9**, Video 7).

Postoperative adverse effects or pharyngonasal regurgitation have not been observed with the folded flap palatoplasty,[143,144,150] apart from one dog reported with soft palate necrosis and 2 dogs with dehiscence.[83,150,151] Whatever technique is chosen, a telescope and high-definition camera system for magnification and illumination of the surgical field (VITOM TM, Karl Storz Endoscopy, Tuttlingen, Germany) are helpful (**Fig. 10**).

Surgical Treatments for Laryngeal Diseases

Everted laryngeal saccules

The excision of ELS has been described using electrocautery, scissors, tonsil snares, or laryngeal biopsy cup forceps.[1,23,39,58,65,77,139,142] In one study reevaluating ELS after single side resection, no regression of the nonremoved site, despite treatment of nares and soft palate, was found. Histopathology of the removed saccules identified edema and inflammation.[127] Altogether, whether resection of the ELS is needed remains questionable. In several recent BOAS outcome studies in which nares and palates were corrected but ELS were either not or rarely addressed, outcomes seemed to be similar to studies in which ELS were excised.[47,105,144,150] Also, complications such as laryngeal webbing owing to secondary intention healing and regrowth might result in the recurrence of the obstruction.[124,125] With this caveat in mind, the authors only recommend removal of ELS when the eversion contributes significantly to the obstruction.

Laryngeal collapse

Because laryngeal collapse is suspected to be secondary to proximal airway obstruction, first address the proximal obstruction areas (ie, nares and soft palate), because this practice may obviate the need to treat the collapse.[2,3,39,41,78,152] In the authors' experience, surgical treatment of laryngeal collapse is considered only when the clinical signs do not improve after appropriate treatment of the nares and soft palate.

Box 1
The folded flap palatoplasty: surgical technique

- The head is restrained, and the mouth kept open. The tongue is pulled rostrally and maintained with a malleable retractor connected to an articulated arm.

- The caudal edge of the soft palate is grasped with forceps and retracted rostrally and dorsally into the oropharynx, until the caudal opening of the nasopharynx can be visualized.

- The contact point on the ventral mucosa of the soft palate is marked, because this point represents the proximal cut of the soft palate.

- The ventral mucosa of the soft palate is then incised in a trapezoidal shape from this mark rostrally to the free edge of the soft palate caudally.

- Laterally, the sides of the trapeze passed just medially to the tonsils.

- The soft tissues under the cut portion of the soft palate are excised together with part of the levator veli palatini muscle.

- The caudal edge of the soft palate is retracted rostrally and is sutured folded on itself with simple interrupted monofilament absorbable sutures.

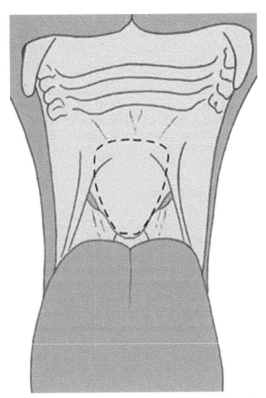

Fig. 7. Folded flap palatoplasty: incision lines in the oral mucosa for the thinning process of soft palate hyperplasia.

Partial laryngectomy, as described elsewhere in this article,[139] has been found to be associated with unacceptably high (50%) mortality rates and is no longer recommended.[142] Laser-assisted partial arytenoidectomy as recommended for the treatment of laryngeal paralysis might provide some relief,[153] but needs to be investigated further. In 1 study, dogs with advanced laryngeal collapses treated with partial cuneiformectomy did not show greater improvement compared with those that did not receive partial cuneiformectomy.[76] Further, handling of the larynx can lead to severe bradycardia secondary to vagal stimulation, which should be balanced against the benefits of partial laryngeal resection. Alternatively, arytenoid lateralization is a valid option for dogs with advanced laryngeal collapse and sufficient mineralization of the laryngeal cartilages.[77,88,154] However, its efficacy is questionable in pugs and dogs suffering from chrondromalacia when the arytenoid cartilages have a tendency to rotate inwardly during inspiration (pugs).[39,41,155] If there is inefficient relief of airway obstruction after these procedures, a permanent tracheostomy can be attempted as a palliative option.[1,23,38,58,77,156,157]

Tonsillectomy and removal of other hyperplastic tissues
Excision of the palatine tonsils has been recommended when they seem to contribute to pharyngeal obstruction[38,58,145] Other surgeons remove them when everted as a part of a multilevel surgery strategy.[76] However, the advantage of tonsillectomy warrants further investigation.[48,65,77] Tonsillectomy does carry the risk of postoperative

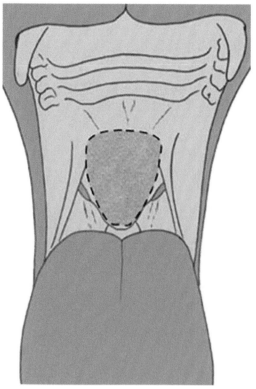

Fig. 8. Folded flap palatoplasty: end of dissection of the soft palate. The yellow area depicts the removed oral part of the soft palate.

hemorrhage and thorough hemostasis is mandatory. Similarly, excision of redundant soft tissues located in the pharynx, especially in its dorsal aspect, has been suggested,[65] but more data are needed to evaluate which of the pharyngeal tissues are involved in the obstruction process and the optimal surgical method to remove the hyperplastic tissue.

Tracheostomy

Although it has been advocated in the past, a preoperative temporary tracheostomy[1,139,158] is not necessary. A temporary postoperative tracheostomy has been reported in the past in 5% to 28% of cases.[38,39,47,150,159] Because the complication rate of a temporary tracheostomy in brachycephalic dogs is very high (86.0%–95.2%),[151,160] it should be reserved for cases not responding to routine postoperative care. The most commonly reported complications are tracheostomy tube obstruction or dislodgement and coughing.[151] Risk factors for temporary tracheostomy tube placement after BOAS surgery was higher age, corticosteroid use, and pneumonia.[161] A modified temporary tracheostomy that included a Penrose drain sling dorsal to the trachea was reported to simplify tracheostomy care, improve tracheostomy outcome, and decrease tube-associated mortality compared with the standard procedure.[162]

A permanent tracheostomy is also associated with a high rate (50%–80%) of major complications (aspiration pneumonia, stoma stenosis, and skinfold occlusion); however, long-term survival with a good quality of life is possible. The reported median

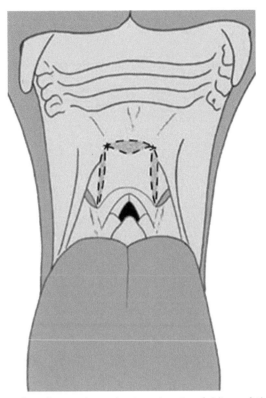

Fig. 9. Folded flap palatoplasty: schematic view showing folding of thinned soft palate upon itself.

survival times were 328[163] and 1825 days,[164] respectively. Acute death at home most likely secondary to tube obstruction was reported in 26% of patients.[163] Older dogs with preoperative administration of corticosteroids or tracheal collapse had a shorter survival time.[164] Dorsal skin resection to prevent skinfold occlusion and intermittent placement of plastic tubes into redilated stomas were found useful long-term

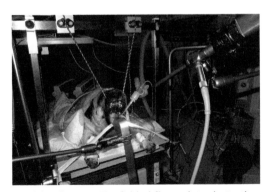

Fig. 10. Surgery setup with telescope. For folded flap palatoplasty, the mouth of the dog is kept open, and the tongue is pushed down using a malleable retractor. Magnification is provided with the Exoscope (VITOM TM, Karl Storz Endoscopy, Tuttlingen, Germany).

treatments of these complications.[165] Overall, a permanent tracheostomy seems to be a valuable salvage procedure for those dogs with severe laryngeal collapse not responsive to more conservative surgeries.[157,163–165]

Surgical Management of Hiatal Hernia

Gastrointestinal clinical signs are reported to improve dramatically after corrective BOAS surgery.[47,83,95] Brachycephalic dogs with persistent regurgitation despite correction of the upper airway obstruction or gastroesophageal reflux secondary to hiatal hernia are potential surgical candidates for hernia repair. Circumferential esophageal hiatal rim reconstruction and esophagopexy were reported to substantially reduce the regurgitation frequency and allowed discontinuation of medical treatment.[166] Mayhew and colleagues[167] (2017) reported surgical treatment of sliding hiatal hernia in 9 brachycephalic dogs applying hiatal plication, esophagopexy, and left-sided incisional gastropexy through a celiotomy. The clinical signs of sliding hiatal hernia improved in most dogs after surgery, but did not resolve consistently.

A laparoscopic technique for the treatment of a sliding hiatal hernia in 18 brachycephalic dogs was recently described. Hiatal plication and esophagopexy was performed with intracorporeal suturing combined with a left-sided laparoscopic or laparoscopic-assisted gastropexy. Regurgitation improved significantly after surgery but did not resolve the clinical signs completely.[168]

Postoperative Care

The challenge during the postoperative period is to enable adequate airflow in a not yet fully awake patient with potentially swollen airway mucosa. It is critical that BOAS-affected dogs are monitored constantly after extubation to determine if ventilation is inadequate.

Several methods can be combined or used independently to help relieve upper airway obstruction or improve ventilation after surgical repair.

- The dog can be recovered with the upper jaw hung up, which allows the lower jaw to drop, which opens the airway further (**Fig. 11**).
- Increasing the oxygen delivery—the placement of a small nasotracheal tube immediately after surgery but before the dog is awake—is a very simple technique of insufflating oxygen, allowing oxygen delivery beyond the rima glottidis.[3,169]
- Stress, panting, and barking should be avoided, because they can lead to life-threatening pharyngeal edema and/or regurgitation. Some authors encourage owners to be present during the recovery phase after the dog has been extubated to minimize stress. This technique seems to decrease the need for hospitalization after recovery and is currently being used by several surgeons (Hervé Brissot, Manuel Jimenez Pelaez, Antoine Bernardé, and Gilles Dupré, personal communication, 2021).
- Life-threatening pharyngeal edema can be treated with nebulized or sprayed adrenaline to avoid tracheostomy.[170,171] Nebulized epinephrine also decreases respiratory clinical signs and might be useful to treat acute respiratory distress.[172]

COMPLICATIONS

The overall major complication rate after BOAS surgery was reported to be 7% and pneumonia was associated with the development of major postoperative

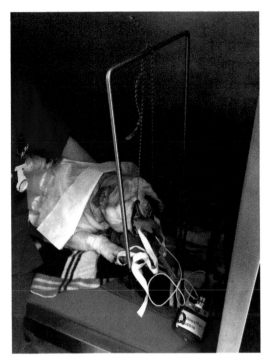

Fig. 11. Patient recovery after BS surgery. Bulldog recovering from anesthesia with the upper jaw hung to help open the mouth to improve oxygenation.

complications.[173] The most important complications after BOAS surgery are airway swelling, regurgitation, and aspiration pneumonia.

Dyspnea secondary to pharyngeal swelling is reported to occur in 1.6% to 23.4% of dogs[83,115,126,174,175]; the treatment options are supplemental oxygen, corticosteroid administration, and nebulization with adrenalin or epinephrine. Reintubation and temporary tracheostomy are further treatment options if the swelling does not resolve. Age, corticosteroid use, and pneumonia were identified as risk factors for temporary tracheostomy.[161] Postoperative regurgitation is reported to occur in 4.7% to 34.5% of brachycephalic dogs,[47,83,115,173,175] and younger dogs and those with a history of regurgitation are reported to be at increased risk.[115] The perioperative administration of metoclopramide and famotidine was found to decrease the risk of postoperative regurgitation from 35% to 9%.[116]

Darcy and colleagues[176] (2018) reported that English and French bulldogs are at high risk for aspiration pneumonia. Preoperative aspiration pneumonia has been identified in 1.6% to 8.3% of dogs[148,173,175] and in 0.8% to 5.5% after surgery.[83,115,148,173,175] Brachycephalic dogs have a 3.77 times higher risk for aspiration pneumonia compared with other dogs, and gastrointestinal clinical signs are risk factors to develop aspiration pneumonia.[176] Postoperative aspiration pneumonia was found associated with temporary tracheostomy and death.[148,161,173]

A brachycephalic risk score for predicting complications following BOAS surgery has been introduced recently.[174]

PROGNOSIS

It is difficult to gain an accurate perspective of the prognosis for individual dogs afflicted with BOAS.[2,38,39,78,97,133,141,146] Most studies evaluating the outcome after

BOAS surgery are retrospective in nature and compare results in different breeds with various combinations of treatments and reconstructive techniques. In addition, these studies compare outcomes with surgical treatments performed at variable patient ages and by different surgeons, using different grading systems.[42,130,143,144] Furthermore, it is difficult to compare the postoperative outcome in these various studies, because there is often a mismatch between the owners' perception of their pets clinical disability and the severity of the clinical signs. In 1 study, younger age has been associated significantly with a poor treatment outcome[76] and with an increased risk of postoperative regurgitation.[115] Another study comparing preoperative and postoperative treatments in different breeds that underwent the same diagnostic workup, treatment, and evaluation methods found no correlations between the severity of laryngeal collapse and overall respiratory signs or prognosis.[83] Yet others identified laryngeal collapse as a negative prognostic indicator for a good outcome after surgery.[76] Despite inherent study limitations, late studies report that around 70% to 90% of BOAS dogs are significantly improved with surgery.[2,42,47,83,105,144] This finding is better than in earlier reports. Similarly, perioperative mortality rates have improved from around 15% in earlier reports[38,97] to less than 4% in more recent studies.[2,42,47,105,144] Postoperative improvement is most often observed immediately after surgery.[42,47] Some studies report the long-term recurrence of clinical signs in up to 100% of cases, although 89% of dogs remain improved compared with their preoperative status.[39] In other studies, clinical grades improved in the first 2 weeks after folded flap palatoplasty[42,83] and remained the same over the following period (mean, 12–22 months), which suggests that more advanced techniques addressing the thickness of the soft palate contribute to better long-term improvement.

CLINICS CARE POINTS

- Perioperative regurgitation and aspiration pneumonia are common complications of brachycephalic obstructive airway surgery. Their incidence can be reduced with omeprazole (1 mg/kg twice daily per os) and metoclopramide (0.2–0.5mg/kg 3 times daily per os) starting 1 to 2 weeks before surgery and should be continued in the postoperative phase.

- Owing to a higher risk for complications during anesthesia all investigations of the airway and corrective surgery should be performed under the same anesthetic.

- The following steps can reduce the increased risk of anesthetic complications:
  ○ Light meal of wet food 3 to 4 hours before anesthesia.
  ○ Continue prokinetics, gastroprotectants, and/or antiemetics.
  ○ Preoxygenate for 3 minutes.
  ○ Lidocaine 2% intravenously during rapid induction.
  ○ Recovery phase: oxygen supplementation, close monitoring for airway obstruction, delay extubation until awake and not tolerating endotracheal tube, avoid stress and consider involving owner to reduce stress.

- Perform rhinoplasty and palatoplasty to address most relevant primary airway obstructions; consider further airway corrections for severe obstructions or if no sufficient improvement.

- If in respiratory distress preoperatively or postoperatively:
  ○ Supplement oxygen.
  ○ Keep mouth open to increase pharyngeal airway space.
  ○ Check body temperature and slowly cool down the patient with wet towels and alcohol applied onto the skin.
  ○ Decrease airway swelling with dexamethasone (0.2 mg/kg IV); can be repeated 1 to 2 times.

- Careful sedation: Butorphanol (0.1–0.2 mg/kg IV start with one-half dose and reassess (dogs are usually so exhausted that they cannot hold head up anymore); acepromazine (0.025 mg/

kg IV, only if not sedated enough with butorphanol and not exhausted—start with one-half dose).

- Nebulize with adrenalin or epinephrine.
- Intubate if the airway obstructs—try extubating when the dog is calm, the airway swelling is decreased, and the temperature is normal.
- If the attempt not successful, repeat endotracheal intubation and/or perform temporary tracheostomy.

SUMMARY

Animals presenting with BOAS suffer multilevel obstruction of the airways and secondary soft tissue collapse. Despite progresses achieved through advanced diagnostic modalities such as CT scans and endoscopy, the main contributor to the increased inspiratory efforts remains to be found. Recent studies suggest that postoperative prognosis is good even in middle-aged dogs.

DISCLOSURE

The authors have nothing to disclose.

SUPPLEMENTARY DATA

Supplementary data related to this article can be found at https://doi.org/10.1016/j.cvsm.2022.01.013.

REFERENCES

1. Hendricks JC. Brachycephalic airway syndrome. Vet Clin North Am Small Anim Pract 1992;22:1145–53.
2. Riecks TW, Birchard SJ, Stephens JA. Surgical correction of brachycephalic syndrome in dogs: 62 cases (1991-2004). J Am Vet Med Assoc 2007;230: 1324–8.
3. Dupré G, Findji L, Oechtering G. Brachycephalic airway syndrome. In: Monnet E, editor. Small animal soft tissue surgery. Ames (IA): Wiley-Blackwell; 2012. p. 167–83.
4. Meola SD. Brachycephalic airway syndrome. Top Companion Anim Med 2013; 28:91–6.
5. Farquharson J, Smith DW. Resection of the soft palate in the dog. J Am Vet Med Assoc 1942;100:427–30.
6. Costa J, Steinmetz A, Delgado E. Clinical signs of brachycephalic ocular syndrome in 93 dogs. Ir Vet J 2021;74(1):3.
7. Niemiec BA. Conditions commonly seen in Brachycephalic breeds. In: Niemiec BA, editor. Breed predispositions to dental and oral disease in dogs. 1st edition. US: Wiley-Blackwell; 2021. chap 4.
8. Brown JD, Podadera J, Ward M, et al. The presence, morphology and clinical significance of vertebral body malformations in an Australian population of French Bulldogs and Pugs. Aust Vet J 2021;99(9):378–87.
9. Conte A, Bernardini M, De Decker S, et al. Thoracic Vertebral Canal Stenosis Associated with Vertebral Arch Anomalies in Small Brachycephalic Screw-Tail Dog Breeds. Vet Comp Orthop Traumatol 2021;34(3):191–9.

10. De Decker S, Packer RMA, Cappello R, et al. Comparison of signalment and computed tomography findings in French Bulldogs, Pugs, and English Bulldogs with and without clinical signs associated with thoracic hemivertebra. J Vet Intern Med 2019;33(5):2151–9.

11. Bertram S, Ter Haar G, De Decker S. Caudal articular process dysplasia of thoracic vertebrae in neurologically normal French bulldogs, English bulldogs, and Pugs: prevalence and characteristics. Vet Radiol Ultrasound 2018;59(4): 396–404.

12. Lackmann F, Forterre F, Brunnberg L, et al. Epidemiological study of congenital malformations of the vertebral column in French bulldogs, English bulldogs and pugs. Vet Rec 2022;190(1):e509.

13. Knowler SP, Galea GL, Rusbridge C. Morphogenesis of canine Chiari malformation and secondary syringomyelia: disorders of cerebrospinal fluid circulation. Front Vet Sci 2018;5:171.

14. Hayes GM, Friend EJ, Jeffery ND. Relationship between pharyngeal conformation and otitis media with effusion in Cavalier King Charles spaniels. Vet Rec 2010;167:55–8.

15. Krainer D, Dupré G. Influence of computed tomographic dimensions of the nasopharynx on middle ear effusion and inflammation in pugs and French bulldogs with brachycephalic airway syndrome. Vet Surg 2021;50(3):517–26.

16. Salguero R, Herrtage M, Holmes M, et al. Comparison between Computed Tomographic Characteristics of the Middle Ear in Nonbrachycephalic and Brachycephalic Dogs with Obstructive Airway Syndrome. Vet Radiol Ultrasound 2016;57(2):137–43.

17. Mielke B, Lam R, Ter Haar G. Computed tomographic morphometry of tympanic bulla shape and position in brachycephalic and mesaticephalic dog breeds. Vet Radiol Ultrasound 2017;58(5):552–8.

18. Matchwick A, Bridges JP, Mielke B, et al. Computed Tomographic Measurement of Trochlear Depth in Three Breeds of Brachycephalic Dog. Vet Comp Orthop Traumatol 2021;34(2):124–9.

19. Stockard CR. The genetic and endocrinic basis for differences in form and behavior. Am Anat Memoir 1941;19:775.

20. Evans HE. The skeleton. In: Evans HE, editor. Millers' anatomy of the dog. Philadelphia: Saunders; 1993. p. 122–218.

21. Schuenemann R, Oechtering GU. Inside the brachycephalic nose: intranasal mucosal contact points. J Am Anim Hosp Assoc 2014;50:149–58.

22. Arrighi S, Pichetto M, Roccabianca P, et al. The anatomy of the dog soft palate. I. Histological evaluation of the caudal soft palate in mesaticephalic breeds. Anat Rec (Hoboken) 2011;294:1261–6.

23. Wykes PM. Brachycephalic airway obstructive syndrome. Probl Vet Med 1991;3: 188–97.

24. Trappler M, Moore K. Canine brachycephalic airway syndrome: pathophysiology, diagnosis, and nonsurgical management. Compend Contin Educvet 2011;33(5):E1–4.

25. Oechtering TH, Oechtering GU, Noller C. Strukturelle Besonderheiten der Nase brachyzephaler Hunderassen in der Computertomographie. Tierarztl Prax 2007; 35:177–87.

26. Heidenreich D, Gradner G, Kneissl S, et al. Nasopharyngeal dimensions from computed tomography of pugs and French bulldogs with brachycephalic airway syndrome. Vet Surg 2016;45(1):83–90.

27. Hussein AK, Sullivan M, Penderis J. Effect of brachycephalic, mesaticephalic, and dolichocephalic head conformations on olfactory bulb angle and orientation in dogs as determined by use of in vivo magnetic resonance imaging. Am J Vet Res 2012;73:946–51.

28. Hennet PR, Harvey CE. Craniofacial development and growth in the dog. J Vet Dent 1992;9:11–8.

29. Hussein AK. MRI mensuration of the canine head: the effect of head conformation on the shape and dimensions of the facial and cranial regions and their components [PhD Thesis]. Glasgow (United Kingdom): University of Glasgow; 2012.

30. Regodon S, Vivo JM, Franco A, et al. Craniofacial angle in dolicho-, meso- and brachycephalic dogs: radiological determination and application. Anat Anz 1993;175(4):361–3.

31. Ginn JA, Kumar MS, McKiernan BC, et al. Nasopharyngeal turbinates in brachycephalic dogs and cats. J Am Anim Hosp Assoc 2008;44:243–9.

32. Billen F, Day M, Clercx C. Diagnosis of pharyngeal disorders in dogs: a retrospective study of 67 cases. J Small Anim Pract 2006;47:122–9.

33. Heidenreich DC, Dupré G. The nasopharyngeal space in brachycephalic dogs: a computed tomographic comparison of Pugs and French Bulldogs. In: Proceedings 24th ECVS annual meeting. Berlin (Germany), July 2-4 2015: Vet Surg; 2015. p. E20, 44(5).

34. Vilaplana Grosso F, Haar GT, Boroffka SA. Gender, weight, and age effects on prevalence of caudal aberrant nasal turbinates in clinically healthy English bulldogs: a computed tomographic study and classification. Vet Radiol Ultrasound 2015;56(5):486–93.

35. Oechtering GU, Pohl S, Schlueter C, et al. A novel approach to brachycephalic syndrome. 1. Evaluation of anatomical intranasal airway obstruction. Vet Surg 2016;45(2):165–72.

36. Schuenemann R, Oechtering G. Inside the brachycephalic nose: conchal regrowth and mucosal contact points after laser-assisted turbinectomy. J Am Anim Hosp Assoc 2014;50(4):237–46.

37. Liu NC, Troconis EL, Kalmar L, et al. Conformational risk factors of brachycephalic obstructive airway syndrome (BOAS) in pugs, French bulldogs, and bulldogs. PLoS One 2017;12(8):e0181928.

38. Harvey CE. Soft palate resection in brachycephalic dogs. II. J Am Anim Hosp Assoc 1982;18:538–44.

39. Torrez CV, Hunt GB. Results of surgical correction of abnormalities associated with brachycephalic airway obstruction syndrome in dogs in Australia. J Small Anim Pract 2006;47:150–4.

40. Grand JG, Bureau S. Structural characteristics of the soft palate and meatus nasopharyngeus in brachycephalic and non-brachycephalic dogs analysed by CT. J Small Anim Pract 2011;52:232–9.

41. Dupré G, Poncet C. Respiratory system - brachycephalic upper airways syndrome. In: Bojrab MJ, editor. Mechanisms of diseases in small animal surgery. 3rd edition. Jackson (WY): Teton New Media; 2010. p. 298–301.

42. Findji L, Dupré G. Folded flap palatoplasty for treatment of elongated soft palates in 55 dogs. Eur J Companion Anim Pract 2009;19:125–32.

43. Pichetto M, Arrighi S, Roccabianca P, et al. The anatomy of the dog soft palate. II. Histological evaluation of the caudal soft palate in brachycephalic breeds with grade I brachycephalic airway obstructive syndrome. Anat Rec (Hoboken) 2011;294:1267–72.

44. Pichetto M, Arrighi S, Gobbetti M, et al. The anatomy of the dog soft palate. III. Histological evaluation of the caudal soft palate in brachycephalic neonates. Anat Rec (Hoboken) 2015;298:618–23.

45. Crosse KR, Bray JP, Orbell G, et al. Histological evaluation of the soft palate in dogs affected by brachycephalic obstructive airway syndrome. N Z Vet J 2015; 63(6):319–25.

46. Oechtering GU, Hueber JP, Kiefer I, et al. Laser assisted turbinectomy (LATE): a novel approach to brachycephalic airway syndrome. In: Proc 16th ECVS Meet. Dublin (Ireland), June 28-30, 2007: Vet Surg; 2007. p. E11, 36(4).

47. Poncet CM, Dupré GP, Freiche VG, et al. Long-term results of upper respiratory syndrome surgery and gastrointestinal tract medical treatment in 51 brachycephalic dogs. J Small Anim Pract 2006;47(3):137–42.

48. Fasanella FJ, Shivley JM, Wardlaw JL, et al. Brachycephalic airway obstructive syndrome in dogs: 90 cases (1991-2008). J Am Vet Med Assoc 2010;237: 1048–51.

49. Fox MW. Developmental abnormalities of the canine skull. Can J Comp Med Vet Sci 1963;27(9):219–22.

50. Jones BA, Stanley BJ, Nelson NC. The impact of tongue dimension on air volume in brachycephalic dogs. Vet Surg 2020;49(3):512–20.

51. Siedenburg JS, Dupré G. Tongue and upper airway dimensions: a comparative study between three popular brachycephalic breeds. Animals (Basel) 2021;11(3).

52. De Bruyn BW, Hosgood G. Abnormal hyoid conformation in French Bulldogs: case report and computed tomographic anatomical comparison. Aust Vet J 2022;100(1–2):63–6.

53. Caccamo R, Buracco P, La Rosa G, et al. Glottic and skull indices in canine brachycephalic airway obstructive syndrome. BMC Vet Res 2014;10:12.

54. Rutherford L, Beever L, Bruce M, et al. Assessment of computed tomography derived cricoid cartilage and tracheal dimensions to evaluate degree of cricoid narrowing in brachycephalic dogs. Vet Radiol Ultrasound 2017;58(6):634–46.

55. Tamura J, Oyama N, Matsumoto S, et al. Unrecognized difficult airway management during anesthesia in two brachycephalic dogs with narrow cricoid cartilage. J Vet Med Sci 2021;83(2):234–40.

56. Coyne BE, Fingland RB. Hypoplasia of the trachea in dogs: 103 cases (19741990). J Am Vet Med Assoc 1992;201(5):768–72.

57. Harvey CE, Fink EA. Tracheal diameter: analysis of radiographic measurements in brachycephalic and nonbrachycephalic dogs. J Am Anim Hosp Assoc 1982; 18:570–6.

58. Aron DN, Crowe DT. Upper airway obstruction. general principles and selected conditions in the dog and cat. Vet Clin North Am Small Anim Pract 1985;15(5): 891–917.

59. Komsta R, Osinski Z, Debiak P, et al. Prevalence of pectus excavatum (PE), pectus carinatum (PC), tracheal hypoplasia, thoracic spine deformities and lateral heart displacement in thoracic radiographs of screw-tailed brachycephalic dogs. PLoS One 2019;14(10):e0223642.

60. Kaye BM, Boroffka SA, Haagsman AN, et al. Computed tomographic, radiographic, and endoscopic tracheal dimensions in English bulldogs with grade 1 clinical signs of brachycephalic airway syndrome. Vet Radiol Ultrasound 2015;56(6):609–16.

61. Regier PJ, Grosso FV, Stone HK, et al. Radiographic tracheal dimensions in brachycephalic breeds before and after surgical treatment for brachycephalic airway syndrome. Can Vet J 2020;61(9):971–6.
62. Milne E, Nuttall T, Marioni-Henry K, et al. Cytological and microbiological characteristics of middle ear effusions in brachycephalic dogs. J Vet Intern Med 2020;34(4):1454–63.
63. Owen MC, Lamb CR, Lu D, et al. Material in the middle ear of dogs having magnetic resonance imaging for investigation of neurologic signs. Vet Radiol Ultrasound 2004;45(2):149–55.
64. Foster A, Morandi F, May E. Prevalence of ear disease in dogs undergoing multidetector thin-slice computed tomography of the head. Vet Radiol Ultrasound 2015;56:18–24.
65. Hobson HP. Brachycephalic syndrome. Semin Vet Med Surg (Small Anim 1995; 10(2):109–14.
66. Kim YJ, Lee N, Yu J, et al. Three-dimensional volumetric magnetic resonance imaging (MRI) analysis of the soft palate and nasopharynx in brachycephalic and non-brachycephalic dog breeds. J Vet Med Sci 2019;81(1):113–9.
67. Sarran D, Caron A, Testault I, et al. Position of maximal nasopharyngeal maximal occlusion in relation to hamuli pterygoidei: use of hamuli pterygoidei as landmarks for palatoplasty in brachycephalic airway obstruction syndrome surgical treatment. J Small Anim Pract 2018;59(10):625–33.
68. Pollard RE, Johnson LR, Marks SL. The prevalence of dynamic pharyngeal collapse is high in brachycephalic dogs undergoing videofluoroscopy. Vet Radiol Ultrasound 2018;59(5):529–34.
69. Rubin JA, Holt DE, Reetz JA, et al. Signalment, clinical presentation, concurrent diseases, and diagnostic findings in 28 dogs with dynamic pharyngeal collapse (2008-2013). J Vet Intern Med 2015;29:815–21.
70. Vodnarek J, Ludewig E, Dupré G. Inter- and Intra-observer agreement in evaluating the nasopharyngeal dimensions in Pugs and French bulldogs by means of fluoroscopic examination 2021. Unpublished data.
71. Hara Y, Teshima K, Seki M, et al. Pharyngeal contraction secondary to its collapse in dogs with brachycephalic airway syndrome. J Vet Med Sci 2020; 82(1):64–7.
72. Noh D, Choi S, Choi H, et al. Dynamic computed tomography evaluation of the nasopharynx in normal Beagle dogs. J Vet Med Sci 2021;83(9):1356–62.
73. Harvey CE. Inherited and congenital airway conditions. J Small Anim Pract 1989;30(3):184–7.
74. Belch A, Matiasovic M, Rasotto R, et al. Comparison of the use of LigaSure versus a standard technique for tonsillectomy in dogs. Vet Rec 2017;180(8):196.
75. Poncet CM, Dupré GP, Freiche VG, et al. Prevalence of gastrointestinal tract lesions in 73 brachycephalic dogs with upper respiratory syndrome. J Small Anim Pract 2005;46:273–9.
76. Liu NC, Oechtering GU, Adams VJ, et al. Outcomes and prognostic factors of surgical treatments for brachycephalic obstructive airway syndrome in 3 breeds. Vet Surg 2017;46(2):271–80.
77. Koch DA, Arnold S, Hubler M, et al. Brachycephalic syndrome in dogs. Comp Cont Ed 2003;25(1):48–55.
78. Pink JJ, Doyle RS, Hughes JML, et al. Laryngeal collapse in seven brachycephalic puppies. J Small Anim Pract 2006;47(3):131–5.
79. Leonard HC. Collapse of the larynx and adjacent structures in the dog. J Am Vet Med Assoc 1960;137:360–3.

80. Wilson FD, Rajendran EI, David G. Staphylotomy in a dachshund. Indian Vet J 1960;37:639–42.
81. Wegner W. Genetisch bedingte zahnanomalien. Prakt Tierarzt 1987;68(5): 19–22.
82. De Lorenzi D, Bertoncello D, Drigo M. Bronchial abnormalities found in a consecutive series of 40 brachycephalic dogs. J Am Vet Med Assoc 2009; 235(7):835–40.
83. Haimel G, Dupré G. Brachycephalic airway syndrome: a comparative study between pugs and French bulldogs. J Small Anim Pract 2015;56(12):714–9.
84. Rudorf H, Barr FJ, Lane JG. The role of ultrasound in the assessment of laryngeal paralysis in the dog. Vet Radiol Ultrasound 2001;42(4):338–43.
85. Bernaerts F, Talavera J, Leemans J, et al. Description of original endoscopic findings and respiratory functional assessment using barometric whole-body plethysmography in dogs suffering from brachy- cephalic airway obstruction syndrome. Vet J 2010;183:95–102.
86. Lecoindre P, Richard S. Digestive disorders associated with the chronic obstructive respiratory syndrome of brachycephalic dogs: 30 cases (1999-2001). Rev Med Vet 2004;155:141–6.
87. Eivers C, Chicon Rueda R, Liuti T, et al. Retrospective analysis of esophageal imaging features in brachycephalic versus non-brachycephalic dogs based on videofluoroscopic swallowing studies. J Vet Intern Med 2019;33(4):1740–6.
88. Ducarouge B. Le syndrome obstructif des voies respiratoies supérieures chez les chiens brachycephales. etude clinique a propos de 27 cas [Thesis]. Lyon (France): University Lyon; 2002.
89. Hardie EM, Ramirez O, Clary EM, et al. Abnormalities of the thoracic bellows: stress fractures of the ribs and hiatal hernia. J Vet Intern Med 1998;12(4): 279–87.
90. Hunt GB, O'Brien C, Kolenc G, et al. Hiatal hernia in a puppy. Aust Vet J 2002; 80(11):685–6.
91. Miles KG, Pope ER, Jergens AE. Paraesophageal hiatal hernia and pyloric obstruction in a dog. J Am Vet Med Assoc 1988;193(11):1437–9.
92. Boesch RP, Shah P, Vaynblat M, et al. Relationship between upper airway obstruction and gastroesophageal reflux in a dog model. J Invest Surg 2005; 18:241–5.
93. White DR, Heavner SB, Hardy SM, et al. Gastroesophageal reflux and eustachian tube dysfunction in an animal model. Laryngoscope 2002;112(6):955–61.
94. Roedler FS, Pohl S, Oechtering GU. How does severe brachycephaly affect dog's lives? Results of a structured preoperative owner questionnaire. Vet J 2013;198:606–10.
95. Kaye BM, Rutherford L, Perridge DJ, et al. Relationship between brachycephalic airway syndrome and gastrointestinal signs in three breeds of dog. J Small Anim Pract 2018;59(11):670–3.
96. Freiche V, Poncet C. Upper airway and gastrointestinal syndrome in brachycephalic dogs. Vet Focus 2007;17(2):4–10.
97. Lorinson D, Bright RM, White RAS. Brachycephalic airway obstruction syndrome - a review of 118 cases. Canine Pract 1997;22:18–21.
98. Reeve EJ, Sutton D, Friend EJ, et al. Documenting the prevalence of hiatal hernia and oesophageal abnormalities in brachycephalic dogs using fluoroscopy. J Small Anim Pract 2017;58(12):703–8.

99. Broux O, Clercx C, Etienne AL, et al. Effects of manipulations to detect sliding hiatal hernia in dogs with brachycephalic airway obstructive syndrome. Vet Surg 2018;47(2):243–51.

100. Vangrinsven E, Broux O, Massart L, et al. Diagnosis and treatment of gastro-oesophageal junction abnormalities in dogs with brachycephalic syndrome. J Small Anim Pract 2021;62(3):200–8.

101. Packer RMA, Hendricks A, Burn CC. Do dog owners perceive the clinical signs related to conformational inherited disorders as 'normal' for the breed? A potential constraint to improving canine welfare. Anim Welfare-The UFAW J 2012; 21:81.

102. Barker DA, Tovey E, Jeffery A, et al. Owner reported breathing scores, accelerometry and sleep disturbances in brachycephalic and control dogs: a pilot study. Vet Rec 2021;189(no-no):e135.

103. Liu N-C, Sargan DR, Adams VJ, et al. Characterisation of brachycephalic obstructive airway syndrome in French Bulldogs using whole- body barometric plethysmography. PLoS One 2015;10:e0130741.

104. Liu NC, Adams VJ, Kalmar L, et al. Whole-body barometric plethysmography characterizes upper airway obstruction in 3 brachycephalic breeds of dogs. J Vet Intern Med 2016;30(3):853–65.

105. Seneviratne M, Kaye BM, Ter Haar G. Prognostic indicators of short-term outcome in dogs undergoing surgery for brachycephalic obstructive airway syndrome. Vet Rec 2020;187(10):403.

106. Erjavec V, Vovk T, Svete AN. Evaluation of oxidative stress parameters in dogs with brachycephalic obstructive airway syndrome before and after surgery. J Vet Res 2021;65(2):201–8.

107. Riggs J, Liu NC, Sutton DR, et al. Validation of exercise testing and laryngeal auscultation for grading brachycephalic obstructive airway syndrome in pugs, French bulldogs, and English bulldogs by using whole-body barometric plethysmography. Vet Surg 2019;48(4):488–96.

108. Villedieu E, Rutherford L, Ter Haar G. Brachycephalic obstructive airway surgery outcome assessment using the 6-minute walk test: a pilot study. J Small Anim Pract 2019;60(2):132–5.

109. Lilja-Maula L, Lappalainen AK, Hyytiainen HK, et al. Comparison of submaximal exercise test results and severity of brachycephalic obstructive airway syndrome in English bulldogs. Vet J 2017;219:22–6.

110. Cook WR. Observations on the upper respiratory tract of the dog and cat. J Small Anim Pract 1964;5:309–29.

111. Ohnishi T, Ogura JH. Partitioning of pulmonary resistance in the dog. Laryngoscope 1969;79(11):1847–78.

112. Negus VE, Oram S, Banks DC. Effect of respiratory obstruction on the arterial and venous circulation in animals and man. Thorax 1970;25(1):1–10.

113. Hueber J. Impulse oscillometric examination of intranasal airway resistance before and after laser assisted turbinectomy for treatment of brachycephalic airway syndrome in the dog [Thesis]. Leipzig (Germany): University of Leipzig; 2008.

114. Lippert JP, Reinhold P, Smith HJ, et al. Geometry and function of the canine nose: how does the function change when the form is changed? Pneumologie 2010;64(7):452–3.

115. Fenner JVH, Quinn RJ, Demetriou JL. Postoperative regurgitation in dogs after upper airway surgery to treat brachycephalic obstructive airway syndrome: 258 cases (2013-2017). Vet Surg 2020;49(1):53–60.

116. Costa RS, Abelson AL, Lindsey JC, et al. Postoperative regurgitation and respiratory complications in brachycephalic dogs undergoing airway surgery before and after implementation of a standardized perianesthetic protocol. J Am Vet Med Assoc 2020;256(8):899–905.

117. Mercurio A. Complications of upper airway surgery in companion animals. Review. Vet Clin North Am Small Anim Pract 2011;41(5):969–80.

118. Gruenheid M, Aarnes TK, McLoughlin MA, et al. Risk of anesthesia-related complications in brachycephalic dogs. J Am Vet Med Assoc 2018;253(3):301–6.

119. Savvas I, Raptopoulos D, Rallis T. A "Light Meal" Three Hours Preoperatively Decreases the Incidence of Gastro-Esophageal Reflux in Dogs. J Am Anim Hosp Assoc 2016;52(6):357–63.

120. Thompson KR, Rioja E. Effects of intravenous and topical laryngeal lidocaine on heart rate, mean arterial pressure and cough response to endotracheal intubation in dogs. Vet Anaesth Analg 2016;43(4):371–8.

121. Downing F, Gibson S. Anaesthesia of brachycephalic dogs. J Small Anim Pract 2018;59(12):725–33.

122. McNally EM, Robertson SA, Pablo LS. Comparison of time to desaturation between preoxygenated and nonpreoxygenated dogs following sedation with acepromazine maleate and morphine and induction of anesthesia with propofol. Am J Vet Res 2009;70(11):1333–8.

123. Doyle CR, Aarnes TK, Ballash GA, et al. Anesthetic risk during subsequent anesthetic events in brachycephalic dogs that have undergone corrective airway surgery: 45 cases (2007-2019). J Am Vet Med Assoc 2020;257(7):744–9.

124. Mehl ML, Kyles AE, Pypendop BH, et al. Outcome of laryngeal web resection with mucosal apposition for treatment of airway obstruction in dogs: 15 cases (19922006). J Am Vet Med Assoc 2008;233:738–42.

125. Matushek KJ, Bjorling DE. A mucosal flap technique for correction of laryngeal webbing. Results in four dogs. Vet Surg 1988;17:318–20.

126. Hughes JR, Kaye BM, Beswick AR, et al. Complications following laryngeal sacculectomy in brachycephalic dogs. J Small Anim Pract 2018;59(1):16–21.

127. Cantatore M, Gobbetti M, Romussi S, et al. Medium term endoscopic assessment of the surgical outcome following laryngeal saccule resection in brachycephalic dogs. Vet Rec 2012;170:518.

128. Liu NC, Genain MA, Kalmar L, et al. Objective effectiveness of and indications for laser-assisted turbinectomy in brachycephalic obstructive airway syndrome. Vet Surg 2019;48(1):79–87.

129. Trader RL. Nose operation. J Am Vet Med Assoc 1949;114:210–1.

130. Huck JL, Stanley BJ, Hauptman JG. Technique and outcome of nares amputation (trader's technique) in immature shih tzus. J Am Vet Med Assoc 2008; 44(2):82–5.

131. Ellison GW. Alapexy: an alternative technique for repair of stenotic nares in dogs. J Am Vet Med Assoc 2004;40(6):484–9.

132. Nelson A. Upper respiratory system. In: Slatter DG, editor. Textbook of small animal surgery. 2nd edition. Philadelphia: Saunders; 1993. p. 733–76.

133. Trostel CT, Frankel DJ. Punch resection alaplasty technique in dogs and cats with stenotic nares: 14 cases. J Am Vet Med Assoc 2010;46(1):5–11.

134. Oechtering GU, Schuenemann R. Brachycephalics-trapped in man-made misery? Proceedings AVSTS Meeting. Cambridge (United Kingdom), October 1-2 2010. p. 28.

135. Tobias KM. Stenotic nares. In: Tobias KM, editor. Manual of soft tissue surgery. Oxford (United Kingdom): Wiley-Blackwell; 2010. p. 401–6.

136. Oechtering GU, Hueber JP, Oechtering TH, et al. Laser assisted turbinectomy (LATE): treating brachycephalic airway distress at its intranasal origin. In: Proceedings ACVS meeting. Chicago (IL), October 17-21 2007: Vet Surg; 2007. p. E18, 36(6).

137. Oechtering GU, Pohl S, Schlueter C, et al. A novel approach to brachycephalic syndrome. 2. Laser-assisted turbinectomy (LATE). Vet Surg 2016;45(2):173–81.

138. Schuenemann R, Oechtering G. Inside the brachycephalic nose: conchal regrowth and mucosal contact points after laser-assisted turbinectomy. J Am Anim Hosp Assoc 2014;50:237–46.

139. Harvey CE, Venker-von Haagan A. Surgical management of pharyngeal and laryngeal airway obstruction in the dog. Vet Clin North Am Small Anim Pract 1975;5:515–35.

140. Bright RM, Wheaton LG. A modified surgical technique for elongated soft palate in dogs. J Am Vet Med Assoc 1983;19:288.

141. Davidson EB, Davis MS, Campbell GA, et al. Evaluation of carbon dioxide laser and conventional incisional techniques for resection of soft palates in brachycephalic dogs. J Am Vet Med Assoc 2001;219(6):776–81.

142. Harvey CE. Review of results of airway obstruction surgery in the dog. J Small Anim Pract 1983;24(9):555–9.

143. Brdecka DJ, Rawlings CA, Perry AC, et al. Use of an electrothermal, feedback-controlled, bipolar sealing device for resection of the elongated portion of the soft palate in dogs with obstructive upper airway disease. J Am Vet Med Assoc 2008;233(8):1265–9.

144. Dunie-Merigot A, Bouvy B, Poncet C. Comparative use of CO2 laser, diode laser and monopolar electrocautery for resection of the soft palate in dogs with brachycephalic airway obstruction syndrome. Vet Rec 2010;167:700–4.

145. Singleton WB. Partial velum palatiectomy for relief of dyspnea in brachycephalic breeds. J Small Anim Pract 1962;3:215–6.

146. Clark GN, Sinibaldi KR. Use of a carbon dioxide laser for treatment of elongated soft palate in dogs. J Am Vet Med Assoc 1994;204(11):1779–81.

147. Brdecka D, Rawlings C, Howerth E, et al. A histopathologlcal comparison of two techniques for soft palate resection in normal dogs. J Am Vet Med Assoc 2007; 43(1):39–44.

148. Kirsch MS, Spector D, Kalafut SR, et al. Comparison of carbon dioxide laser versus bipolar vessel device for staphylectomy for the treatment of brachycephalic obstructive airway syndrome. Can Vet J 2019;60(2):160–6.

149. Dupré G, Findji L. Nouvelle technique chirurgicale: La palatoplastie modifiee chez le chien. Nouveau Prat Vet 2004;20:553–6.

150.. Findji L, Dupré GP. Folded flap palatoplasty for treatment of elongated soft palates in 55 dogs. Vet Med Austria/Wien Tierärztl Mschr 2008;95:56–63.

151. Stordalen MB, Silveira F, Fenner JVH, et al. Outcome of temporary tracheostomy tube-placement following surgery for brachycephalic obstructive airway syndrome in 42 dogs. J Small Anim Pract 2020;61(5):292–9.

152. Seim HB. Surgical management of brachycephalic syndrome. Proceedings north American veterinary conference. Orlando (FL), January 16-21, 2010.

153. Olivieri M, Voghera S, Fossum T. Video-assisted left partial arytenoidectomy by diode laser photoablation for treatment of canine laryngeal paralysis. Vet Surg 2009;38:439–44.

154. White RN. Surgical management of laryngeal collapse associated with brachycephalic airway obstruction syndrome in dogs. J Small Anim Pract 2012;53: 44–50.

155. Tokunaga S, Ehrhart EJ, Monnet E. Histological and mechanical comparisons of arytenoid cartilage between 4 brachycephalic and 8 non-brachycephalic dogs: a pilot study. PLoS One 2020;15(9):e0239223.
156. Hedlund CS. Brachycephalic syndrome. In: Bojrab MJ, Ellison GW, Slocum B, editors. Current techniques in small animal surgery. 4th edition. Baltimore (MD): Williams & Wilkins; 1998. p. 357–62.
157. Gobbetti M, Romussi S, Buracco P, et al. Long-term outcome of permanent tracheostomy in 15 dogs with severe laryngeal collapse secondary to brachycephalic airway obstructive syndrome. Vet Surg 2018;47(5):648–53.
158. Orsher R. Brachycephalic airway disease. In: Bojrab M, editor. Disease mechanisms in small animal surgery. 2nd edition. Philadelphia: Lea & Febiger; 1993. p. 369–70.
159. Harvey CE, O'Brien JA. Upper airway obstruction surgery 7: tracheotomy in the dog and cat: analysis of 89 episodes in 79 animals. J Am Anim Hosp Assoc 1982;18:563–6.
160. Nicholson I, Baines S. Complications associated with temporary tracheostomy tubes in 42 dogs (1998 to 2007). J Small Anim Pract 2012;53:108–14.
161. Worth DB, Grimes JA, Jimenez DA, et al. Risk factors for temporary tracheostomy tube placement following surgery to alleviate signs of brachycephalic obstructive airway syndrome in dogs. J Am Vet Med Assoc 2018;253(9): 1158–63.
162. Bird FG, Vallefuoco R, Dupré G, et al. A modified temporary tracheostomy in dogs: outcome and complications in 21 dogs (2012 to 2017). J Small Anim Pract 2018;59(12):769–76.
163. Occhipinti LL, Hauptman JG. Long-term outcome of permanent tracheostomies in dogs: 21 cases (2000-2012). Can Vet J 2014;55(4):357–60.
164. Grimes JA, Davis AM, Wallace ML, et al. Long-term outcome and risk factors associated with death or the need for revision surgery in dogs with permanent tracheostomies. J Am Vet Med Assoc 2019;254(9):1086–93.
165. Bernardé A, Matres-Lorenzo L, Carcia-Rodriguez M. Long-term management of stenosis after tube-less permanent tracheostomy in brachycephalic dogs:19 cases 2021. Unpublished data.
166. Hosgood GL, Appelgrein C, Gelmi C. Circumferential esophageal hiatal rim reconstruction for treatment of persistent regurgitation in brachycephalic dogs: 29 cases (2016-2019). J Am Vet Med Assoc 2021;258(10):1091–7.
167. Mayhew PD, Marks SL, Pollard R, et al. Prospective evaluation of surgical management of sliding hiatal hernia and gastroesophageal reflux in dogs. Vet Surg 2017;46(8):1098–109.
168. Mayhew PD, Balsa IM, Marks SL, et al. Clinical and videofluoroscopic outcomes of laparoscopic treatment for sliding hiatal hernia and associated gastroesophageal reflux in brachycephalic dogs. Vet Surg 2021;50(Suppl 1):O67–77.
169. Senn D, Sigrist N, Fortere F, et al. Retrospective evaluation of postoperative nasotracheal tubes for oxygen supplementation in dogs following surgery for brachycephalic syndrome: 36 cases (2003-2007). J Vet Em Crit Care Med 2011;3:1–7.
170. Debuigne M, Chesnel M. Life-threatening pharyngeal oedema secondary to severe per-anaesthetic regurgitation in a French bulldog: management with topical adrenaline and nasotracheal tube. Vet Rec Case Rep 2021;9(4):e2179.
171. Ellis J, Leece EA. Nebulized Adrenaline in the Postoperative Management of Brachycephalic Obstructive Airway Syndrome in a Pug. J Am Anim Hosp Assoc 2017;53(2):107–10.

172. Franklin PH, Liu NC, Ladlow JF. Nebulization of epinephrine to reduce the severity of brachycephalic obstructive airway syndrome in dogs. Vet Surg 2021;50(1):62–70.
173. Ree JJ, Milovancev M, MacIntyre LA, et al. Factors associated with major complications in the short-term postoperative period in dogs undergoing surgery for brachycephalic airway syndrome. Can Vet J 2016;57(9):976–80.
174. Tarricone J, Hayes GM, Singh A, et al. Development and validation of a brachycephalic risk (BRisk) score to predict the risk of complications in dogs presenting for surgical treatment of brachycephalic obstructive airway syndrome. Vet Surg 2019;48(7):1253–61.
175. Lindsay B, Cook D, Wetzel JM, et al. Brachycephalic airway syndrome: management of post-operative respiratory complications in 248 dogs. Aust Vet J 2020;98(5):173–80.
176. Darcy HP, Humm K, Ter Haar G. Retrospective analysis of incidence, clinical features, potential risk factors, and prognostic indicators for aspiration pneumonia in three brachycephalic dog breeds. J Am Vet Med Assoc 2018; 253(7):869–76.

Fluid Therapy for the Emergent Small Animal Patient: Crystalloids, Colloids, and Albumin Products

Elisa Mazzaferro, DVM, MS, PHD[a], Lisa L. Powell, DVM[b,*]

KEYWORDS

- Intravenous fluids • Crystalloids • Colloids • Albumin • Volume resuscitation
- Dehydration

KEY POINTS

- Fluid therapy is essential in the treatment of emergent veterinary patients and includes crystalloid solutions, blood component therapy, concentrated albumin solutions, and synthetic colloids.
- Bolus intravenous fluid therapy can restore perfusion and stabilize critically ill and injured patients for further diagnostics and treatment.
- Synthetic colloids help maintain colloid osmotic pressure and improve blood pressure but should be used with caution in coagulopathic patients, those with cardiac disease, and potentially those with renal dysfunction.
- Concentrated albumin solutions may have a role in the treatment of critically ill veterinary patients with severe hypoalbuminemia (eg, septic peritonitis); further prospective, comparative studies are needed to fully elucidate the role of albumin solutions in dogs and cats.
- The pros and cons of the use of human serum albumin and canine serum albumin will be reviewed.

TOTAL BODY WATER AND FLUID COMPARTMENTS WITHIN THE BODY

A discussion of intravenous (IV) fluid administration is incomplete without an understanding of total body water (TBW) and fluid balance between the various compartments within the body. Approximately 60% of a healthy animal's total body weight is water. This value can change slightly depending on age, lean body mass, degree of leanness or obesity, and gender. TBW has been estimated as approximately 534 mL/kg to 660 mL/kg in healthy dogs and cats.[1]

---

[a] Cornell University Veterinary Specialists, 880 Canal Street, Stamford, CT 06902, USA;
[b] BluePearl Veterinary Partners, 7717 Flying Cloud Drive, Eden Prairie, MN 55344, USA
* Corresponding author.
E-mail address: ervet1@gmail.com

Vet Clin Small Anim 52 (2022) 781–796
https://doi.org/10.1016/j.cvsm.2022.01.008
vetsmall.theclinics.com
0195-5616/22/© 2022 Elsevier Inc. All rights reserved.

Conceptually, the body can be divided into the intracellular and extracellular compartments. Fluid located within cells is known as intracellular fluid and contributes approximately two-thirds (66%) to TBW. Extracellular fluid (ECF) is that located outside of cells and contributes approximately one-third (33%) to TBW; the ECF can be further subdivided into the intravascular and interstitial compartments. Fluid contained within blood vessels is intravascular fluid. The intravascular fluid contains plasma water, cellular components, proteins, and electrolytes. The interstitial extravascular compartment is the space located outside of the blood vessels. Intravascular fluid contributes only 8% to 10% of TBW, and interstitial fluid contributes 24% of TBW. A small amount of fluid is known as transcellular fluid and is located within the gastrointestinal tract, joints, cartilage, and cerebrospinal space.[1] Total intravascular fluid volume has been estimated as 80 mL/kg to 90 mL/kg in dogs and cats. Of that, the fluid component, or intravascular plasma water volume, has been estimated as approximately 45 mL/kg to 50 mL/kg.[1]

GOALS OF FLUID THERAPY

Administration of IV fluids requires an understanding of the type of fluid lost, the presence of underlying disease processes, an animal's hydration and intravascular volume status, acid-base and electrolyte derangements, an animal's ability to retain fluid within the intravascular space, and determinants of resuscitation endpoints when treating dehydration or various forms of hypovolemia. An understanding of electrolyte and protein composition within the body is also essential to help maintain homeostasis and to use the variety of crystalloid fluids that are available to treat specific abnormalities. Thus, the goals of fluid therapy are to replenish interstitial, intracellular, and intravascular fluid deficits; to correct and maintain electrolyte and acid-base derangements; and to maintain normal TBW in the face of excessive loss or lack of adequate intake.

CRYSTALLOID FLUIDS

A crystalloid fluid contains water and various forms of electrolytes (including salt) or sugar crystals (**Table 1**).[1,2] Some crystalloid fluids also contain buffers (eg, acetate, gluconate, and lactate) that are metabolized to bicarbonate to increase serum pH. Crystalloid fluids are categorized according to their osmolality relative to that of plasma. An isotonic crystalloid fluid has an osmolality similar to or equal to that of plasma and the extracellular compartment (eg, approximately 300 mOsm/L). Fluids with tonicity lower than that of the extracellular space are called hypotonic fluids (eg, 0.45% dextrose and 5% dextrose in water [D5W]) and can cause fluid influx into red blood cells (RBCs) and hemolysis.[1,2] Fluids with tonicity greater than that of the ECF compartment (eg, >300 mOsm/L) are called hypertonic solutions (eg, 7.2% and 23.4% hypertonic saline) and can be used to expand intravascular fluid volume in a hypovolemic animal by pulling water from the interstitial into the intravascular space. It has been estimated that approximately 80% of an isotonic crystalloid fluid administered IV leaves the intravascular compartment and moves to the interstitial compartment within 1 hour of infusion.[3]

Isotonic fluids have sodium concentrations similar to that of plasma and the ECF compartment.[1,2,4] Water and sodium are intimately associated within the body's fluid compartments. Wherever sodium goes, water must follow. For this reason, the concentration of sodium in a crystalloid fluid becomes important when selecting a particular fluid to treat a specific disease state. Other important components of isotonic crystalloid fluids to consider include the presence or absence of buffers or various electrolytes (calcium, magnesium, potassium, chloride, and so forth).

Table 1
Various crystalloid fluids and their components

Fluid	Osmolarity	Buffer	Sodium	Chloride	Potassium	Calcium	Magnesium	Glucose
Normosol-R	296	Acetate 27 Gluconate 23	140	98	5	0	3	0
PlasmaLyte-A	294	Acetate 27	140	98	5	0	3	0
0.9% Saline	308	0	154	154	0	0	0	0
LRS	272	Lactate 28	130	109	4	3	0	0
D5W	252	0	0	0	0	0	0	50 g/L
0.45% NaCl 1 2.5% dextrose	280	0	77	77	0	0	0	25 g/L
Normosol-M 1 5% dextrose	364	Acetate 16	40	40	13	0	3	50 g/L
PlasmaLyte-M	363	Acetate 16	40	40	13	0	3	110
PlasmaLyte-56	110	Acetate 16	40	40	13	0	3	0
3% NaCl	1026	0	513	513	0	0	0	0
7% NaCl	2567	0	1283	1283	0	0	0	0

Fluids used to replace intravascular and interstitial volume deficit should contain 130 mEq/L to 154 mEq/L of sodium. Several solutions are used for replacement of fluid volume, electrolyte abnormalities, and correction of acid-base abnormalities, including Normosol-R, PlasmaLyte-A, normal (0.9%) saline, and lactated Ringer solution (LRS) (also called Hartmann solution).

Maintenance crystalloid solutions contain lower concentrations of sodium and other compounds compared with the extracellular space[1,2,4] and are used primarily to replace sensible fluid losses that can be measured and insensible fluid losses that can be estimated.[3] An example of a maintenance isotonic crystalloid fluid is 0.45% sodium with 2.5% dextrose, PlasmaLyte-M, and PlasmaLyte 56.

HYPERTONIC SALINE

Hypertonic sodium (eg, 7.2% and 23.4% NaCl) contains the highest concentration of sodium (eg, 1283 mEq/L of sodium and approximately 4000 mEq/L). Infusion of hypertonic saline should only be considered in a hypovolemic patient with normal interstitial and intracellular hydration (ie, only lacking fluid within the intravascular space). Infusion of hypertonic saline increases intravascular sodium concentration, and the intravascular space has a higher osmolality compared with the interstitial and intracellular space. To maintain fluid equilibrium, water diffuses down a concentration gradient by osmosis, from an area of higher water concentration (lower osmolality). After infusion of hypertonic saline, water moves from the intracellular and interstitial space into the intravascular space and causes intravascular volume expansion at the expense of the interstitium. The effect is short-lived for 20 to 30 minutes unless the hypertonic saline is administered concurrently with a colloid to retain the fluid within the intravascular space.[5,6] Hypertonic saline (23.4%) can be diluted with a synthetic colloid at a ratio of 1 part hypertonic saline with 2.5 parts colloid, which creates a 7.5% solution.[7] Hypertonic saline in combination with a synthetic colloid (dogs: 5–10 mL/kg of the combination; cats: 2 mL/kg of the combination; total dose in either species should not exceed 1 mL/kg/min as a bolus)[7] can also be used to initially treat hypovolemic shock, provided a patient is not clinically dehydrated.

After correction of intravascular hypovolemia, replacement crystalloid fluids must be administered after administration of hypertonic saline (with or without colloids) to replenish that fluid borrowed from the interstitial and intracellular compartments to rehydrate them. Potential complications of hypertonic saline administration include rapid respiratory rate, hypotension, bradycardia, and hypernatremia.[1,7]

SODIUM

Sodium is the major extracellular cation (ie, positive charged molecule) in the body. Normal sodium concentrations are 140 mEq/L 150 mEq/L for dogs and 150 mEq/L to 160 mEq/L for cats.[8] The sodium content of most isotonic crystalloid fluids ranges from 130 mEq/L to 140 mEq/L. Normal (0.9%) saline is the isotonic crystalloid fluid with the highest sodium concentration (154 mEq/L) and is used as a replacement fluid. In the realm of isotonic crystalloid fluids, LRS contains the lowest concentration of sodium (130 mEq/L) relative to plasma. Conditions that promote hyperaldosteronemia and sodium retention, such as congestive heart failure and hepatic failure, may benefit from infusion of lower concentrations of sodium.

Maintenance fluids can be used to replace daily ongoing sodium losses. Fluids, such as Plasmalyte-M and Plasmalyte 56, contain approximately 40 mEq/L sodium. If such fluids were used as replacement solutions, a patient's serum sodium could be decreased and lead to a state of hyponatremia.

Rapid changes in serum sodium concentration can be detrimental, depending on the how quickly an animal's sodium balance and serum sodium concentration become deranged. Diarrhea, heat-induced illness, hyperthermia, and lack of access to water can cause varying degrees of hypernatremia. Hypernatremia largely is characterized by a free water deficit, a deficit of fluid in excess of electrolytes. Ideally, serum sodium concentration should not be lowered by more than 15 mEq in a 24-hour period. Similarly, syndromes, such as hypoadrenocorticism, can cause decreases in serum sodium concentration. Overzealous administration of sodium-containing fluids, such as normal (0.9%) saline, can result in cerebral edema and central pontine myelinolysis.[9]

CHLORIDE

Chloride is a major extracellular anion (ie, negative charged molecule). Chloride can be lost in vomitus caused by an upper gastrointestinal obstruction, from administration of diuretics (eg, furosemide) or from loss in diarrheic feces. The presence of a hypochloremic metabolic alkalosis is typically less common in veterinary medicine and is often characteristic of the causes discussed previously. Normal (0.9%) saline contains supraphysiologic concentrations of chloride (154 mEq/L) and is used as a chloride replacement fluid in cases of hypochloremia. Other isotonic crystalloid fluids contain varying concentrations of chloride (55–103 mEq/L). Although chloride is important, consideration of sodium and other electrolyte concentrations is more important when selecting a replacement fluid for a specific disease state.

POTASSIUM

Potassium is the major intracellular cation. Serum potassium can become elevated due to severe dehydration, hypoadrenocorticism, metabolic acidosis, diabetic ketoacidosis (DKA), renal failure, or obstructive uropathies. Most replacement and maintenance crystalloid fluids contain minimal supplementation of potassium (eg, 4 mEq/L of potassium in LRS) and typically need to be supplemented in the form of potassium chloride. In animals with hyperkalemia, it is ideal to avoid the administration of a potassium-containing fluid whenever possible; however, studies have shown that as long as the underlying disease mechanism is promptly treated, the small amount of potassium with replacement or maintenance fluids is rarely consequential.[10] Administration of IV fluids alone dilutes serum potassium, as intravascular fluid volume is replenished, even if the fluid contains small amounts of potassium. In animals with hypokalemia, potassium supplementation is commensurate with the degree of hypokalemia.[5,8] It is advisable to not exceed administration of more than 0.5 mEq/kg/h of potassium IV.

MAGNESIUM

Magnesium is required for regulation and normal functioning of the sodium-potassium-ATPase pump. Some maintenance fluids (eg, PlasmaLyte and Normosol) contain trace amounts of magnesium. In general, most healthy patients do not require additional supplementation of magnesium. In animals with refractory hypokalemia (eg, DKA), animals with endocrine diseases predisposing them toward significant electrolyte changes (eg, DKA), or in critically ill patients, magnesium should be supplemented (eg, 0.75 mEq/kg/d or 0.375 mmol/kg/d) in addition to potassium, because both electrolytes follow similar physiologic paths within the body. Total body magnesium is a function of absorption and loss as well as redistribution throughout body compartments. Any physiologic condition that can cause a lack of intake and absorption, increased loss in diarrheic feces, renal tubular loss, or redistribution can cause hypomagnesemia. For example, in animals with DKA and whole-body magnesium depletion secondary to glucose/osmotic diuresis, administration of insulin and dextrose for treatment causes magnesium to rapidly shift to the intracellular space and result in a serum ionized hypomagnesemia. Although the crystalloid fluids contain small quantities of magnesium, the amount is insufficient to replenish a whole-body magnesium deficit in some populations of critically ill patients.

CALCIUM

Calcium is an important cation that is necessary for normal muscle conduction and coagulation. Calcium is present in small amounts in LRS (3 mEq/L) and typically does not need to be supplemented in healthy patients above this amount. In cases of puerperal tetany (eg, eclampsia), however, LRS may be the preferred fluid as adjunct therapy to those that do not contain calcium and to those that promote calcium excretion (0.9% NaCl). In addition, the preemptive use of a calcium-containing fluid, such as LRS, may be beneficial in helping to prevent hypocalcemia during the postoperative period after surgical removal of the parathyroid gland.

Hypercalcemia can be seen due to a variety of causes. Administration of a calcium-containing fluid is contraindicated in hypercalcemic patients if other crystalloid fluids are available. Normal (0.9%) saline is the treatment of choice in cases of hypercalcemia not only because the fluid does not contain calcium but also because the higher sodium content (eg, 154 mEq/L) promotes calciuresis at the Na_2Ca exchanger.[11]

BUFFERS

A buffer is a compound that is converted or metabolized in the body to bicarbonate to help maintain normal physiologic blood pH. The most common buffers found in IV fluids include lactate, acetate, and gluconate. Medical conditions that cause metabolic acidosis (lactic acidosis secondary to poor perfusion, DKA, uremia, ethylene glycol toxicosis, salicylate toxicosis, and so forth) should ideally be treated with a crystalloid fluid that contains a buffer. Certain medical conditions, however, may warrant the judicious use or the more appropriate use of certain buffers. In cases of hepatic dysfunction, the liver's ability to convert lactate to bicarbonate may be diminished; therefore, LRS is relatively contraindicated. Acetate and gluconate, commonly found in Normosol-R or PlasmaLyte, are buffers that are metabolized to bicarbonate in the liver and muscle tissue. Therefore, in patients with LSA or whose liver function is suboptimal, crystalloid fluids that contain acetate and gluconate may be preferable to lactate-containing solutions. Acetate, which has been reported to potential hypotension with large, massive infusions (eg, dialysis),[12] should ideally be avoided in patients requiring large, rapid boluses (eg, anesthetic-induced hypotension).

Normal (0.9%) saline contains no buffers and is known as an acidifying crystalloid fluid because it promotes excretion of bicarbonate by the renal tubules.[5] In cases of a hypochloremic metabolic alkalosis, an acidifying solution, such as 0.9% saline without additional buffers, is preferred, to avoid administration of additional sources of bicarbonate and to replenish chloride ions lost in the vomitus.

DEXTROSE

Dextrose-containing fluids, such as D5W and 0.45% sodium chloride with 2.5% dextrose, are not common fluid choices in the dehydrated patient, and their use is typically limited to patients with severe hypernatremia, patients who cannot tolerate a large amount of sodium (eg, heart failure), or during treatment of conditions that cause hyperaldosteronism (hepatic failure, cardiac disease, and so forth). Dextrose-containing fluids are largely hypotonic compared with plasma; D5W is analogous to infusing a free water solution, once the dextrose is rapidly metabolized by the body. The remaining fluid redistributes within the intravascular, interstitial, and intracellular fluid compartments. Because free water alone is severely hypotonic (eg, 0 Osm/L) relative to plasma (eg, 300 Osm/L), infusion of free water causes rapid and severe hemolysis; hence, sterile water is not used. The addition of 5% dextrose (50 mg of dextrose/mL) makes the fluid isoosmolar and brings the tonicity of the fluid up to a safe acceptable range. The dextrose in these fluids is quickly metabolized but is insufficient to meet an animal's daily metabolic caloric requirements.

MAINTENANCE FLUID REQUIREMENTS

Many estimates of the maintenance fluid requirements for healthy dogs and cats have been recommended. In general, the estimates have been extrapolated from those recommended for humans or have been suggested based on experiments performed on healthy dogs and cats. The most recent swing of the fluid pendulum has been based on data obtained from calorimetry analysis in which fluid requirements are extrapolated from an animal's resting energy expenditure (REE) and lean body mass.[13,14] An animal's metabolic water requirements are equivalent to the number of basal calories required. During metabolism of 1 kcal of energy, 1 mL of water is consumed. By calculating the REE, or daily caloric requirements, a patient's daily fluid requirements for metabolic purposes can be calculated by the following linear formula: REE = mL $H_2O^* = [(30 \times$ body weight [kg]) + 70], where * denotes requirement for a 24-hour period.

   This formula is accurate for animals weighing greater than 2 kg and less than 100 kg. One caveat is that the REE is applicable to a healthy animal that is euvolemic, resting, and in a postprandial state. This formula denotes a starting point for dehydrated or hypovolemic animals or those with excessive fluid losses. Because some patients may become dehydrated when this formula is used, frequent evaluation of hydration status (body weight, evidence of hemodilution, urine specific gravity, and so forth) is essential during hospitalization. As a rule of thumb, 1 mL of water is equivalent to 1 g of body weight. Therefore, loss of 1 kg is equivalent to a loss of 1 L of water. Careful weighing of the animal on a regular basis allows clinicians to determine whether additional ongoing losses are occurring, allowing for accurate correction of interstitial and intracellular dehydration. One caveat is that if an animal is leaking fluid into the interstitial space or body cavitary effusions, fluid, and thus body weight, will increase and can confound accurate evaluation of hydration deficits based on body weight alone. For this reason, changes in body weight should always be considered with other physical examination parameters and diagnostic modalities such as cavitary ultrasound scans when formulating a fluid therapy plan.

DEHYDRATION

Dehydration refers to the fluid deficit within the interstitial and intracellular fluid compartments. The extent of dehydration can be estimated based on subjective guidelines of skin turgor, mucous membrane dryness, and sunken appearance of the eyes within the orbit (**Table 2**). Once degree of dehydration is determined, the volume of fluid that must be administered to replace the fluid deficit can be calculated by the following formula:

Table 2	
Subjective parameters used to estimate the degree of interstitial dehydration	
Estimated Degree of Dehydration	**Clinical Signs**
<5%	History of vomiting or diarrhea or other fluid loss, normal mucous membranes, unable to detect <5% on physical examination
5%	History of vomiting or diarrhea or other fluid loss, tachy or dry mucous membranes
7%	History of vomiting or diarrhea or other fluid loss, dry mucous membranes, increased skin tenting, tachycardia, normal pulse quality, and arterial blood pressure
10%	History of vomiting or diarrhea or other fluid loss, dry mucous membranes, increased skin tenting, tachycardia, weak pulses, hypotension
12%	History of vomiting or diarrhea or other fluid loss, dry mucous membranes, sunken eyes, increased skin tenting, tachycardia or bradycardia, weak to absent pulses, hypotension, cold extremities, hypothermia

Dehydration (%) x body weight in kg x 1000 = milliliters fluid deficit.

The fluid deficit then should be added to the animal's maintenance fluid requirements and replaced over a 6-hour to 24-hour period, depending on a patient's stability and ability to handle the volume administered. There is no absolute correct method of replacing an animal's fluid deficit, as long as the deficit is considered in the calculation of the total amount of fluids that need to be administered to a dehydrated patient. Frequent weighing and calculation of urine, vomit, and diarrhea fluid output (again, knowing that 1 mL of fluid weighs 1 g) allow a clinician to determine whether a patient's fluid deficit and maintenance needs are met or whether IV crystalloid dose needs to be adjusted.

HYPOVOLEMIA

Hypovolemia denotes loss of fluid from the intravascular space and is semantically different than dehydration. This fluid loss may be relative or absolute, meaning that in conditions of vasodilation (eg, sepsis or an anesthetized patient), there is a relative intravascular fluid deficit. Absolute intravascular fluid deficits occur as a result of fluid loss, such as that associated with hemorrhage or excessive ongoing losses (vomiting, diarrhea, renal loss, and so forth), where fluid efflux from the interstitial space to compensate for intravascular fluid loss has been depleted. Likewise, if an isoosmolar fluid is lost (eg, blood), there is no osmotic gradient drive to pull fluid from the interstitial space into the intravascular space. Clinical signs of hypovolemia are manifested as abnormalities of perfusion and include tachycardia, peripheral vasoconstriction with cool extremities, hypothermia, prolonged capillary refill time, hypotension, pallor, and mental dullness. When an animal presents in hypovolemic shock, the location of the fluid deficit, the presence of electrolyte abnormalities, and whether interstitial or intracellular dehydration is a component of a fluid deficit or if the deficit is associated with the intravascular space alone must be considered. With hypovolemia, rapid fluid replacement is imperative to improve perfusion parameters. Previously, recommendations for the treatment of hypovolemic shock (eg, shock volume) in dogs and cats have been reported as 90 mL/kg and 44 mL/kg, respectively,[4,8,13,14] which represents the blood volume of a patient. Because administration of large volume of crystalloids can dilute coagulation factors, platelets, and RBCs, more recently, the use of smaller aliquots is recommended rather than replacing the whole blood volume at once **Table 3**.

Table 3
Relative indications and relative contraindication for use of various isotonic, hypotonic, and hypertonic crystalloid fluids

Fluid	Indications	Relative Contraindications
Normosol-R	Replacement, metabolic acidosis, anorexia, vomiting, hypovolemic shock, diarrhea, renal failure	Hyperkalemia, metabolic alkalosis
PlasmaLyte-A	Replacement, metabolic acidosis, anorexia, vomiting, hypovolemic shock, diarrhea, renal failure	Hyperkalemia, metabolic alkalosis
0.9% NaCl	Replacement, hypovolemic shock, anorexia, vomiting, diarrhea, metabolic alkalosis, hyperkalemia, hypercalcemia acute hyponatremia, chronic hypernatremia, renal failure	Cardiac disease, liver disease, metabolic acidosis
LRS	Replacement, hypovolemic shock, vomiting, diarrhea, hypocalcemia, metabolic acidosis, renal failure	Hypercalcemia, hyperkalemia, liver failure
D5W	Drug carrier, correction of hypernatremia and free water deficit, congestive heart failure	Does not provide sufficient calories to be used as a form of parenteral nutrition
0.45% NaCl + 2.5% dextrose	Maintenance, replacement of insensible losses, correction of free water deficit	Not to be used as a replacement fluid
Normosol-M	Replacement of insensible losses	Hyponatremia, not to be used as a replacement fluid
PlasmaLyte-M	Replacement of insensible losses	Hyponatremia, not to be used as a replacement fluid
3% NaCl	Intravascular volume expansion, hypovolemic shock	Interstitial dehydration, hypernatremia
7% NaCl	Intravascular volume expansion, hypovolemic shock	Interstitial dehydration, hypernatremia

Ideally, it is preferred to administer a one-fourth of the shock volume (eg, 20–30 mL/kg for dogs and 10–15 mL/kg for cats over 20 minutes) and reassess a patient's perfusion parameters. If normalizing, then moving to maintenance fluid rates and performing diagnostics can be considered to assess and treat the primary cause of the problem. If a patient fails to respond (eg, perfusion parameters have still not normalized), additional aliquots (eg, one-fourth shock bolus) of crystalloid fluids should be readministered once or twice more; additional therapy may warrant the use of a colloid thereafter. Once stabilized, a continuous rate of infusion of fluids should be maintained, because 80% of a crystalloid fluid volume infused leaved the intravascular space within 1 hour of infusion, if not administered along with a colloid.[3]

COLLOID OSMOTIC PRESSURE

COP is the pressure exerted on membranes primarily due to the presence of albumin. Normal plasma COP in dogs and cats has been reported as 16.7 mm Hg to 28.9 mm Hg and 21 mm Hg to 34 mm Hg, respectively.[15–17] Normal whole-blood COP in dogs and cats has been reported as 17.9 mm Hg to 27.1 mm Hg and 21 mm Hg to 34 mm Hg, respectively.[15,16] The traditional Starling's law was thought to govern the movement of fluid between the intracellular and extracellular (intravascular and interstitial) space:

$$J_v = K_f[(P_c - P_i) - \sigma(\pi_c - \pi_i)]$$

where J_v is net fluid movement between compartments, K_f is filtration coefficient, P_c is capillary hydrostatic pressure, P_i is interstitial hydrostatic pressure, σ is reflection coefficient, π_c is COP, and π is interstitial osmotic pressure.

The filtration coefficient *(Kf)* is a measure of how well a tissue allows fluid to efflux and is a product of the surface area of the tissue and how permeable the capillary wall is to water (also referred to as hydraulic conductivity). The reflection coefficient (σ) is a measure of protein permeability in the membrane. Technological advances in the field of electron microscopy has allowed visualization and a better understanding of the micromolecular structure of the endothelium and its role in transcompartmental fluid exchange. A simplified explanation of the endothelial glycocalyx (EG) is that it is a complex matrix of glycoproteins and proteoglycans firmly adhered to the luminal endothelial membrane. The surface of the EG has a net negative charge and that attracts positively charged cells, ions, and macromolecules (namely, albumin) to its surface and deflects negatively charged cells such as red and white blood cells.[18] The space in between the endothelial cell and the EG is known as the sub-EG space. With albumin's attraction to the EG, fluid flux across the EG barrier is largely prevented during states of health.[18,19] During states of critical illness, such as hypervolemia, sepsis, cardiac disease, hyperglycemia, systemic inflammatory response syndrome, and ischemia, damage to the EG occurs that results in dysfunction.[18] Treatment of the conditions that lead to EG dysfunction, therefore, is of utmost importance, rather than consideration of a patient's COP alone to prevent abnormal intercompartmental fluid flux during conditions of critical illness.

COLLOID SOLUTIONS

Colloid solutions contain high-molecular-weight (MW) particles, thereby increasing plasma COP and more efficiently holding fluid within the intravascular space. Colloids can be further classified as natural or synthetic. Natural colloid solutions include blood products (eg, plasma and whole blood) and concentrated albumin. Synthetic colloids include dextrans and hydroxyethyl starches (HESs).

NATURAL COLLOIDS

Blood products include whole blood, component therapy (eg, plasma), and concentrated albumin solutions. Packed RBCs (pRBCs) have a lower COP (eg, 5 mm Hg) and are not considered a true colloid compared with whole blood (eg, because the plasma proteins have been separated out of the solution). If an anemic patient is euvolemic (eg, due to hemolysis of RBCs), pRBC transfusion is most appropriate, because the risk of hypervolemia can be avoided.

Plasma transfusions, with a COP of 20 mm Hg, are most appropriate in patients with coagulation abnormalities rather than hypoproteinemic patients. Although the COP of fresh frozen plasma or frozen plasma is comparable to normal plasma, the volume of plasma needed to significantly increase albumin by 1 mg/dL is large (eg, 45 mL/kg, IV) compared with the volume necessary to correct a coagulopathy (eg, 6–20 mL/kg, IV); this is usually cost prohibitive and increases the risk of fluid overload and triggering for future transfusion reactions. Recent studies have reported the use of constant rate infusions of cryopoor plasma to be effective at raising COP and albumin concentrations in dogs with critical illness.[20–22]

Whole-blood transfusions are indicated when both plasma and RBCs are required for transfusion. Fresh whole blood also contains platelets; however, the number of platelets is not sufficient to support patients with severe thrombocytopenia. Also, platelet function within a unit of whole blood is negated once the unit has been refrigerated. In patients with severe thrombocytopenia hemorrhaging into life-threatening tissue (eg, brain or lung), a whole-blood transfusion or the use of lyophilized platelets may be indicated to attempt hemostasis.

Concentrated albumin solutions, including 25% HSA and CSA, have been used in critically ill canine and feline patients to help support blood pressure and to aid in the treatment of significant hypoalbuminemia.[23] Studies have been published assessing the utility of HSA in the treatment of critically ill, hypoalbuminemic dogs and cats.[24–28] The initial studies were descriptive and retrospective in nature and preceded the availability of concentrated canine albumin for use in clinical practice. Studies assessing the use of HSA in healthy dogs have been published, however, and have unmasked the occurrence of hypersensitivity reactions in some dogs, including immediate anaphylactoid reactions and delayed events, including urticaria, vasculitis, lethargy, edema, and death postinfusion.[29,30] In addition, a study evaluating dogs that had received HSA revealed the presence of HSA autoantibodies in all dogs, increasing the risk for type III hypersensitivity reactions.[31] Previously, in critically ill dogs and cats receiving HSA, there were few reported hypersensitivity reactions, which may be due to their immunoparalyzed state.[25–28] In these studies, dogs and cats with higher serum albumin levels were more likely to survive compared with those with lower serum albumin concentration. Despite the lack of adverse reactions in the Vigano studies, more recent publications have documented adverse sequelae including glomerulonephritis, acute kidney injury, oligoanuria, and death in critically ill dogs following administration of HSA.[32,33]

More recently, CSA has been produced and available through a national veterinary blood bank (Animal Blood Resources International, Dixon, California, and Stockbridge, Michigan; abrint.net). This is considered to be a better, safer option with less risk for hypersensitivity reaction than with the human product. CSA is a lyophilized product and is currently sold in 5-g bottles at an estimated $275 per bottle. The published dose, based on company safety studies in healthy beagles, is 800 mg/kg to 844 mg/kg over 6 hours (Animal Blood Resources International, package insert, lyophilized canine albumin; abrint.net). Canine albumin also has been administered to healthy beagle dogs without adverse reactions.[34] The use of CSA has been evaluated in a prospective, blinded, comparative study in dogs with septic peritonitis.[35] This study showed that CSA was safe in this population of dogs and caused an initial increase in serum albumin that was significantly different than the untreated dogs. At the time of discharge or death, however, there was no significant difference in serum albumin levels between the 2 groups. Some limitations to the study included a small population (n = 14 total dogs), and dogs receiving CSA were only administered 1 dose (eg, after surgical intervention for septic peritonitis). It is unknown if multiple dosing, if indicated, would improve albumin levels for a longer period of time, providing a prolonged duration of effect. In addition, the study was not powered to assess outcome, so it is still not known if there is a survival benefit or decreased hospitalization when dogs with septic peritonitis are administered CSA. It is unknown if transfusing concentrated albumin solutions actually improves survival or if albumin is simply a marker of improved clinical outcome.

Based on these studies, the use of HSA should only be considered for critically ill veterinary patients with a life-threatening hypoalbuminemia (eg, septic peritonitis) if CSA or plasma products are not available. It should not be routinely used for patients with a low COP; rather, a safer synthetic colloid, such as an HES, can be used if cardiac or renal dysfunction or coagulopathies are not present. If considering use of an albumin source (rather than a synthetic colloid), the alternative use of CSA over HSA seems a safer option for use in dogs; however, it is unclear if the use of concentrated albumin products decreases hospitalization time or improves survival compared with dogs with similar disease that do not receive albumin products. A comparative, prospective veterinary study is required to more fully answer these questions.

SYNTHETIC COLLOIDS

Synthetic colloids, such as dextrans and HESs, are fluids that can be used to increase blood pressure and support COP. The HESs (eg, hetastarch, tetrastarch, and pentastarch) are most commonly used, because dextrans were found to induce anaphylaxis and acute kidney injury in humans. In veterinary medicine, the use of synthetic colloids in the form of HES are most common, because they are readily available, inexpensive, and carry fewer potential side effects compared with administration of human albumin.

HESs are esterified amylopectin-containing starches that remain in the intravascular space after administration due to its high MW. The differences between hetastarch, pentastarch, and tetrastarch are the average MW of the particles and the degree of substitution of glucose units on the starch particle with a hydroxyethyl group. Hetastarch (450 kDa) has the highest average MW, with pentastarch (260 kDa) and tetrastarch (130 kDa) having lower MWs. The MW of the product and the degree of substitution (hetastarch 0.5, pentastarch 0.45, and tetrastarch 0.4) determine the exerted COP of the fluid and the degradation time. The higher the substitution with hydroxyethyl groups, the longer the fluid persists in the intravascular space. Therefore, hetastarch lasts approximately 24 hours after administration, whereas pentastarch and tetrastarch last approximately 12 hours. Serum a-amylase degrades the HESs, and elimination occurs through the kidneys. When describing HES solutions, 3 numbers are used: the concentration of the HES solution, the MW, and the degree of substitution of hydroxyethyl groups/glucose unit. Some key factors describing HES solutions include the following:

1. The concentration of HES solutions, commonly 6%, is isoosmolar.
2. The higher the average MW of the HES solution, the longer the solution lasts, because larger molecules are more slowly degraded.
3. The degree of substitution of hydroxyethyl groups per glucose molecule is reported as a decimal percent. For example, hetastarch has a degree of substitution between 0.6 and 0.75, meaning that 60% to 75% of the glucose molecules contain a hydroxyethyl group at either the carbon-2 or carbon-6 position. The higher the degree of substitution, the longer the colloidal effects last, because the molecules are metabolized more slowly.

Side effects can also be seen with synthetic colloids and include influencing in vitro coagulation, increasing the potential for volume overload due to the efficacy of expanding intravascular volume and promoting acute kidney injury (AKI) in some patients.[36] Although a small cohort of retrospective studies have documented changes in serum creatinine and AKI with HES use,[36,37] it seems that the number of days on HES therapy, and not dose alone, was associated with an increase in grade of AKI 10 days after HES administration.[37] A prospective postmortem evaluation of 53 dogs who succumbed to critical illness documented cumulative HES dose, and presenting serum creatinine concentration was predictive of postmortem renal tubular injury.[38] Other prospective studies have not supported an increase in urinary biomarkers of AKI or in-hospital mortality in dogs.[39–42] A prospective internet-based survey with 1134 responders from 42 countries has documented a significant decrease in use of HES for colloid support, with concerns over use with coagulopathies, impaired renal function, and hypertension.[43] At this time, more prospective studies are required to further elucidate the absolute and relative safety of synthetic colloids in critically ill small animal patients; however, more recent use of natural colloids such as fresh frozen and cryopoor plasma and concentrated albumin products may be safer alternatives for improving cardiovascular stability and oncotic support in dogs and cats with critical illness.

Coagulation abnormalities are more likely with the higher MW HES and at doses of greater than 20 mL/kg/d and include decreased circulating factor VIII and von Willebrand factor, platelet dysfunction, and decreased fibrin clot stabilization.[44] Clinical manifestation of coagulation abnormalities secondary to the use of high MW HES has not been reported in the veterinary literature. Synthetic colloid administration may be safer and more effective than using concentrated human albumin solutions for the treatment of low COP due to lower risk of immune reactions and increased effectiveness as a colloid due to its variation in size (eg, molecules larger than albumin may not leak through vessels).

SUMMARY

Fluid therapy is essential in the treatment of emergent veterinary patients and includes crystalloid solutions, blood component therapy, concentrated albumin solutions, and synthetic colloids. Bolus IV fluid therapy can restore perfusion and stabilize critically ill and injured patients for further diagnostics and treatment. Synthetic colloids help to maintain COP and improve blood pressure but should be used with caution in coagulopathic patients or those with cardiac disease or renal dysfunction. Concentrated albumin solutions may have a role in the treatment of critically ill veterinary patients with severe hypoalbuminemia (eg, septic peritonitis); however, canine albumin is considered the safest option; further prospective, comparative studies are needed to fully elucidate the role of albumin solutions in dogs and cats.

CLINICS CARE POINTS

- Crystalloid fluid therapy is an essential treatment modality for the support of ill veterinary patients, including therapy for dehydration, cardiovascular shock, and support for ongoing fluid losses.
- Sytnthetic colloid therapy is associated with coagulopathies and may contribute to renal dysfunction. These risks should be considered prior to use in veterinary patients.
- Concentrated albumin solutions can be effective for the support of colloid oncotic pressure in hypoalbuminemic veterinary patients.

DISCLOSURE

The authors have nothing to disclose.

REFERENCES

1. Wellman ML, DiBartola SP, Kohn CW. Applied physiology of body fluids in dogs and cats. In: DiBartola SP, editor. Fluid, electrolyte and acid-base disorders in small animal practice. 3rd edition. St Louis (MO): Saunders- Elsevier; 2006. p. 3–26.
2. Rudloff E, Kirby R. Fluid therapy: crystalloids and colloids. Vet Clin North Am Small Anim Pract 1998;28(2):297–328.
3. Griffel MI, Kaufman BS. Pharmacology of colloids and crystalloids. Crit Care Clin 1992;8(2):235–53.
4. DiBartola SP, Bateman S. Introduction to fluid therapy. In: DiBartola SP, editor. Fluid, electrolyte, and acid-base disorders. 3rd edition. St Louis (MO): Saunders-Elsevier; 2006. p. 325–44.
5. Mathews KA. The various types of parenteral fluids and their indications. Vet Clin North Am Small Anim Pract 1998;28(3):483–513.
6. Silverstein DC, Aldrich J, Haskins SC, et al. Assessment of changes in blood volume in response to resuscitative fluid administration in dogs. J Vet Emerg Crit Care 2005;15(3):185–92.
7. Rozanski E, Rondeau M. Choosing fluids in traumatic hypovolemic shock: the role of crystalloids, colloids and hypertonic saline. J Am Anim Hosp Assoc 2002; 38(6):499–501.
8. Wingfield WE. Chapter 13 fluid and electrolyte therapy. In: Wingfield WE, Raffe MR, editors. The veterinary ICU book. Jackson Hole (WY): Teton Newmedia; 2002. p. 170.
9. MacMillan KL. Neurological complications following treatment of canine hypoadrenocorticism. Can Vet J 2003;44(6):490–2.
10. Drobatz KJ, Cole SG. The influence of crystalloid fluid type on acid-base and electrolyte status of cats with urethral obstruction. J Vet Emerg Crit Care 2008; 18(4):355–61.
11. Rose BD. Ch 3: the proximal tubule. In: Clinical physiology of acid-base and electrolyte disorders. 4th edition. New York: Mc-Graw-Hill, Inc; 1994. p. 87.
12. Graefe U, Milutinovich J, Follette WC, et al. Less dialysis-induced morbidity and vascular instability with bicarbonate in dialysate. Ann Intern Med 1978;88:332–6.
13. Walton RS, Wingfield WE, Ogilvie GK, et al. Energy expenditure in 104 Postoperative and traumatically injured dogs with indirect calorimetry. Vet Emerg Crit Care 1996;6(2):71–9.
14. O'Toole E, Miller CW, Wilson BA, et al. Comparison of the standard predictive equation for calculation of resting energy expenditure with indirect calorimetry in hospitalized and healthy dogs. J Am Vet Med Assoc 2004;225(1):58–64.
15. Culp AM, Clay ME, Baylor IA, et al. Colloid osmotic pressure and total solids measurements in normal dogs and cats. Abstract in: Proceedings of the 4th International Veterinary Emergency and Critical Care Symposium. San Antonio, Texas: Veterinary Emergency and Critical Care Society; 1994. p. 705.
16. Odunayo A, Kerl ME. Comparison of whole blood and plasma colloid osmotic pressure in healthy dogs. J Vet Emerg Crit Care (San Antonio) 2011;21(3): 236–41.
17. Brown SA, Dusza K, Boehmer J. Comparison of measured and calculated values for colloid osmotic pressure in hospitalized animals. Am J Vet Res 1994;55(7): 910–4.
18. Alphonsus CS, Rodseth RN. The endothelial glycocalyx: a review of the vascular barrier. Anaesthesia 2014;69:777–84.

19. Jdelicka J, Becker BF, Chappell D. Endothelial glycocalyx. Crit Care Clin 2020;36: 217–32.

20. Culler CA, Jazbik C, Guillaumin J. Comparison of albumin, colloid osmotic pressure, von Willebrand factor and coagulation factors in canine cryopoor plasma, cryoprecipitate and fresh frozen plasma. J Vet Emerg Crit Care 2017;27(6): 638–44.

21. Culler CA, Balakrishnan A, Yaxley PE, et al. Clinical use of cryopoor plasma continuous rate infusion in critically ill, hypoalbuminemic dogs. J Vet Emerg Crit Care 2019;29:314–20.

22. Ropski MK, Guillaumin J, Monnig AA, et al. Use of cryopoor plasma for albumin replacement and continuous antimicrobial infusion for treatment of septic peritonitis in a dog. J Vet Emerg Crit Care 2017;27(3):348–56.

23. Mazzaferro EM, Edwards T. Update on albumin therapy in critical illness. Vet Clin Small Anim 2020;50:1289–305.

24. Horowitz FFB Read RL, Powell LL. A retrospective analysis of 25% human serum albumin supplementation in hypoalbuminemic dogs with septic peritonitis. Can Vet J 2015;56:591–7.

25. Trow A, Rozanski E, de Laforcade A, et al. Evaluation of the use of human albumin in critically ill dogs: 73 cases (2003-2006). J Vet Intern Med 2008;233:607–12.

26. Mathews K, Barry M. The use of 25% human serum albumin: outcome and efficacy in raising serum albumin and systemic blood pressure in critically ill dogs and cats. J Vet Emerg Crit Care 2005;15:110–8.

27. Vigano F, Perissinotto L, Bosco V. Administration of 5% human serum albumin in critically ill small animal patients with hypoalbuminemia: 418 dogs and 170 cats (1994-2008). J Vet Emerg Crit Care 2010;20:237–43.

28. Vigano F, Blasi C, Carminato N, et al. Prospective review of clinical hypersensitivity reactions after administration of 5% human serum albumin in 40 critically ill cats. Top Companion Anim Med 2019;35:38–41.

29. Cohn L, Kerl M, Lenox C, et al. Response of healthy dogs to infusions of human serum albumin. Am J Vet Res 2007;68:657–63.

30. Francis AH, Martin L, Haldorson G, et al. Adverse reactions suggestive of type III hypersensitivity in six healthy dogs given human albumin. J Am Vet Med Assoc 2007;320:873–9.

31. Martin L, Luther T, Alperin D, et al. Serum antibodies against human albumin in critically ill and healthy dogs. J Am Vet Med Assoc 2008;232:1004–9.

32. Powell C, Thompson L, Murtaugh R. Type III hypersensitivity reaction with immune complex deposition in 2 critically ill dogs administered human serum albumin. J Vet Emerg Crit Care 2013;23(6):598–604.

33. Mazzaferro EM, Balakrishnan A, Hackner SG, et al. Delayed Type-III hypersensitivity reaction with acute kidney injury in two dogs following administration of concentrated human albumin during treatment of hypoalbuminemia secondary to septic peritonitis. J Vet Emerg Crit Care 2020;30(5):574–80.

34. Enders B, Musulin S, Holowaychuk M, et al. Repeated infusion of lyophilized canine albumin safely and effectively increases serum albumin and colloid osmotic pressure in healthy dogs. J Vet Emerg Crit Care 2018;28(S1):S5.

35. Craft EM, Powell LL. The use of canine-specific albumin in dogs with septic peritonitis. J Vet Emerg Crit Care 2012;22(6):631–9.

36. Hayes G, Benedicenti L, Mathews K. Retrospective cohort study on the incidence of acute kidney injury and death following hydroxyethyl starch (HES 10%, 250/ 0.5/5:1) administration in dogs (2007-2010). J Vet Emerg Crit Care 2016;26: 35–40.

37. Sigrist NE, Kalin N, Dreyfus A. Changes in serum creatinine concentration and acute kidney injury (AKI) grade in dogs treated with hydroxyethyl starch 130/0.4 from 2013-2016. J Vet Int Med 2017;31:434–41.
38. Schmid SM, Cianciolo RE, Drobatz KJ, et al. Postmorten renal tubular injury in 53 dogs. J Vet Emerg Crit Care 2019;29(3):279–87.
39. Boyd CJ, Sharp CR, Claus MA, et al. Prospective randomized controlled blinded clinical evaluation of biomarkers of acute kidney injury following 6% hydroxyethyl starch 130/0.4 or Hartmann's solution in dogs. J Vet Emerg Crit Care 2021;31:306–14.
40. Bruno B, Troia R, Dondi F, et al. Stage 1 Biomarkers of kidney injury in dogs undergoing constant rate infusion of hydroxyethyl starch 130/0.4. Animals (Basel) 2021;1199:2555.
41. Sigrist NE, Kalin N, Dreyfus A. Effects of hydroxyethyl starch 130/0.4 on serum creatinine concentration and the development of acute kidney injury in nonazotemic cats. J Vet Int Med 2017;31(6):1749–56.
42. Boyd CJ, Claus MA, Raisis AL, et al. Evaluation of biomarkers of kidney injury following 4% succinylated gelatin and 6% hydroxyethyl starch 130/0.4 administration in a canine hemorrhagic shock model. J Vet Emerg Crit Care 2019;29:132–42.
43. Yozova ID, Howard J, Sigrist N, et al. Current trends in volume replacement therapy and the use of synthetic colloids in small animals – An internet based survey (2016). Front Vet Sci 2017;4:140.
44. Chan DL. Colloids: current recommendations. Vet Clin North Am Small Anim Pract 2008;38(3):587–93.

Glucocorticoids, Cyclosporine, Azathioprine, Chlorambucil, and Mycophenolate in Dogs and Cats

Clinical Uses, Pharmacology, and Side Effects

Katrina R. Viviano, DVM, PhD, Dip. ACVIM, Dip. ACVCP*

KEYWORDS

- Immunosuppression • Steroids • Feline • Canine

KEY POINTS

- Provide an update on the clinical uses of the primary (glucocorticoids) and secondary (cyclosporine, azathioprine (dogs), chlorambucil, and mycophenolate) immunosuppressive drugs used in the management of immune-mediated diseases in dogs and cats.
- Highlight the common immunosuppressive drugs used in dogs and cats, including their mechanisms of action, pharmacokinetics, pharmacodynamics, and side effects that may impact their clinical use.
- Call attention to areas whereby new information may aid clinicians in using these immunosuppressive drugs. For example, high dose glucocorticoids and gastrointestinal bleeding, cyclosporine and therapeutic drug monitoring, and the emerging use of mycophenolate in dogs and cats.

INTRODUCTION

The body's immune system is essential for protecting it from various pathogens and other external insults. The immune system is tightly regulated and maintained through the complex interactions between the cells and mediators of both the innate and adaptive immune systems.

Immune-mediated diseases arise from the dysregulation of either the innate or adaptive immune systems or both.[1] The complexity of immune dysregulation is incompletely understood but is likely multifactorial, including inherent genetic factors and environmental triggers (ie, infectious agents, drugs, vaccines, or neoplasia). In some patients, the immune system may be appropriately or inappropriately triggered

Department of Medical Sciences, School of Veterinary Medicine, University of Wisconsin-Madison, 2015 Linden Drive, Madison, WI, USA
* Corresponding Author.
E-mail address: katrina.viviano@wisc.edu

Vet Clin Small Anim 52 (2022) 797–817
https://doi.org/10.1016/j.cvsm.2022.01.009
0195-5616/22/© 2022 Elsevier Inc. All rights reserved.

subsequently, leading to lymphocyte dysfunction. For example, failure of lymphocyte selection or the generation of antibodies or T cells directed toward self-antigens.[2] The inappropriately stimulated immune system produces a marked local or systemic inflammatory response leading to tissue destruction and clinical disease.

Some of the more common systemic inflammatory diseases with an immune-mediated etiology in dogs and cats included protein-losing enteropathy (PLE)/inflammatory bowel disease (IBD), immune-mediated anemias (immune-mediated hemolytic anemia (IMHA), precursor-directed immune-mediated anemia (PIMA)), immune-mediated thrombocytopenia (IMT), and immune-mediated polyarthritis (IMPA).[3] Despite the varying and incompletely understood pathogenic mechanisms or triggers among this group of diseases, immune dysfunction is central to tissue injury and the rationale for using immunomodulatory or immunosuppressive therapies. The treatment goals are to induce disease remission by inhibiting inflammation and modulating lymphocyte function while minimizing adverse drug effects.

This article focuses on the common immunosuppressive drugs used in dogs and cats, centering on updated or emerging drug information and how it may impact our clinical prescribing. Much of the use of these immunosuppressive drugs in dogs and cats is extrapolated from their use in people with similar immune-mediated disorders or organ transplant recipients. However, new information is constantly emerging to further our understanding and optimize the use of these immunosuppressive drugs in dogs and cats.

FIRST-LINE IMMUNOSUPPRESSIVE DRUGS
Glucocorticoids

Clinical Uses in Dogs and Cats: Glucocorticoids remain the mainstay of first-line treatment of inflammatory and immune-mediated diseases in dogs and cats despite their long list of clinically limiting side effects. The advantages of glucocorticoids are their systemic impact on both the innate and acquired immunity and their relatively rapid onset of action, thereby maintaining their role in the acute management of inflammatory/immune-mediated diseases. The use of glucocorticoids is in the treatment of a variety of canine and feline immune-mediated diseases including immune-mediated anemias, IMT, IMPA, and IBD.[4]

Despite the variety of immune-mediated diseases treated with glucocorticoids, the treatment goals are similar. During acute illness, using immunosuppressive doses to achieve clinical remission is followed by slowly tapering the dose of glucocorticoids to the lowest dose to control the inflammatory or immune-mediated disease targeted. On a case-by-case basis, glucocorticoids may be combined with other immunosuppressive agents to treat inflammatory or immune-mediated diseases in dogs and cats, especially in patients who are nonresponsive to glucocorticoids alone or have a severe life-threatening presentation.

Primary Mechanism of Action(s): Glucocorticoids affect most, if not all, cells of the body through their binding to the intracellular cytoplasmic glucocorticoid receptor.[5–7] Once the glucocorticoid-receptor complex translocates to the nucleus, it binds DNA glucocorticoid response elements influencing gene transcription.[8] The cellular effects of glucocorticoids are considered dose-dependent. At anti-inflammatory doses, glucocorticoids inhibit phospholipase A2 and the release of pro-inflammatory cytokines as well as stabilize granulocyte cell membranes. At immunosuppressive doses, glucocorticoids target macrophage function by downregulating Fc receptor expression, decreasing responsiveness to antibody-sensitized cells, and decreasing antigen processing.[9-12] Glucocorticoids suppress T cell function, induce apoptosis of T cells, and with chronic use, inhibit B cell antibody production in some patients.[7,13]

Pharmacokinetics (PKs)/Pharmacodynamics (PDs): Available glucocorticoids vary in their potency, route of administration, and duration of action.[14,15] The most common intermediate-acting systemic glucocorticoids used in veterinary medicine include prednisone/prednisolone (**Table 1**). Prednisone is a prodrug metabolized to its active form, prednisolone. Cats achieve higher plasma concentrations (4–5 times higher AUC) when administered oral prednisolone versus prednisone[16], suggesting that cats either have lower prednisone absorption and/or decreased prednisone conversion to prednisolone.

Alternative forms of glucocorticoids may be preferred in specific patient populations. In patients with severe malabsorption, injectable dexamethasone sodium phosphate may provide improved bioavailability as well as clinical response. Also, dexamethasone lacks mineralocorticoid activity minimizing sodium and water retention, which may be clinically significant in treating patients with underlying cardiovascular disease or diseases associated with fluid retention (eg, hypoalbuminemia, portal hypertension). The potency of dexamethasone is 4 to 10 times that of prednisone; therefore, a dose reduction is necessary when prescribing dexamethasone.[17,18]

In some patients, locally delivered glucocorticoids may be advantageous. Budesonide is an oral, locally active, high potency glucocorticoid formulated to exploit the pH differential between the proximal and distal small intestine, targeting budesonide's action to the distal intestinal tract. At the level of the enterocyte, budesonide is absorbed and delivered by the portal system to the liver. Approximately 80% to 90% of the absorbed budesonide undergoes first-pass metabolism, minimizing its systemic bioavailability. Some systemic absorption occurs, as evidenced by the blunted response to ACTH stimulation testing in dogs treated with budesonide at 3 mg/m^2 for 30 days.[19,20]

Budesonide is used in the management of Crohn's disease in people[21] and IBD in dogs.[22] In dogs with inflammatory enteropathies, a double-blinded, randomized trial compared glucocorticoid induction treatment with prednisone versus budesonide.[23] Over the 6 weeks of the study, there were no significant differences in disease remission rates, defined as greater than 75% reduction in the baseline canine IBD activity index, or side effects between the 2 glucocorticoids treatments.

In dogs and cats with inflammatory respiratory disease, locally delivered inhaled fluticasone may control clinical signs in patients with glucocorticoid responsive inflammatory airway disease, which minimizes the adverse systemic side effects of glucocorticoid treatment.[24-26]

Side Effects/Drug Interactions: The wide cellular/tissue distribution of the glucocorticoid receptor makes significant systemic effects unavoidable.[27] Adverse effects include the iatrogenic hyperadrenocorticism, adrenal gland suppression, gastrointestinal (GI) ulceration, insulin resistance and secondary diabetes mellitus, muscle catabolism, delayed wound healing, opportunistic infections, and behavior changes. Clinical signs of hyperadrenocorticism are more common in dogs, including polydipsia, polyuria, polyphagia, weight gain, and increased panting. In addition, some dogs experience elevated serum alkaline phosphatase activity secondary to the induction of the steroid-induced isoenzyme.[28] In cats, the development of diabetes mellitus can be associated with glucocorticoid treatment, especially over long durations or the use of long-acting glucocorticoid formulations.

The co-administration of glucocorticoid with nonsteroidal anti-inflammatory drugs (NSAIDs) is contraindicated due to the significant risk of GI ulceration or perforation.[29] However, steroids treatment alone can result in GI ulceration, especially in dogs treated with high doses or for long durations. Some dogs develop clinical signs associated with GI blood loss or anemia requiring aggressive glucocorticoid dose reductions. In healthy dogs, glucocorticoid treatment with prednisone (2 mg/kg/d) for 28 days resulted in endoscopic evidence of gastric ulceration after 14 days of treatment.[30] Interestingly, no dogs had clinical signs or biochemical changes associated with gastric ulcers over the 28 days of the glucocorticoid administration. However, the results of this study highlight that glucocorticoid-associated gastric ulceration can occur as early as 14 days into treatment and likely goes undetected based on bloodwork and clinical monitoring. In addition, it highlights the importance of monitoring and clinical vigilance during steroid treatment. When prescribing steroids, especially high doses consider a modest (25%) glucocorticoid dose reduction with the first 7 to 14 days, in patients with stable disease followed by a slower glucocorticoid taper based on the clinical status of the patient's underlying immune-mediated disease.[4]

Steroid side effects are common and best avoided by maintaining vigilance in your glucocorticoid therapeutic plan along with close monitoring. In patients with intolerable or life-threatening glucocorticoid side effects or those that lack any clinically significant response to steroids with 7 to 14 days are cases whereby alternative immunosuppressive drugs need consideration; continued high dose and long-duration steroids are unlikely to achieve a favorable clinical outcome.

Clinical care points

- *Glucocorticoids:* Because of the risk of GI bleeding in dogs, judicious use, including close monitoring for side effects (**Table 1**), is necessary to optimize clinical use, especially high-dose or long treatment durations. Glucocorticoid-associated gastric ulceration can occur as early as 14 days into treatment and may go clinically undetected. Concurrent use with NSAIDs is contraindicated.

SECOND-LINE IMMUNOSUPPRESSIVE DRUGS
Cyclosporine

Clinical Uses in Dogs and Cats: The initial use of cyclosporine in human and veterinary medicine was in the management of transplant recipients,[31,32] but cyclosporine uses continue to expand to include the treatment of inflammatory and immune-mediated diseases.[33] Specifically in veterinary medicine, cyclosporine is considered first-line therapy for perianal fistulas[34–38] keratoconjunctivitis sicca (KCS or dry eye),[39] and in some patients with atopic dermatitis.[40–42]

The use of cyclosporine in treating other inflammatory or immune-mediated diseases remains mainly as a second-line immunosuppressive drug. Examples include its use in the treatment of feline and canine IBD,[33,43,44] immune-mediated anemias,[4,45–47] IMT,[48,49] and IMPA.[50–52]

Primary Mechanism of Action(s): Cyclosporine binds to cytoplasmic cyclophilin, an immunophilin or highly conserved protein that acts as a protein-folding enzyme expressed in high concentration in T lymphocytes.[53–55,] The cyclosporine–cyclophilin complex binds and blocks the function of calcineurin, a serine/threonine phosphatase activated by increased intracellular calcium concentrations following T cell receptor activation. Calcineurin functions to dephosphorylate the nuclear factor of activated T cells (NFAT), enabling it to translocate into the nucleus, bind the nuclear transcription factor AP-1, and induce the transcription of genes for T cell activation. The cyclosporine–cyclophilin complex prevents the dephosphorylation of NFAT, decreasing the expression of IL-2 and other cytokines preventing further T cell activation. Decreased IL-2 concentrations attenuate the clonal proliferation of T and B lymphocytes. Cyclosporine also decreases the production of IL-3, IL-4, tissue necrosis factor-alpha (TNF-α), and interferon-gamma (INF-γ), altering the function of granulocytes, macrophages, NK cells, eosinophils, and mast cells. In small animal veterinary species, cyclosporine is reported *in vitro* and *in vivo* to decrease lymphocyte cytokine production in both canine and feline lymphocytes.[60,64–66]

Pharmacokinetics (PKs)/Pharmacodynamics (PDs): A patient's clinical response to cyclosporine can be challenging to predict due to inter-and intra-patient variability in drug exposure. Patient variability in response to cyclosporine is partly due to species or formulation differences and differences in the drug's PKs and PDs.[56] Patient factors that impact cyclosporine's PKs include gastric contents (presence or absence of food), intrinsic liver function, and concurrently administered medications.[57]

Despite the microemulsion formulation improving the intestinal absorption of cyclosporine, the disposition of orally administered cyclosporine remains variable. One recommendation to optimize the oral absorption of the veterinary-approved microemulsion of cyclosporine is to administer the capsules on an empty stomach. The standard recommendation is to administer cyclosporine capsules either 2 hours before or after a meal.[40,58]

Therapeutic drug monitoring (TDM) may guide cyclosporine's therapeutic use in some clinical patients. For example, patients who experience unexpected side effects or lack a clinical response to cyclosporine may benefit from TDM. The assay methods available to quantify cyclosporine concentrations vary and are dependent on the compartment analyzed (plasma vs whole blood) and analytical method used (immunoassay vs high-performance liquid chromatography (HPLC)).[59] For PK assessments, whole blood cyclosporine concentrations determined by HPLC are the recommended compartment to sample and preferred quantification method.[56] Other important information needed as part of TDM is the patient's clinical history, concurrent medications, and the timing of the blood collection. Cyclosporine concentrations 2 hours after dosing represent cyclosporine peak concentrations. Cyclosporine concentrations just before the next dose represent cyclosporine trough concentrations. Peak concentrations may be more representative of treatment efficacy whereby trough concentrations may help assess excessive whole blood concentrations or toxicity.[56]

In veterinary medicine, the targeted blood concentrations of cyclosporine necessary to effectively treat immune-mediated diseases are not as clearly established as in transplant medicine. For example, extrapolated from transplant medicine trough whole blood cyclosporine levels between 400 and 600 ng/mL and peak concentrations of 800 and 1400 ng/mL have been recommended as the therapeutic target in veterinary medicine for efficacy and safety.[60–62] Interestingly, a suggested therapeutic goal for cyclosporine in the treatment of immune-mediated cytopenias in people is a whole blood trough cyclosporine concentration between 150 and 250 ng/mL for a maximum of 3 to 4 months followed by maintenance therapy with the minimum dosage to maintain remission.[63]

Limited clinical therapeutic data are available for cyclosporine in treating immune-mediated diseases in dogs and cats. In one retrospective study in cats with pure red cell aplasia, cyclosporine combined with glucocorticoids resulted in clinical improvement. In 5 cats trough cyclosporine concentrations were available that ranged from 96 to 368 ng/mL (median 218).[47] Others have recommended cyclosporine trough concentrations of 250 ng/mL for IBD and 100 to 600 ng/mL for perianal fistulas.[56] However, trough levels may not reliably predict clinical response.

Recent work has investigated monitoring a patient's immune response to cyclosporine by determining the percentage of T cell suppression compared with a normal individual of the same species through the assessment of IL-2 expression. Available PD assays report lymphocyte suppression as a range from low to marked, providing a PD measure of cyclosporine's effect on the patient's immune system.[56] PD monitoring is currently limited to people and dogs and not yet available in cats.[56,67,]

The clinical use of cyclosporine PD testing is conducted in collaboration with other patient information and cyclosporine whole blood concentrations to aid clinicians in tailoring cyclosporine treatment. Ideally, the goal is to dose cyclosporine to control the patient's underlying immune-mediated disease yet minimize toxicity and side effects. For example, a dog with IMHA who lacks a clinical response to cyclosporine with a concurrently low cyclosporine blood concentration and low lymphocyte suppression may benefit from a cyclosporine dose increase. Alternatively, a dog with stable IMHA and marked lymphocyte suppression or high cyclosporine concentrations may suggest a patient that would benefit from a cyclosporine dose reduction.

TDM offers a way to integrate a patient's clinical response with their whole blood cyclosporine concentrations and associated lymphocyte response. TDM is recommended once cyclosporine concentrations reach steady-state, approximately 5 to 7 days, an estimate based on the variable cyclosporine half-life in dogs.[56] In dogs, the concurrent assessment of peak whole blood cyclosporine concentrations (2 hours after dosing) with cyclosporine PD testing is recommended. However, research continues to explore additional immunosuppressive markers that parallel cyclosporine's clinical response, including the use of drug exposure,[68,69] T cell cytokine expression,60[,70] and lymphocyte-specific proliferation.[71]

Side Effects/Drug Interactions: Historically, the use of cyclosporine has centered around its glucocorticoid "sparing effects," relative rapid onset of immunosuppression, and potential for less systemic adverse effects. Mild GI upset following oral cyclosporine administration is the most common side effect. The GI signs associated with cyclosporine can be managed in some dogs and cats and may not require drug discontinuation. GI upset can be transient or responsive to dose reduction. Other approaches to control cyclosporine GI upset include concurrent treatment with metoclopramide or maropitant or administering cyclosporine as frozen capsules.[58,72,73]

Severe systemic cyclosporine side effects requiring drug discontinuation include gingival hyperplasia, opportunistic infections, hepatotoxicity, anaphylaxis,[47] thromboembolic complications,[74] and lymphoproliferative disorders.[75–77] Gingival hyperplasia may require cyclosporine discontinuation in some patients. However, in a small case series, treatment with azithromycin improved gingival hyperplasia in 6 dogs treated with long-term cyclosporine for the treatment of atopy (n = 5) or perianal fistulas (n = 1).[78] Some of the reported opportunistic infections associated with cyclosporine administration include bacterial infections (pyelonephritis, pneumonia, pyoderma, pyometra, pericarditis, and septic arthritis), fungal infections especially when concurrently treated with glucocorticoids, and protozoal infections (toxoplasmosis, neosporosis).[61,79–84]

Cyclosporine is a substrate of cytochrome P450 enzyme CYP3A. Drug–drug interactions may result when drugs that inhibit or induce CYP3A are concurrently administered with cyclosporine. Cyclosporine is also a substrate of the drug transporter, P-glycoprotein, which also influences its disposition and leads to potential drug interactions or unexpected adverse effects.[56] For example, higher than expected cyclosporine-induced immunosuppression occurred in a dog heterozygous for the MDR-1 mutation, a case report highlighting the role of TDM to tailor treatment in patients treated with cyclosporine.[85] Other clinically relevant drug interactions reported in dogs as a result of the decreased cyclosporine metabolism and increased cyclosporine blood levels include its co-administered with azole antifungals,[32,38,86,87] clarithromycin,[88] and grapefruit juice.[89,90] The co-administration of cyclosporine with ketoconazole is often used therapeutically to decrease the dose and cost of cyclosporine while maintaining therapeutic blood levels.[32,38] The presumed mechanism of this exploited drug interaction is via the inhibition of CYP3A and/or P-glycoprotein efflux.[91] In cats, decreased cyclosporine concentrations occurred with cyclosporine co-administrated with phenobarbital (CYP3A and P-glycoprotein inducer).[92]

CLINICAL CARE POINTS

- *Cyclosporine:* Therapeutic drug monitoring may help guide use in patients that experience unexpected side effects or lack a clinical response to cyclosporine (**Table 1**). The concurrent assessment of peak whole blood cyclosporine concentrations (2 hours after dosing) with cyclosporine PD testing is recommended in dogs.

Azathioprine

Clinical Uses in Dogs: Uses of azathioprine in people are for the treatment of immune-mediated disease and in organ transplant medicine.[93] Its treating immune-mediated diseases in dogs, azathioprine's use is partly due to its glucocorticoid "sparing effect," which enables sustained disease remission while tapering or following glucocorticoid withdrawal. Its effectiveness in the treatment of acute immune-mediated illness is limited based on its delayed efficacy of days to weeks.[94,95] Few controlled studies evaluating the use of azathioprine in treating immune-mediated disease in dogs are available; therefore, its use is reliant on published retrospective studies and consensus recommendations provided in treatment guidelines, for example, in the treatment of IMHA.[4,96–98]

Primary Mechanism of Action(s): Azathioprine is a thiopurine that is a prodrug of 6-mercaptopurine (6-MP).[99,100] In the liver and other peripheral tissues (eg, erythrocytes), 6-MP is enzymatically oxidized to inactive metabolites 6-thiouric acid via xanthine oxidase or methylated via thiopurine methyltransferase (TPMT) to 6-methylmercaptopurine (6-MMP). The 6-thioguanine nucleotides (6-TGNs) arise via hypoxanthine phosphoribosyltransferase (HPRT), the active metabolites responsible for the therapeutic and cytotoxic effects of azathioprine. 6-TGNs compete with endogenous purines for incorporation into RNA and DNA, creating nonfunctional DNA and RNA and disrupting mitosis. Azathioprine targets cell-mediated immunity, specifically lymphocytes, due to its lack of a salvage pathway for purine biosynthesis. Through its inhibition of de novo purine synthesis, azathioprine interferes with lymphocyte proliferation, reduces lymphocyte numbers, and decreases T cell-dependent antibody synthesis.

Pharmacokinetics (PKs)/Pharmacodynamics (PDs): In people, TPMT activity is variable and correlates with clinical outcomes including therapeutic efficacy and toxicity. Due to genetic polymorphisms, some individuals have increased or decreased TMPT activity. Decreased TMPT activity is associated with an increased risk of azathioprine-induced myelosuppression due to increased substrate availability for HRPT and the generation of cytotoxic 6-TGNs.

TPMT activity is variable in dogs with a 9-fold difference reported, including lower TMPT activity in giant schnauzers and higher TMPT activity in Alaskan malamutes.[101] Compared with dogs or people, cats have decreased TMPT activity that increases their risk of toxicity and the rationale to avoid using azathioprine in cats.[102,103]

Side Effects/Drug Interactions: The most common side effects attributed to azathioprine administration and subsequent drug withdrawal in people and dogs include GI upset (vomiting and diarrhea), myelosuppression, hepatotoxicity, and pancreatitis.[104,105]

Myelosuppression correlates with low TMPT activity in people. Dogs seem to have similar TMPT activity compared with people. In people and dogs, azathioprine myelosuppression is a delayed response that is reversible following drug withdrawal. Dose-dependent neutropenia and thrombocytopenia occur in dogs within the first 3 months of treatment, which parallels the reports of myelosuppression in people.[96,106–108] The estimated prevalence of myelosuppression is 8% to 13% in dogs.

In dogs, the estimated prevalence of azathioprine hepatotoxicity was 15%, as reported in a recent retrospective study.[107] The median time after starting azathioprine to hepatotoxicity, defined by a $\geq$ 2-fold increase in alanine aminotransferase (ALT) was 2 weeks. Interestingly, despite the increases in ALT, no dogs experienced clinical signs of hepatotoxicity or biochemical markers of liver failure. Due to the risk of hepatitis and hepatic necrosis before and after the initiation of azathioprine therapy, liver enzymes monitoring is recommended. In people, hepatotoxicity correlates with increased erythrocyte 6-MMP concentrations.[109] In rats, liver necrosis associated with azathioprine administration results in oxidative damage, glutathione depletion, and marked increases in alanine transaminase activity (ALT).[110]

Allopurinol, a xanthine oxidase inhibitor, results in a significant increase in 6-TGNs concentrations, increasing the risk of azathioprine toxicity (ie, myelosuppression). In people, historically concurrent treatment with azathioprine and allopurinol was considered contraindicated or minimally required a significant azathioprine dose reduction to avoid this drug–drug interaction.[111] Interestingly, in people with high TPMT activity and IBD nonresponsive to azathioprine therapy, the concurrent administration of allopurinol with azathioprine increases 6-TGN concentrations and induced disease remission.[112–114]

CLINICAL CARE POINTS

- *Azathioprine*: Use in cats is not recommended. In some dogs, azathioprine-associated myelosuppression or hepatotoxicity may limit its clinical use; therefore, monitoring is recommended (**Table 1**).

Chlorambucil

Clinical Uses in Dogs and Cats: Prospective clinical studies evaluating the use of chlorambucil as an immunosuppressive agent are lacking. Most of the published studies in cats focus on the use of chlorambucil as a chemotherapeutic agent in the treatment of lymphoma.[115–117]

Despite the lack of data, chlorambucil is the cytotoxic drug of choice in cats. Its role as second-line immunosuppressive therapy in cats is most common in the treatment of IBD that is either severe or poorly responsive to prednisolone therapy.[118–120] In a recent case series of cats with idiopathic IMT chlorambucil was successful as a second-tier drug in one cat that failed to achieve remission with prednisone alone.[49]

In dogs, chlorambucil is less commonly used in the treatment of immune-mediated disease. In a retrospective study, prednisone combined with chlorambucil was compared with prednisone combined with azathioprine in dogs with PLE.[121] Prednisone/chlorambucil was suggested to be more efficacious in achieving disease remission relative to prednisone/azathioprine. Clinical markers of disease improvement included serum albumin concentrations, weight gain, and median survival.

Primary Mechanism of Action(s): Chlorambucil is a nitrogen mustard derivative and prodrug converted in the liver to its active metabolite, phenylacetic acid. It is a cell-cycle nonspecific, cytotoxic, alkylating agent capable of cross-linking DNA.

Chlorambucil targets B cells and is considered a slow-acting immunosuppressive agent that may require 2 weeks to reach therapeutic efficacy.

Pharmacokinetics (PKs)/Pharmacodynamics (PDs): Limited information is available regarding the PKs or PDs of chlorambucil in cats. Information from other species describes chlorambucil as a highly protein-bound drug that undergoes liver metabolism. The active metabolite phenylacetic acid mustard is further metabolized in the liver to inactive metabolites that are excreted in the urine.[122]

Side Effects/Drug Interactions: In cats, chlorambucil has fewer side effects than azathioprine. Cytotoxic myelosuppression and GI toxicity are associated with chlorambucil administration. Myelosuppression is considered mild and generally occurs 7 to 14 days following the start of therapy. Neurotoxicity (ie, reversible myoclonus) has been reported in a cat in association with a chlorambucil overdose.[123] In a case series, acquired Fanconi syndrome occurred in 4 cats treated with glucocorticoids and chlorambucil for underlying primary GI disease (IBD, n = 2; small cell lymphoma, n = 2).[124]

CLINICAL CARE POINTS

- *Chlorambucil:* More commonly used immunosuppressive drug in cats compared with dogs (**Table 1**). In cats, side effects can include myelosuppression, reversible myoclonus, and acquired Fanconi syndrome.

Mycophenolate

Clinical Uses in Dogs and Cats: Mycophenolate use in treating immune-mediated disease in veterinary medicine continues to increase. Its initial use in dogs was primarily extrapolated from its use as an immunosuppressant in people to prevent allograft rejection in transplant patients,[125–127] and the treatment of immune-mediated diseases.[128–130] The role of mycophenolate as an immunosuppressive agent in veterinary medicine continues to expand with an increasing number of manuscripts, initially as case reports or cases series but more recently multiple retrospective studies have been published describing its use in dogs and cats. Canine diseases reported to be treated with mycophenolate alone or combined with other immunosuppressive agents include immune-mediated anemias,[4,131–133] IMT,[134,135] IMPA,[136] myasthenia gravis,[137,138] meningoencephalomyelitis,[139,140] immune-mediated glomerulonephritis,[141] and immune-mediated skin disease.[142,143]

A retrospective study in dogs with IMT evaluated for the duration of hospitalization and survival (30-day and 60-day) found no difference between the dogs treated with combination glucocorticoids and cyclosporine or glucocorticoids and mycophenolate.[135] Interestingly, the dogs treated with glucocorticoids and mycophenolate experienced less adverse effects. Others have reported glucocorticoids combined with mycophenolate was efficacious in treating IMHA in dogs, with similar outcomes when compared with other immunosuppressive protocols.[131,132]

The use of mycophenolate in cats with immune-mediated disease is beginning to emerge in the literature. The available case reports in cats suggest mycophenolate may be effective and well-tolerated when combined with prednisolone. For example, mycophenolate was successfully in 2 cats with refractory IMHA and a cat with IMPA[144,145]

Primary Mechanism of Action(s): Mycophenolate is the prodrug of mycophenolic acid (MPA), a potent, selective, noncompetitive, reversible inhibitor of inosine-5'-monophosphate dehydrogenase (IMPDH), specifically the type II isoform of IMPDH.[54,130] IMPDH catalyzes the rate-limiting step of the *de novo* biosynthesis of guanosine nucleotides that converts inosine monophosphate to guanosine mono-phosphate. The IMPDH type II isoform is more susceptible to MPA than the type I iso-form (expressed in many cell types) and more abundant in activated lymphocytes. In addition, T and B lymphocytes are entirely dependent on the *de novo* pathway for pu-rine synthesis, differentiation, proliferation, and immunoglobulin production. Myco-phenolate action and immunosuppressive effects are selective for lymphocytes via the depletion of guanosine and deoxyguanosine nucleotides.

Pharmacokinetics (PKs)/Pharmacodynamics (PDs): Work in healthy dogs suggests the PK of mycophenolate in dogs likely parallels that of people with some patient to patient variability.[146–149] For use in people, mycophenolate is available as an immediate-release formulation of mycophenolate mofetil (MMF) or as enteric-coated mycophenolate acid (EC-MPS) formulated to target small intestinal drug absorption. In people, the enteric-coated formulation may minimize the MMF-associated GI intolerance. A modified release mycophenolate formulation for potential development in dogs showed similar lymphocyte inhibition to immediate release MMF in healthy beagles.[149]

Mycophenolate's active metabolite, MPA, undergoes enterohepatic recirculation, contributing to drug–drug interactions and altered drug exposure. The excreted MPA-7-O-glucuronide metabolite undergoes hydrolysis to MPA following biliary excretion in the GI tract. MPA is highly protein binding (82%–97%) that may impact the concentration of free drug available in patients with hypoalbuminemia[150] Myco-phenolate's hepatic metabolism to the active (MPA) and inactive metabolites occur in part via glucuronidation in dogs and people.[148,151] In healthy cats, a recent PK study documented that cats can biotransform MMF to MPA.[152,153] *Ex vivo* studies suggest mycophenolate to MPA metabolism in cats is likely via glucosidation.[154] In healthy cats, the plasma disposition of MMF was variable as reported in other species.[152]

In people, MPA exposure targets for either transplant recipients or lupus patients include the area under the curve (AUC0-12h) ranging from 30 to 60 mg h/L.[151] Other studies targeted plasma MPA concentrations of 1 to 5 μg/mL.[155,156] In transplant pa-tients, there is a reported 10-fold variation in drug exposure.[151] Factors that may impact drug exposures include underlying liver and kidney function, drug–drug inter-actions, and genetic factors. In people, PD monitoring focuses on IMPDH inhibition; IMPDH catalytic activity is inversely related to MPA concentrations. A similar approach for TDM of mycophenolate in dogs and cats is limited to research studies. However, with more experience and continued studies, specific PK and PD targets may be iden-tified in dogs and cats to assist clinical use.

Side Effects/Drug Interactions: Side effects reported in people treated with myco-phenolate include GI upset, opportunistic infections, allergic reactions, neutropenia, and lymphoma.[130,157] GI upset is the most commonly reported side effect that is dose-dependent and reversible with dose reduction or drug discontinuation.[158,159]

Limited information is available about the side effects of mycophenolate in dogs and cats. The primary side effect reported in dogs treated with oral mycophenolate is diar-rhea that can limit its use in some dogs.[132,136,137,146] Of the published studies in dogs treated with mycophenolate, lower mycophenolate doses (mean 15 mg/kg/d) seemed to be better tolerated.[160] Allergic reactions have been reported with the administration of parenteral mycophenolate in dogs.[161]

In healthy cats, GI side effects associated with mycophenolate occurred when dosed at 15 mg/kg q8 hours in 3/3 cats, 15 mg/kg q12 hours in 2/3 cats and no GI side effects in the 3 cats treated at 10 mg/kg q12 hours.[152] A single case report described the potential for hepatotoxicity and pancreatitis in a cat with IMHA treated with mycophenolate.[162]

Drug interactions reported in people treated with mycophenolate that resulted in decreased mycophenolate bioavailability may also be clinically relevant in veterinary patients. Consider possible drug–drug interactions in patients nonresponsive to mycophenolate receiving concurrent medications. The concurrent administration of mycophenolate with either fluoroquinolones or metronidazole may reduce the enterohepatic circulation of mycophenolate.[163] If an enteric-coated formulation of oral mycophenolate is not used, the higher gastric pH achieved with proton pump inhibitors may reduce the dissolution of mycophenolate and decreases drug exposure.[164]

Cyclosporine decreases mycophenolate exposure via the inhibition of the enterohepatic recirculation of mycophenolate due to reduced biliary excretion of the glucuronide metabolite by multidrug resistance protein 2 transporter (MRP-2).[165] Glucocorticoids induce the uridine diphosphate-glucuronosyltransferase (UGT) enzyme system increasing the metabolism of mycophenolate.[166] The concurrent use of mycophenolate with azathioprine is not recommended based on the increased risk for bone marrow suppression.[130]

CLINICAL CARE POINTS

- *Mycophenolate:* Increased clinical use in dogs and emerging uses in cats (**Table 1**). Diarrhea is a clinically important side effect that seems to be dose-dependent. Limiting dosages to 10 mg/kg q12 hours in dogs and cats seems to minimize mycophenolate-associated diarrhea.

Table 1
A comparison of the mechanism of action, common starting immunosuppressive dosage(s), and side effects/drug interactions of the more common immunosuppressive therapies used in treating immune-mediated or inflammatory diseases of dogs and cats

Drug	MOA	Dosage(s)	Side Effects/Drug Interactions
Glucocorticoids Prednisone Prednisolone	Via the intracellular cytoplasmic GC receptor, binds DNA glucocorticoid response elements influencing gene transcription	Canine/Feline:* Immunosuppression: 2 mg/kg/day PO; for dogs > 30 kg maximum dose of 60 mg/day; Anti-inflammatory: 0.5 to 1 mg/kg/day PO; for dogs > 30 kg maximum dose of 40 mg/day.	Polydipsia, polyuria, polyphagia Gastrointestinal ulceration Diabetes mellitus Delayed wound healing Behavior changes
Cyclosporine	Calcineurin inhibitor	Canine/Feline: 4–5 mg/kg PO q12 hr	GI upset, gingival hyperplasia, hepatotoxicity, opportunistic infections, anaphylaxis (IV) Potential drug interactions – ketoconazole, clarithromycin,

(continued on next page)

Table 1
(continued)

Drug	MOA	Dosage(s)	Side Effects/Drug Interactions
			grapefruit juice, phenobarbital
Azathioprine	Thiopurine analog – disrupts DNA/RNA synthesis	Canine: 2 mg/kg PO q24 hr × 7 d than 1 mg/kg PO q48 hr	GI upset, myelosuppression, hepatic necrosis Potential drug interactions - allopurinol
Chlorambucil	Alkylating agent – cell cycle nonspecific	Feline IBD: 2 mg/cat PO q48–72 h or 20 mg/m^2 PO q14 d[119]	GI upset, myelosuppression
Mycophenolate	Purine synthesis inhibitor	Canine: 7.5–10 mg/kg PO q12 hr[150]	Diarrhea, weight loss, allergic reaction Potential drug interactions -FQ, metronidazole, PPIs, GC, cyclosporine

Abbreviations: FQ, fluoroquinolones; GC, glucocorticoids; GI, gastrointestinal; MOA, mechanism of action; PPIs, proton pump inhibitors.

FOOTNOTE: *If dexamethasone, sodium phosphate is desired instead of prednisone/prednisolone, dosing is determined based on the patient's calculated prednisone/prednisolone dose; dividing the prednisone mg dose by 7 to account for dexamethasone's higher potency. For example, in a 20 kg dog treated with 2 mg/kg/day (40 mg/day) of prednisone, the calculated daily dexamethasone, sodium phosphate dose would be 5.7 mg.

SUMMARY

The treatment of immune-mediated disease in dogs and cats continues to evolve as new therapies are introduced or adapted from human medicine. Glucocorticoids remain the first-line treatment of many cats and dogs with immune-mediated or inflammatory diseases.

Often second-line therapies are introduced due to the patient's lack of response to glucocorticoids, intolerable side effects associated with glucocorticoids, or may be introduced early in the disease treatment due to the patient's severe life-threatening clinical presentation. The incorporation of cyclosporine, mycophenolate, azathioprine (dogs), or chlorambucil into our treatment protocols in dogs and cats with immune-mediated diseases continues to increase as second-line therapies. However, their use is clinician and patient-dependent. **Table 1** summarizes these common immunosuppressive drugs used in dogs and cats.

New drugs continue to emerge for patients with refractory disease or intolerable side effects associated with the standard immunosuppressive therapies. As we adopt emerging immunosuppressive therapeutics for veterinary patients, our knowledge of their therapeutic efficacy and potential for side effects remains limited. Ultimately, any immunosuppressive treatment protocol goals are to initially achieve disease remission while minimizing side effects, followed by a gradual taper of drug(s) to the lowest dose(s) to maintain disease remission or, in some cases, successful drug withdrawal.

DISCLOSURE

The author has nothing to disclose.

REFERENCES

1. Kuchroo VK, Ohashi PS, Sartor RB, et al. Dysregulation of immune homeostasis in autoimmune diseases. Nat Med 2012;18:42–7.
2. Davidson A, Diamond B. Autoimmune diseases. N Engl J Med 2001;345: 340–50.
3. Gershwin LJ. Autoimmune diseases in small animals. Vet Clin North Am Small Anim Pract 2010;40:439–57.
4. Swann JW, Garden OA, Fellman CL, et al. ACVIM consensus statement on the treatment of immune-mediated hemolytic anemia in dogs. J Vet Intern Med 2019;33:1141–72.
5. Cain DW, Cidlowski JA. Immune regulation by glucocorticoids. Nat Rev Immunol 2017;17:233–47.
6. Ferguson D, Hoenig M. Glucocorticoids, Mineralocorticoids, Adrenolytic Drugs. In: Riviere JE,Papich MG, editor. Veterinary Pharmacology and Therapeutics. 10th edition. Ames (IA): Wiley-Blackwll; 2018. p. 729–62.
7. Zen M, Canova M, Campana C, et al. The kaleidoscope of glucorticoid effects on immune system. Autoimmun Rev 2011;10:305–10.
8. Ashwell JD, Lu FW, Vacchio MS. Glucocorticoids in T cell development and function*. Annu Rev Immunol 2000;18:309–45.
9. Al-Ghazlat S. Immunosuppressive therapy for canine immune-mediated hemolytic anemia. Compend Contin Educ Vet 2009;31:33–41.
10. Buttgereit F, Scheffold A. Rapid glucocorticoid effects on immune cells. Steroids 2002;67:529–34.
11. Friedman D, Netti F, Schreiber AD. Effect of estradiol and steroid analogues on the clearance of immunoglobulin G-coated erythrocytes. J Clin Invest 1985;75: 162–7.
12. Gernsheimer T, Stratton J, Ballem PJ, et al. Mechanisms of response to treatment in autoimmune thrombocytopenic purpura. N Engl J Med 1989;320: 974–80.
13. Miller E. Immunosuppressive therapy in the treatment of immune-mediated disease. J Vet Intern Med 1992;6:206–13.
14. Viviano KR. Update on immunosuppressive therapies in dogs and cats. Vet Clin North Am Small Anim Pract 2013;43:1149–70.
15. Plumb DC. Plumb's veterinary drugs. Tulsa (OK): Educational Concepts, LLC (dba Brief Media); 2015.
16. Graham-Mize C, Rosser E. Bioavailability and activity of prednisone and prednisolone in the feline patient [abstract]. Vet Dermatol 2004;15:7.
17. Ballard PL, Carter JP, Graham BS, et al. A radioreceptor assay for evaluation of the plasma glucocorticoid activity of natural and synthetic steroids in man. J Clin Endocrinol Metab 1975;41:290–304.
18. Cantrill HL, Waltman SR, Palmberg PF, et al. In vitro determination of relative corticosteroid potency. J Clin Endocrinol Metab 1975;40:1073–7.
19. Stroup ST, Behrend EN, Kemppainen RJ, et al. Effects of oral administration of controlled-ileal-release budesonide and assessment of pituitary-adrenocortical axis suppression in clinically normal dogs. Am J Vet Res 2006;67:1173–8.

20. Tumulty JW, Broussard JD, Steiner JM, et al. Clinical effects of short-term oral budesonide on the hypothalamic-pituitary-adrenal axis in dogs with inflammatory bowel disease. J Am Anim Hosp Assoc 2004;40:120–3.

21. De Cassan C, Fiorino G, Danese S. Second-generation corticosteroids for the treatment of Crohn's disease and ulcerative colitis: more effective and less side effects? Dig Dis 2012;30:368–75.

22. Pietra M, Fracassi F, Diana A, et al. Plasma concentrations and therapeutic effects of budesonide in dogs with inflammatory bowel disease. Am J Vet Res 2013;74:78–83.

23. Dye TL, Diehl KJ, Wheeler SL, et al. Randomized, controlled trail of budesondie and prednisone for the treatment of idiopathic inflammatory bowel disease. J Vet Intern Med 2013;27:1385–91.

24. Bexfield NH, Foale RD, Davison LJ, et al. Management of 13 cases of canine respiratory disease using inhaled corticosteroids. J Small Anim Pract 2006;47:377–82.

25. Cohn LA, DeClue AE, Cohen RL, et al. Effects of fluticasone propionate dosage in an experimental model of feline asthma. J Feline Med Surg 2010;12:91–6.

26. Leemans J, Kirschvink N, Clercx C, et al. Effect of short-term oral and inhaled corticosteroids on airway inflammation and responsiveness in a feline acute asthma model. Vet J 2012;192:41–8.

27. Galon J, Franchimont D, Hiroi N, et al. Gene profiling reveals unknown enhancing and suppressive actions of glucocorticoids on immune cells. FASEB J 2002;16:61–71.

28. Pettersson H, Ekstrand C, Hillstrom A, et al. Effect of 1 mg/kg oral prednisolone on biochemical analytes in ten dogs: a cross-over study. Comp Clin Pathol 2021;30:519–28.

29. Boston SE, Moens NM, Kruth SA, et al. Endoscopic evaluation of the gastroduodenal mucosa to determine the safety of short-term concurrent administration of meloxicam and dexamethasone in healthy dogs. Am J Vet Res 2003;64:1369–75.

30. Whittemore JC, Mooney AP, Price JM, et al. Clinical, clinicopathologic, and gastrointestinal changes from aspirin, prednisone, or combination treatment in healthy research dogs: A double-blinded randomized trial. J Vet Intern Med 2019;33:1977–87.

31. Calne RY, White DJ, Thiru S, et al. Cyclosporin A in patients receiving renal allografts from cadaver donors. Lancet 1978;2:1323–7.

32. McAnulty JF, Lensmeyer GL. The effects of ketoconazole on the pharmacokinetics of cyclosporine A in cats. Vet Surg 1999;28:448–55.

33. Makielski K, Cullen J, O'Connor A, et al. Narrative review of therapies for chronic enteropathies in dogs and cats. J Vet Intern Med 2019;33:11–22.

34. Griffiths LG, Sullivan M, Borland WW. Cyclosporin as the sole treatment for anal furunculosis: preliminary results. J Small Anim Pract 1999;40:569–72.

35. Hardie RJ, Gregory SP, Tomlin J, et al. Cyclosporine treatment of anal furunculosis in 26 dogs. J Small Anim Pract 2005;46:3–9.

36. Mathews KA, Sukhiani HR. Randomized controlled trial of cyclosporine for treatment of perianal fistulas in dogs. J Am Vet Med Assoc 1997;211:1249–53.

37. O'Neill T, Edwards GA, Holloway S. Efficacy of combined cyclosporine A and ketoconazole treatment of anal furunculosis. J Small Anim Pract 2004;45:238–43.

38. Patricelli AJ, Hardie RJ, McAnulty JE. Cyclosporine and ketoconazole for the treatment of perianal fistulas in dogs. J Am Vet Med Assoc 2002;220:1009–16.

39. Moore CP. Immunomodulating agents. Vet Clin North Am Small Anim Pract 2004;34:725–37.
40. Guaguere E, Steffan J, Olivry T, et al. a new drug in the field of canine dermatology. Vet Dermatol 2004;15:61–74.
41. Olivry T, Foster AP, Mueller RS, et al. Interventions for atopic dermatitis in dogs: a systemic review of randomised controlled trials. Vet Dermatol 2010;21:4–22.
42. Steffan J, Favrot C, Mueller R. A systemic review and meta-analysis of the efficacy and safety of cyclosporin for the treatment of atopic dermatitis in dogs. Vet Dermatol 2006;17:3–16.
43. Allenspach K, Rufenacht S, Sauter S, et al. Pharmacokinetics and clinical efficacy of cyclosporine treatment of dogs with steroid-refractory inflammatory bowel disease. J Vet Intern Med 2006;20:239–44.
44. Webb CB. Feline inflammatory bowel disease. NAVC Clin Br 2012;11–4.
45. Black V, Adamantos S, Barfield D, et al. Feline non-regenerative immune-mediated anemia: Features and outcome in 15 cases. J Feline Med Surg 2016;18: 597–602.
46. Grundy SA, Barton C. Influence of drug treatment on survival of dogs with immune-mediated hemolytic anemia: 88 cases (1989-1999). J Am Vet Med Assoc 2001;218:543–6.
47. Viviano KR, Webb JL. Clinical use of cyclosporine as an adjunctive therapy in the management of feline idiopathic pure red cell aplasia. J Feline Med Surg 2011;13:885–95.
48. Nakamura RK, Tompkins E, Bianco D. Therapeutic options for immune-mediated thrombocytopenia. J Vet Emerg Crit Care (San Antonio) 2012;22: 59–72.
49. Wondratschek C, Weingart C, Kohn B. Primary immune-mediated thrombocytopenia in cats. J Am Anim Hosp Assoc 2010;46:12–9.
50. Inkpen H. Student paper communicaton: chronic progressive polyarthritis in a domestic shorthair cat. Can Vet J 2015;56:621–3.
51. Oohashi E, Yamanda K, Oohashi M, et al. Chronic progressive polyarthritis in a female cat. J Vet Med Sci 2010;72:511–4.
52. Rhoades AC, Vernau W, Kass PH, et al. Comparison of the efficacy of prednisone and cyclosporine for treatment of dogs with primary immune-mediated polyarthritis. J Am Vet Med Assoc 2016;248:395–404.
53. Stahelin H. Cyclosporin A. Historical background. Prog Allergy 1986;38:19–27.
54. Halloran PF. Molecular mechanisms of new immunosuppressants. Clin Transplant 1996;10:118–23.
55. Whitley NT, Day MJ. Immunomodulatory drugs and their application to the management of canine immune-mediated disease. J Small Anim Pract 2011;52: 70–85.
56. Archer TM, Fellman CL, Stokes JV, et al. Pharmacodynamic monitoring of canine T-cell cytokine responses to oral cyclosporine. J Vet Intern Med 2011;25:1391–7.
57. Aronson LR, Stumhofer JS, Drobatz KJ, et al. Effect of cyclosporine, dexamethasone, and human CTLA4-Ig on production of cytokines in lymphocytes of clinically normal cats and cats undergoing renal transplantation. Am J Vet Res 2011;72:541–9.
58. Cridge H, Kordon A, Pinchuk LM, et al. Effects of cyclosporine on feline lymphocytes activated in vitro. Vet Immunol Immunopathol 2020;219:109962.
59. Fellman CL, Stokes JV, Archer TM, et al. Cyclosporine A affects the in vitro expression of T cell activation-related molecules and cytokines in dogs. Vet Immunol Immunopathol 2011;140:175–80.

60. Archer TM, Booth DM, Langston VC, et al. Oral cyclosporine treatment in dogs: A review of the literature. J Vet Intern Med 2014;28:1–20.
61. Whalen RD, Tata PN, Burckart GJ, et al. Species differences in the hepatic and intestinal metabolism of cyclosporine. Xenobiotica 1999;29:3–9.
62. Steffan J, Strehlau G, Maurer M. Cyclosporin A pharmacokinetics and efficacy in the treatment of atopic dermatitis in dogs. J Vet Pharmacol Ther 2004;27:231–8.
63. Trifilio SM, Scheetz M, Borensztajn J, et al. Variability of cyclosporine concentrations by HPLC and TDX monoclonal assay methods, application of a correction factor, and description of a novel clinical approach to determine the practical consequences of changing assay technique. Clin Transpl 2012;27(1):154–61.
64. Dedeaux A, Grooters A, Wakamatu-Utsuki N, et al. Opportunitic fungal infections in small animals. J Am Anim Hosp Assoc 2018;54:327–37.
65. Nam HS, McAnulty JF, Kwak HH, et al. Gingival overgrowth in dogs associated with clinically relevant cyclosporine blood levels: observations in a canine renal transplantation model. Vet Surg 2008;37:247–53.
66. Teramura M, Kimura A, Iwase S, et al. Treatment of severe aplastic anemia with antithymocyte globulin and cyclosporin A with or without G-CSF in adults: a multicenter randomized study in Japan. Blood 2007;110:1756–61.
67. Colombo S, Sartori R. Ciclosporin and the cat. Current understanding and review of clinical use. J Feline Med Surg 2018;20:244–55.
68. Mehl ML, Kyles AE, Craigmill AL, et al. Disposition of cyclosporine after intravenous and multi-dose oral administration in cats. J Vet Pharmacol Ther 2003;26: 349–54.
69. Nashan B, Cole E, Levy G, et al. Clinical validation studies of Neoral C(2) monitoring: a review. Transplantation 2002;73:S3–11.
70. Fellman CL, Archer TM, Wills RW, et al. Effects of cyclosporine and dexamethasone on canine T cell expression of interleukin-2 and interferon-gamma. Vet Immunol Immunopathol 2019;216:109892.
71. Nafe LA, Dodam JR, Reinero CR. Ex vivo immunosuppression of canine t lymphocyte-specific proliferation using dexamethasone, cyclosporine, and active metabolites of azathioprine and leflunomide in a flow cytometric assay. Can J Vet Res 2012;78(3):168–75.
72. Bachtel JC, Pendergraft JS, Rosychuk RAW, et al. Comparision of the stability and pharmacokinetics in dogs of modified ciclosporin capsulte stored at -20oC and room temperature. Vet Dermatol 2015;26:228–e250.
73. Whitehouse W, Viviano K. Update in feline therapeutics: clinical use of 10 emerging therapies. J Feline Med Surg 2015;17:220–34.
74. Thomason J, Lunsford K, Stokes J, et al. The effects of cyclosporine on platelet function and cyclooxygenase expression in normal dogs. J Vet Intern Med 2012; 26:1389–401.
75. Namikawa K, Maruo T, Honda M, et al. Gingivial overgrowth in a dog that received long-term cyclosporine for immune-mediated hemolytic anemia. Can Vet J 2012;53:67–70.
76. Robson D. Review of the pharmacokinetics, interactions and adverse reactions of cyclosporine in people, dogs and cats. Vet Rec 2003;152:739–48.
77. Schmiedt CW, Grimes JA, Holzman G, et al. Incidence and risk factors for development of malignant neoplasia after feline renal transplantation and cyclosporine-based immunosuppression. Vet Comp Oncol 2009;7:45–53.
78. Diesel A, Moriello K. Medical managment of cyclosporine-induced gingival overgrowth using oral azithromycin in six dogs. Vet Sci 2015;2:13–22.

79. Dowling SR, Webb J, Foster JD, et al. Opportunistic fungal infections in dog treated with ciclosporin and glucocoriticoids: Eight cases. J Small Anim Pract 2016;57:105–9.

80. Galgut BI, Janardhan KS, Grondin TM. Detection of Neospora caninum tachyzoites in cerebropinal fluid of a dog following prednisone and cyclosporin therapy. Vet Clin Pathol 2010;39:386–90.

81. High EJ, Olivry T. The prevalence of bacterial infection during cyclosporine therapy in dogs: a critically appraised topic. Can Vet J 2020;61:1283–9.

82. Lappin MR, VanLare KA, Seewald W, et al. Effect of oral administration of cyclosporine on Toxoplasma gondii infection status of cats. Am J Vet Res 2015;76: 351–7.

83. Mohri T, Takashima K, Yamane T. Purulent pericarditis in a dog administered immune-suppressive drugs. J Vet Med Sci 2009;71:669–72.

84. Radowicz SN, Power HT. Long-term use of cyclosporine in the treatment of canine atopic dermatitis. Vet Dermatol 2005;16:18–86.

85. Mackin AJ, Riggs C, Beatty T, et al. Excessive cyclosporine-associated immunosuppression in a dog heterozygous for the MDR1 (ABCB1-1Δ) mutation. J Am Anim Hosp Assoc 2020;56:190–5.

86. Katayama M, Igarashi H, Fukai K, et al. Fluconazole decreases cyclosporine dosage in renal transplanted dogs. Res Vet Sci 2010;89:124–5.

87. Katayama M, Katayama R, Kamishina H. Effects of multiple oral dosing of itraconazole on the pharmacokinetics of cyclosporine in cats. J Feline Med Surg 2010;12:512–4.

88. Katayama M, Nishijima N, Okamura Y, et al. Interaction of clarithromycin with cyclosporine in cats: pharmacokinetic study and case report. J Feline Med Surg 2012;14:257–61.

89. Amatori FM, Meucci V, Giusiani M, et al. Effect of grapefruit juice on the pharmacokinetics of cyclosporine in dogs. Vet Rec 2004;154:180–1.

90. Radwanski NE, Cerundolo R, Shofer FS, et al. Effects of powdered whole grapefruit and metoclopramide on the pharmacokinetics of cyclosporine in dogs. Am J Vet Res 2011;72:687–93.

91. Trepanier LA. Cytochrome P450 and its role in veterinary drug interactions. Vet Clin North Am Small Anim Pract 2006;36:975–85, v.

92. Hoshino Y, Inden T, Otaka R, et al. Interaction of cyclosporine with phenobarbital in cats: a preliminary study. J Vet Med Sci 2019;81:1621–3.

93. Kruh J, Foster CS. Corticosteroid-sparing agents: conventional systemic immunosuppressants. Dev Ophthalmol 2012;51:29–46.

94. Harkin KR, Phillips D, Wilkerson M. Evaluation of azathioprine on lesion severity and lymphocyte blastogenesis in dogs with perianal fistulas. J Am Anim Hosp Assoc 2007;43:21–6.

95. Ogilvie GK, Felsburg PJ, Harris CW. Short-term effect of cyclophosphamide and azathioprine on selected aspects of the canine blastogenic response. Vet Immunol Immunopathol 1988;18:119–27.

96. Piek CJ, Junius G, Dekker A, et al. Idiopathic immune-mediated hemolytic anemia: treatment outcome and prognostic factors in 149 dogs. J Vet Intern Med 2008;22:366–73.

97. Reimer ME, Troy GC, Warnick LD. Immune-mediated hemolytic anemia: 70 cases (1988-1996). J Am Anim Hosp Assoc 1999;(35):384–91.

98. Weinkle TK, Center SA, Randolph JF, et al. Evaluation of prognostic factors, survival rates, and treatment protocols for immune-mediated hemolytic anemia in dogs: 151 cases (1993-2002). J Am Vet Med Assoc 2005;226:1869–80.

99. Aarbakke J, Janka-Schaub G, Elion GB. Thiopurine biology and pharmacology. Trends Pharmacol Sci 1997;18:3–7.
100. Elion GB. The george Hitchings and Gertrude Elion Lecture. The pharmacology of azathioprine. Ann N Y Acad Sci 1993;685:400–7.
101. Kidd LB, Salavaggione OE, Szumlanski CL, et al. Thiopurine methyltransferase activity in red blood cells of dogs. J Vet Intern Med 2004;18:214–8.
102. Beale KM, Altman D, Clemmons RR, et al. Systemic toxicosis associated with azathioprine administration in domestic cats. Am J Vet Res 1992;53:1236–40.
103. Salavaggione OE, Yang C, Kidd LB, et al. Cat red blood cell thiopurine S-methyltransferase: companion animal pharmacogenetics. J Pharmacol Exp Ther 2004;308:617–26.
104. Houston DM, Taylor JA. Acute pancreatitis and bone marrow suppression in a dog given azathioprine. Can Vet J 1991;32:496–7.
105. Schwab M, Schaffeler E, Marx C, et al. Azathioprine therapy and adverse drug reactions in patients with inflammatory bowel disease: impact of thiopurine S-methyltransferase polymorphism. Pharmacogenetics 2002;12:429–36.
106. Hassankhani M, Aldavood SJ, Khosravi A, et al. The effects of prolonged azathioprine adminitration on blood cells, lymphocytes, and immunoglobulins of Iranian mixed-breed dogs. Iran J Vet Med 2017;11:361–76.
107. Wallisch K, Trepanier LA. Incidence, timing, and risks factors of azathioprine hepatotoxicosis in dogs. J Vet Intern Med 2015;29:513–8.
108. Chun JY, Kang B, Lee YM, et al. Adverse events associated with azathioprine treatment in korean pediatric inflammatory bowl disease patients. Pediatr Gastroenterol Hepatol Nutr 2013;16:171–7.
109. Dubinsky MC, Lamothe S, Yang HY, et al. Pharmacogenomics and metabolite measurement for 6-mercaptopurine therapy in inflammatory bowel disease. Gastroenterology 2000;118:705–13.
110. El-Beshbishy HA, Tork OM, El-Bab MF, et al. Antioxidant and antiapoptotic effects of green tea polyphenols against azathioprine-induced liver injury in rats. Pathophysiology 2011;18:125–35.
111. Berns A, Rubenfeld S, Rymzo WT Jr, et al. Hazard of combining allopurinol and thiopurine. N Engl J Med 1972;286:730–1.
112. Ansari A, Elliott T, Baburajan B, et al. Long-term outcome of using allopurinol cotherapy as a strategy for overcoming thiopurine hepatotoxicity in treating inflammatory bowel disease. Aliment Pharmacol Ther 2008;28:734–41.
113. Govani SM, Higgins PD. Combination of thiopurines and allopurinol: adverse events and clinical benefit in IBD. J Crohns Colitis 2010;4:444–9.
114. Sparrow MP, Hande SA, Friedman S, et al. Allopurinol safely and effectively optimizes tioguanine metabolites in inflammatory bowel disease patients not responding to azathioprine and mercaptopurine. Aliment Pharmacol Ther 2005; 22:441–6.
115. Barrs VR, Beatty JA. Feline alimentary lymphoma: 2. Further diagnostics, therapy and prognosis. J Feline Med Surg 2012;14:191–201.
116. Kiselow MA, Rassnick KM, McDonough SP, et al. Outcome of cats with low-grade lymphocytic lymphoma: 41 cases (1995-2005). J Am Vet Med Assoc 2008;232:405–10.
117. Lingard AE, Briscoe K, Beatty JA, et al. Low-grade alimentary lymphoma: clinicopathological findings and response to treatment in 17 cases. J Feline Med Surg 2009;11:692–700.
118. Jergens AE. Feline idiopathic inflammatory bowel disease: what we know and what remains to be unraveled. J Feline Med Surg 2012;14:445–58.

119. Trepanier L. Idiopathic inflammatory bowel disease in cats. Rational treatment selection. J Feline Med Surg 2009;11:32–8.

120. Willard MD. Feline inflammatory bowel disease: a review. J Feline Med Surg 1999;1:155–64.

121. Dandrieux JRS, Noble PJM, Scase TJ, et al. Comparison of a chlorabmucil-prednisolone combination with an azathioprine-prednisolone combination for treatment of chronic enteropathy with concurrent protein-losing enteropathy in dogs: 27 cases (2007-2010). J Am Vet Med Assoc 2013;242:1705–14.

122. Ehrsson H, Walllin I, Simonsson B, et al. Effect of food on pharmacokinetics of chlorambucil and its main metabolite, phenylacetic acid mustard. Eur J Clin Pharmacol 1984;27:111–4.

123. Benitah N, de Lorimier LP, Gaspar M, et al. Chlorambucil-induced myoclonus in a cat with lymphoma. J Am Anim Hosp Assoc 2003;39:283–7.

124. Reinert NC, Feldman DG. Acquired Fanconi syndrome in four cats treated with chlorambucil. J Feline Med Surg 2016;18:1034–40.

125. Czaja AJ. Diagnosis, pathogenesis, and treatment of autoimmune hepatitis after liver transplantation. Dig Dis Sci 2012;57:2248–66.

126. Danovitch GM. Mycophenolate mofetil: a decade of clinical experience. Transplantation 2005;80:S272–4.

127. Ritter ML, Pirofski L. Mycophenolate mofetil: effects on cellular immune subsets, infectious complications, and antimicrobial activity. Transpl Infect Dis 2009;11:290–7.

128. Drosos AA. Newer immunosuppressive drugs: their potential role in rheumatoid arthritis therapy. Drugs 2002;62:891–907.

129. Juel VC, Massey JM. Myasthenia gravis. Orphanet J Rare Dis 2007;2:44.

130. Orvis AK, Wesson SK, Breza TS Jr, et al. Mycophenolate mofetil in dermatology. J Am Acad Dermatol 2009;60:183–99 [quiz: 200-182].

131. Wang A, Smith JR, Creevy KE. Treatment of canine idiopathic immune-mediated haemolytic anaemia with mycophenolate mofetil and glucocorticoids: 30 cases (2007 to 2011). J Small Anim Pract 2013;54:399–404.

132. West LD, Hart JR. Treatment of idiopathic immune-mediated hemolytic anemia with mycophenolate mofetil in five dogs. J Vet Emerg Crit Care (San Antonio) 2014;24:226–31.

133. Yuki M, Sugimoto N, Otsuka H, et al. Recovery of a dog from aplastic anaemia after treatment with mycophenolate mofetil. Aust Vet J 2007;85:495–7.

134. Yau VK, Bianco D. Treatment of five haemodynamically stable dogs with immune-mediated thrombocytopenia using mycophenolate mofetil as single agent. J Small Anim Pract 2014;55:330–3.

135. Cummings FO, Rizzo SA. Treatment of presumptive primary immune-mediated thrombocytopenia with mycophenolate mofetil versus cyclosporine in dogs. J Small Anim Pract 2017;58:96–102.

136. Fukushima K, Lappin M, Legare M, et al. A retrospective study of adverse effects of mycophenolate mofetil administration to dogs with immune-mediated disease. J Vet Intern Med 2021;35:2215–21.

137. Dewey CW, Cerda-Gonzalez S, Fletcher DJ, et al. Mycophenolate mofetil treatment in dogs with serologically diagnosed acquired myasthenia gravis: 27 cases (1999-2008). J Am Vet Med Assoc 2010;236:664–8.

138. Abelson AL, Shelton GD, Whelan MF, et al. Use of mycophenolate mofetil as a rescue agent in the treatment of severe generalized myasthenia gravis in three dogs. J Vet Emerg Crit Care (San Antonio) 2009;19:369–74.

139. Barnoon I, Shamir MH, Aroch I, et al. Retrospective evaluation of combined my-cophenolate mofetil and prednisone treatment for meningoencephalomyelitis of unknown etiology in dogs: 25 cases (2005-2011). J Vet Emerg Crit Care (San Antonio) 2016;26:116–24.

140. Woolcock AD, Wang A, Haley A, et al. Treatment of canine meningoencephalo-myelitis of unknown aetiology with mycophenolate mofetil and coritcosteroids: 25 cases (2007-2012). Vet Med Sci 2016;(2):125–35.

141. Segev G, Cowgill LD, Heiene R, et al. Consensus receommendations for immu-nosuppressive treatment of dogs with glomerular disease based on established pathology. J Vet Intern Med 2013;27:S44–54.

142. Ackermann AL, May ER, Frank LA. Use of mycophenolate mofetil to treat immune-mediated skin disease in 14 dogs - a retrospective evaluation. Vet Der-matol 2017;28:195, e144.

143. Ginel PJ, Blanco B, Lucena R, et al. Steroid-sparing effect of mycophenolate mofetil in the treatment of a subepidermal blistering autoimmune disease in a dog. J S Afr Vet Assoc 2010;81:253–7.

144. Bacek LM, Macintire DK. Treatment of primary immune-mediated hemolytic ane-mia with mycophenolate mofetil in two cats. J Vet Emerg Crit Care (San Antonio) 2011;21:45–9.

145. Tamura Y, Nagamoto T, Segawa K, et al. Successful treatment and long-term follow up of idiopathic immune-mediated polyarthritis with mycophenolate mofe-til in a cat. J Feline Med Surg Open Rep 2020;6. 2055116920963995.

146. Chanda SM, Sellin JH, Torres CM, et al. Comparative gastrointestinal effects of mycophenolate mofetil capsules and enteric-coated tablets of sodium-mycophenolic acid in beagle dogs. Transpl Proc 2002;34:3387–92.

147. Langman LJ, Shapiro AM, Lakey JR, et al. Pharmacodynamic assessment of mycophenolic acid-induced immunosuppression by measurement of inosine monophosphate dehydrogenase activity in a canine model. Transplantation 1996;61:87–92.

148. Machka C, Lange S, Werner J, et al. Everolimus in combination with mycophe-nolate mofetil as pre- and post-transplantation immunosuppression after non-myeloablative hematopoietic stem cell transplantation in canine littermates. Biol Blood Marrow Transpl 2014;20:1301–6.

149. Klotsman M, Sathyan G, Anderson WH. Single-dose pharmacokinetics of myco-phenolic acid following administration of immediate-release mycophenolate mo-fetil in healthy Beagle dogs. J Vet Pharmacol Ther 2021;44.

150. Klotsman M, Sathyan G, Anderson WH, et al. Mycophenolic acid in patients with immune-mediated inflammatory diseases: From humans to dogs. J Vet Pharma-col Ther 2019;42:127–38.

151. Rahman ANA, Tett SE, Staatz CE. Clinical pharmacokinetic and pharmacody-namics of mycophenolate in patients with autoimmune disease. J Clin Pharma-cokinet 2013;52:303–31.

152. Slovak JE, Hwang JK, Rivera SM, et al. Pharmacokinetics of mycophenolic acid and its effect on CD4+ and CD8+ T cells after oral administration of mycophe-nolate mofetil to healthy cats. J Vet Intern Med 2019;33:2020–8.

153. Slovak JE, Rivera SM, Hwang JK, et al. Pharmacokinetics of mycophenolic acid after intravenous administration of mycophenolate mofetil in healthy cats. J Vet Intern Med 2017;31:1827–32.

154. Slovak JE, Mealey K, Court MH. Comparative metabolism of mycophenolic acid by glucuronic acid and glucose conjugation in human, dog, and cat liver micro-somes. J Vet Pharmacol Ther 2017;40:123–9.

155. Gajarski RJ, Crowley DC, Zamberlan MC, et al. Lack of correlation between MMF dose and MPA level in pediatric and young adult cardiac transplant patients: Does the MPA level matter? Am J Transpl 2004;4:1495–500.
156. Dipchand AI, Pietra B, McCrindle BW, et al. Mycophenolic acid levels in pediatric heart transplant recipients receiving mycophenolate mofetil. J Heart Lung Transpl 2001;20:1035–43.
157. Behrend M. Adverse gastrointestinal effects of mycophenolate mofetil: aetiology, incidence and management. Drug Saf 2001;24:645–63.
158. Arns W, Breuer S, Choudhury S, et al. Enteric-coated mycophenolate sodium delivers bioequivalent MPA exposure compared with mycophenolate mofetil. Clin Transpl 2005;19:199–206.
159. Staatz CE, Tett SE. Pharmacology and toxicology of mycophenolate in organ transplant recipients: An update. Arch Toxicol 2014;88:1351–89.
160. Lacerda RP, Pena Gimenez MT, Laguna F, et al. Corneal grafting for the treatment of full-thickness corneal defects in dogs: A review of 50 cases. Vet Ophthalmol 2017;20:222–31.
161. Dewey CW, Booth DM. Pharmacokinetics of single-dose oral and intravenous mycophenolate mofetil adminstraton in normal dogs (abstract). J Vet Intern Med 2001;15:304.
162. Kopke MA, Galloway PEJ. Suspected hepatopathy and pancreatitis associated with mycophenolate mofetil use in a cat with immune-mediated hemolytic anemia. JFMS Open Rep 2020;6. 2055116920905038.
163. Naderer OJ, Dupuis RE, Heinzen EL, et al. The influence of norfloxacin and metronidazole on the disposition of mycophenolate mofetil. J Clin Pharmacol 2005;45:219–26.
164. Gabardi S, Olyaei A. Evaluation of potential interactions between mycophenolic acid derivatives and proton pump inhibitors. Ann Pharmacother 2012;46: 1054–64.
165. Manitpisitkul W, McCann E, Lee S, et al. Drug interactions in transplant patients: what everyone should know. Curr Opin Nephrol Hypertens 2009;18:404–11.
166. Lam S, Partovi N, Ting LS, et al. Corticosteroid interactions with cyclosporine, tacrolimus, mycophenolate, and sirolimus: fact or fiction? Ann Pharmacother 2008;42:1037–47.

Asymptomatic Canine Degenerative Valve Disease

Diagnosis and Current and Future Therapies

Sonya G. Gordon, DVM, DVSc*, Ashley B. Saunders, DVM,
Sonya R. Wesselowski, DVM, MS

KEYWORDS

- Chronic • Mitral valve • Myxomatous • Preclinical • Stage B2 • Treatment

KEY POINTS

- Asymptomatic mature dogs with systolic heart murmurs characteristic of mitral regurgitation should undergo diagnostics to establish a diagnosis and accurately stage the disease severity.
- Treatment is not recommended in dogs with Stage B1 degenerative valve disease.
- Treatment with pimobendan is recommended in dogs with Stage B2 degenerative valve disease characterized by sufficient left heart enlargement.
- Follow-up and client communication regarding monitoring for the development of clinical signs remains a cornerstone of therapy in all stages of degenerative valve disease.
- Left mainstem bronchial compression and pulmonary hypertension represent common sequelae of degenerative valve disease that can complicate the diagnosis of congestive heart failure.

INTRODUCTION

Degenerative valve disease (DVD) is the leading cause of heart disease and heart failure in dogs and has many recognized aliases, including myxomatous mitral valve disease, chronic degenerative valvular disease, endocardiosis of the atrioventricular valves, and mitral valve disease.[1,2] Older small-breed dogs are predisposed, but large breeds are also at risk as they age.[1] Although dogs of any breed can develop DVD, some breeds, such as the Cavalier King Charles spaniel (CKCS), are known to suffer from a higher incidence overall and may be affected at younger ages, although their typical course of progression is not different from other small-breed dogs.[3,4] Affected large-breed dogs may experience more rapid progression.[5] The etiology of DVD remains unknown, but there is likely a genetic component in some breeds, such as the CKCS.[2,3]

Department of Small Animal Clinical Sciences, College of Veterinary Medicine and Biomedical Sciences, Texas A&M University, College Station, TX 77843-4474, USA
* Corresponding author.
E-mail address: sgordon@cvm.tamu.edu

Vet Clin Small Anim 52 (2022) 819–840
https://doi.org/10.1016/j.cvsm.2022.01.010
0195-5616/22/© 2022 Elsevier Inc. All rights reserved.

vetsmall.theclinics.com

The underlying pathophysiology of DVD is characterized primarily by myxomatous degeneration of the mitral valve and associated chordae tendineae with concurrent involvement of the tricuspid valve in approximately 30% of cases.[1] The degenerating mitral ± tricuspid valves become incompetent, leading to increasing volumes of regurgitation, commensurate volume overload, and associated atrial and ventricular chamber enlargement. Degeneration of the mitral valve is typically most severe, leading to progressive left atrial and left ventricular enlargement.

DVD is most often identified during the long asymptomatic stage and progresses slowly over years; however, individual dogs may experience more rapid progression. Initial detection of DVD is usually related to the identification of a left apical systolic murmur characteristic of mitral regurgitation (MR) in a dog with no past or present clinical signs attributable to congestive heart failure (CHF). A staging scheme for DVD was introduced in the 2009 American College of Veterinary Internal Medicine (ACVIM) consensus statement,[6] with a revised version published in 2019[7] (**Table 1**). These guidelines provide an outline for diagnosis, treatment, and monitoring recommendations in dogs across the DVD severity spectrum. In the original guidelines, dogs in stage B1 were defined as asymptomatic dogs with normal left heart size whereas stage B2 encompassed asymptomatic dogs with evidence of left-sided cardiomegaly (atrial, ventricular, or both). The revised guidelines have now opted to refine the criteria for delineating stage B1 from stage B2 with the inclusion criteria from the EPIC (Evaluation of Pimobendan In dogs with preclinical myxomatous mitral valve disease and Cardiomegaly) clinical trial[8] (**Box 1**) due to strong evidence produced from this trial that dogs meeting or exceeding these physical examination, echocardiographic, and radiographic criteria experienced a significant and clinically relevant delay in the onset of CHF, among other benefits, with chronic administration of pimobendan.

Table 1
Degenerative Valve Disease Staging Scheme

A	• Dogs, who based on signalment (age, breed/weight), have an increased risk of developing DVD.		
B	• Dogs in Stage B have never suffered from any signs or symptoms attributable to CHF due to DVD. • This is the asymptomatic or preclinical Stage of DVD. • All dogs with Stage B DVD have a characteristic MR murmur without sufficient cardiac chamber enlargement	B1	• Normal heart size • Cardiac enlargement < that required for a diagnosis of B2
		B2	• Sufficient left-sided cardiac chamber enlargement
C	• Stage C stands for CHF (cardiogenic pulmonary edema) • Dogs with past or current signs or symptoms of CHF in the presence of a characteristic MR murmur and obvious cardiac chamber enlargement. • Dogs with Stage C can be 'stable' on CHF therapies or suffer from 'active' signs or symptoms of CHF.		
D	• This is the end or refractory Stage of CHF due to DVD. • Dogs in this Stage typically progress from Stage C (i.e., do not jump from Stage B to D) • Stage D dogs continue to suffer from persistent or intermittent clinical signs or symptoms that limit their quality of life despite appropriate therapies		

Abbreviations: CHF, congestive heart failure; DVD, degenerative valve disease; MR, mitral regurgitation
Adapted from the 2019 ACVIM Consensus Statement[7]

In this article, we focus on stage B1 and B2 DVD, the asymptomatic stage of DVD when dogs have no current or previous clinical signs or symptoms attributable to CHF. We will discuss the diagnosis of these two stages and how this has evolved as a result of new evidence and publication of the 2019 ACVIM consensus statement. We will also address current and future therapies, including the impact of recent evidence on the current recommendations for asymptomatic DVD. Finally, a few special considerations in stage B DVD will be highlighted.

DIAGNOSIS OF STAGE B1 AND B2 DVD

Asymptomatic dogs with left apical systolic murmurs characteristic of MR should undergo baseline diagnostics to establish the etiology of the murmur and stage of the disease. Given the treatment implication now tied to the diagnosis of stage B2 DVD versus stage B1 DVD, accurate identification of these two stages has become more clinically important. As outlined in **Box 1**, the EPIC inclusion criteria that now define stage B2 require both radiographic and echocardiographic evidence of left-sided cardiomegaly, including a radiographic vertebral heart size[9] (VHS) greater than 10.5 (**Fig. 1**B), 2-dimensional left atrial–aortic ratio[10] (2DLA:Ao) of 1.6 or greater (**Fig. 2**), and normalized left ventricular internal diameter in diastole[11] (LVIDDN) of 1.7 or greater (**Fig. 3**), in addition to a characteristic left apical systolic heart murmur of moderate-to-loud intensity ($\geq$grade 3/6).[8] In keeping with these criteria, both radiographs and an echocardiogram should ideally be part of the screening process for asymptomatic dogs with DVD. This allows a definitive diagnosis of DVD to be made and for accurate staging according to both radiographic and echocardiographic indices. Additionally, obtaining baseline two-view radiographs in a dog with asymptomatic DVD is beneficial from a monitoring perspective and serves as a point of comparison for future radiographs if clinical signs have developed and CHF is suspected.

Although echocardiography is ideal, availability and expense put this diagnostic test out of reach for many clients. In these cases, reliance on radiographic assessment of cardiac size with VHS has often been used in combination with signalment and physical examination findings. Although a VHS of 10.5 or greater is considered to exceed the 95% confidence interval of the normal reference range,[9] reliance on this cutoff alone to identify cardiac enlargement has the potential to be inaccurate. Furthermore, there are known breed-related differences in normal VHS reference ranges, with much

---

Box 1
Summary of EPIC study inclusion criteria:

- Asymptomatic small-breed dog

- No concurrent or prior treatment with cardiac medications such as an ACE inhibitor

- No evidence of a serious systemic disease expected to limit the dogs survival or require treatment with a cardiovascular medication during the study (for example, dogs requiring amlodipine for treatment of systemic hypertension were not eligible for inclusion).

- Heart murmur characteristic of MR ($\geq$3/6)

- Radiographic cardiomegaly (VHS > 10.5) (see **Fig. 1**)

- Echocardiographic criteria:
  - Evidence of DVD (MR and valvular changes), and
  - Left atrial enlargement 2-dimensional left atrial-aortic ratio (2DLA:Ao) $\geq$ 1.6[10] and (see **Fig. 2**)
  - Normalized left ventricular internal dimension (LVIDDN) $\geq$ 1.7 (see **Fig. 3**)
    - Calculation of LVIDDN[11]

higher normal VHS ranges reported in some breeds, including the CKCS.[12,13] With this in mind, it is prudent to use a higher VHS cutoff if recommendations for treatment are based solely on history, physical examination, and thoracic radiographs. The ACVIM consensus statement recommends a VHS cutoff of 11.5 or greater for this indication.[7] This cutoff was initially based on the results of previous studies, demonstrating that dogs with asymptomatic DVD and a VHS of 11.5 to 12.5[14,15] had a significant increase in risk of developing left-sided CHF in the near (6–12 months) future. In addition, the median VHS of dogs in the EPIC study was approximately 11.5.[8] Subsequently, additional studies comparing radiographic and echocardiographic heart size have produced data supporting the 11.5 VHS cutoff as having good specificity for identifying DVD dogs meeting echocardiographic criteria for stage B2 in both mixed populations of dogs and in CKCS specifically[16] (including two unpublished datasets of the authors), although other studies have reported higher VHS cutoffs ranging between 11.7 and 12.25 as having optimal specificity (ie, minimizing the rate of false positives) for identifying stage B2.[17–19] An additional factor to consider is the rate of progression of heart enlargement. Relatively large increases in heart size, even if the VHS is less than 11.5, are known to be associated with an increased risk of CHF in dogs with DVD.[15] Therefore, another criterion to consider is an increase in VHS from one recheck to the next, with an increase in VHS of 0.5 or more in 6 months being a supported benchmark for recommending pimobendan treatment.[20] Use of a VHS of 11.5 or

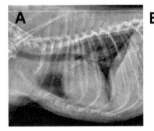 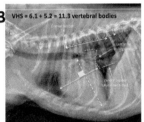 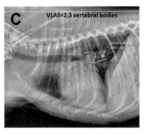

Fig. 1. Accurate measurement of VHS and VLAS is an important aspect of staging DVD, which helps to determine therapeutic recommendations and can be used to monitor disease progression. (*A*) Right lateral radiograph from a dog with asymptomatic DVD. (*B*) Measurement of VHS: *Step 1-VHS.* Identify the long axis of the heart (*dashed line*) beginning at the bottom of the carina (*dashed circle*) and ending at the apex. *Step 2-VHS.* Identify the short axis of the heart (*solid line*) at the level of the ventral border of the caudal vena cava and perpendicular (90°) to the long axis. This is typically the widest portion of the heart but may not be in dogs with severe left atrial enlargement. *Step 3-VHS.* Identify the 4th thoracic vertebra (T4) and place two lines equal in length to the long- and short-axis lines at the beginning of T4 parallel to the vertebrae. *Step 4-VHS.* Determine the length of both lines to the nearest 0.1 thoracic vertebra and add them together. The sum of both lines is the VHS. Note: The vertebral disc space is considered to be part of the vertebra that precedes it and should be taken into account when estimating to the nearest 0.1 thoracic vertebra. The normal canine VHS reference range is 8.7 to 10.5.[9] (*C*) Measurement of VLAS: *Step 1-VLAS.* Identify the bottom of the carina (as per Step 1-VHS). *Step 2-VLAS.* Identify the intersection of the dorsal border of the caudal vena cava and the caudal aspect of the cardiac silhouette. *Step 3-VLAS.* Join the landmarks identified in Steps 2 and 3. *Step 4-VLAS.* Identify the 4th thoracic vertebra (T4) and place a line equal in length of the line drawn in Step-3-VLAS parallel to the vertebrae. *Step 4-VLAS.* Determine the length of the line to the nearest 0.1 thoracic vertebra. This is the VLAS. Note: The vertebral disc space is considered to be part of the vertebra that precedes it and should be taken into account when estimating to the nearest 0.1 thoracic vertebra. The normal canine VLAS reference range is 1.4 to 2.2[23].

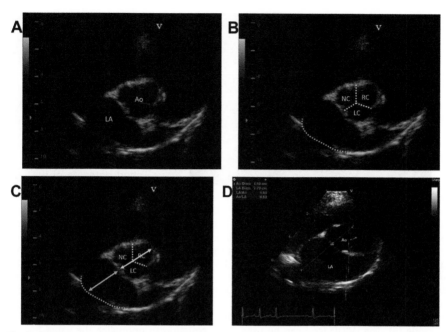

Fig. 2. There are a variety of methods to measure the left atrium (LA). The EPIC study evaluated the LA from a 2-dimensional image acquired from the right parasternal short-axis window at the level of the aortic valve, an image routinely acquired in basic echocardiographic exams. The LA is measured at maximum size (the end of systole or soon after the T wave ends on simultaneous ECG), which is the first frame in which aortic valve closure can be seen. Incorrectly measuring the LA in diastole (close to the next QRS) can lead to underestimation of LA size. The aorta (Ao) is measured from inside edge along the junction of the noncoronary (NC) and left coronary (LC) cusps according to the published Swedish method.[10] The LA dimension is measured from inside edge to inside edge on the same line as the Ao, as if the line used to measure the aorta is extended through the LA. It is important when measuring the LA to be careful not to overestimate its size by measuring beyond the wall of the LA (*dashed green line*) into a pulmonary vein. The LA:Ao is derived from dividing the Ao dimension into the LA dimension. An LA:Ao of 1.6 or greater was used to select dogs for the EPIC trial. The normal reference range for LA:Ao when measured by the Swedish method is 0.9 to 1.3. (*A–C*) demonstrate the landmarks that are required to measure the LA:Ao by the Swedish method in a dog with normal left atrial size (LA:Ao = 1.2). Panel D demonstrates measurements in a dog with DVD and left atrial enlargement (LA:Ao = 1.6).

greater will improve the specificity (positive predictive value) of significant heart enlargement and guard against overtreatment of possible stage B1 dogs. However, based on the reported interobserver and intraobserver variability of VHS measurement, repeated measures of VHS to assess rate of disease progression should ideally be performed by the same observer.[21] The authors and the Cardiac Education Group (CEG) recommend that in dogs with a VHS between 10.6 and 11.4, an echocardiogram is needed to confirm eligibility for pimobendan treatment. The CEG is a group of board-certified veterinary cardiologists from both academia and private practice that offer independent recommendations for the evaluation and treatment of canine and feline heart disease (**Box 2; Table 2**).

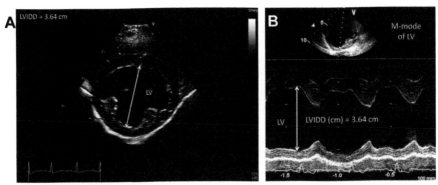

Fig. 3. There are a variety of methods to measure the left ventricle (LV) and thus many ways to assess for LV enlargement. The EPIC study evaluated the LV from an M-mode image acquired from the right parasternal short-axis window at the level of the tips of the mitral valve. This is a common image routinely acquired in basic echocardiographic exams. A standard measurement from this image includes the internal dimension of the LV in diastole (LVIDD), which is the maximum size of the LV chamber. Alternatively, the LVIDD can be measured from a 2D image taken from the same image that would be used for an M-mode. For this method of measurement of LVIDD, a loop is saved and the largest chamber size is selected for measurement by scrolling slowly through the loop. The 2D method (A) may be easier and more accurate when the image is difficult to align properly for M-mode (B). The LVIDD (cm) can be used in an equation to normalize the value for the dog's weight (kg). This is the normalized LVIDD index (LVIDDN).[11] It is important that the LVIDD measurement is in centimeters (not millimeters as it is sometimes reported) and the weight is in kilograms when calculating the LVIDDN. In this example, the LVIDD is 3.64 cm in a dog that weighs 8 kg. The calculated LVIDDN is 1.98. The formula to calculate the LVIDDN = [LVIDD (cm)]/[weight (kg)$^{0.294}$]. The reference range for LVIDDN is 1.27 to 1.85. An LVIDD of 1.7 or greater was used to select dogs for the EPIC study. The reason for selection of an LVIDDN that was not above the upper normal reference range is related to a previous study that demonstrated dogs with DVD and an LVIDDN of 1.7 or greater had a worse clinical outcome than dogs with and LVIDDN less than 1.7 despite that fact that it was within the reported normal range.

Although VHS is an objective radiographic assessment of global heart size, a measurement called vertebral left atrial size (VLAS) has been more recently described and is intended to assess specifically for left atrial enlargement (**Fig. 1**C).[22] A normal canine reference interval of 1.4 to 2.2 vertebral bodies has been proposed for VLAS,[23] though breed-specific reference intervals are beginning to be explored for this measurement, as they were for VHS, with breed-related differences likely to be clinically relevant.[16,24] Multiple studies have investigated the correlations between VLAS and echocardiographic evidence of left atrial enlargement, with optimal specificity cutoffs for predicting stage B2 status ranging between 2.8 and 3.1.[17–19,22,25] At this time, the ACVIM consensus statement considers a VLAS of 3 or greater as likely predictive of stage B2 status.[7]

Future Directions for Staging DVD

Newer studies have begun to explore the utility of prediction models that can incorporate demographic information alongside diagnostic test variables to help veterinarians predict the likelihood of stage B2 DVD in the absence of an echocardiogram. These models have the potential to optimize recommendations

> **Box 2**
> **Recommendations for Pimobendan initiation in Stage B2 DVD when an Echocardiogram is NOT available:**
>
> - Asymptomatic small-breed dog, and
> - Heart murmur characteristic of MR ($\geq$3/6), and
> - VHS $\geq$ 11.5 , or
> - Progressive increase in VHS of $\geq$ 0.5 VHS units over 6 months, or
> - VLAS >3.0

for confirmatory echocardiography by identifying only those dogs at high risk of stage B2 DVD. Additionally, in those dogs in which echocardiography is entirely out of reach, increased confidence in a decision to start pimobendan therapy may be obtained using this approach. Initial work has shown that these types of models are superior to any single diagnostic used in isolation. Incorporation of physical examination variables, electrocardiogram (ECG) variables, and radiographic measurements produced excellent discriminatory ability in one prediction model that assessed large-breed dogs with clinically important DVD[16] whereas physical examination, history, and blood test variables, including the cardiac biomarker N-terminal pro B-type natriuretic peptide (NT-proBNP), showed very good ability to predict stage B2 status in another model derived from DVD dogs weighing between 2 and 25 kg.[26] A similar study in CKCS has also been carried out, with breed-specific prediction models outperforming non–breed-specific models and showing excellent discriminatory ability for predicting stage B2 status when physical examination, radiographic measurements, ECG variables, and cardiac biomarkers are used together.[27] Importantly, all of these models take advantage of combining multiple pieces of information to improve the accuracy of predicting stage B2 status. This multipronged approach can help to safeguard against the odds that a single spurious result will lead to misclassification of any individual dog, potentially resulting in unnecessary referral or inappropriate initiation of medication. Although these prediction models hold a great degree of promise, full use of the models will require a web-based or smartphone application interface in which an individual dog's demographic information and available diagnostic test results can be input to predict the likelihood of stage B2 status for that specific dog. This work is currently underway by several groups including that of the authors.

GENERAL MANAGEMENT MEASURES FOR STAGE B1 AND B2
Additional recommended diagnostic tests

Once a diagnosis of stage B1 or B2 is reached, it is prudent to complete the diagnostic workup including measurement of indirect systemic blood pressure (BP)[7,28] and routine blood work $\pm$ urinalysis.

Client communication

Client communication should emphasize the typical slow progression of DVD (often many years) while highlighting that some dogs may progress more quickly making it important that they return for scheduled recheck examinations and learn how to recognize signs of possible disease progression. Possible signs of DVD progression

Table 2
Treatment Recommendations for Dogs with Asymptomatic Degenerative Valve Disease

	Tx	Diagnostic Criteria for Treatment[c]	Medication(s)	Other recommendations
• *Asymptomatic* older small breed dog • Systolic heart murmur characteristic of DVD • Normal systemic blood pressure	No	• VHS < 10.5 • VHS: between 10.5-11.4 and no Echo available • Echo LA:Ao < 1.6 (even if LVIDN ≥ 1.7 and VHS > 10.5) • Echo LVDDN < 1.7 (even if LA:Ao ≥ 1.6 and VHS >10.5)	None at this time	VHS < 10.5 and murmur ≤ grade 3/6: recheck q 12 months All others: recheck q 6-8 months, HRR q 1 week

	Yes[a,b]	[d]Echo LA:Ao (2D) ≥ 1.6 & LVIDDN ≥ 1.7 +/- VHS ≥10.5
		• No Echo available
		  o Systolic MR murmur ≥ 3/6 and
		    ■ VHS ≥ 11.5 or VLAS ≥ 3.0
		    ■ Progressive ↑ in radiographic heart size
		      • ↑ VHS by ≥ 0.5 in 6 months (even if VHS < 11.5)
			[d]Initiate Pimobendan
			What about RAASi
			• Acceptable to continue RAASi if dog already receiving
			• Initiate ACEI if there is clear evidence of progressive ↑ in heart size (↑ VHS by ≥ 0.5 in 6 months) despite pimobendan treatment
			• Consider addition of RAASi if pimobendan treatment is declined
				All: recheck q 6-12 months, HRR q 1 week
				VHS > 12.5: recheck q 4-6 months, HRR q 1 week

This summary table reflects the opinions of the authors and is based on the results of the EPIC study[8], CEG recommendations[20] and the 2019 ACVIM Consensus statement[7].

Tx=treatment recommended, VHS=radiographic vertebral heart size, VLAS=vertebral left atrial size (Fig1): Echo=echocardiogram with emphasis on 2D left atrial size and left ventricular internal dimension in diastole: LA:Ao=Left atrial to aortic ratio as measured from a 2 dimensional short axis image (Fig 2); LVIDDN =normalized left ventricular internal diameter in diastole (Fig 3): RAASi-=renin angiotensin aldosterone system inhibition with an angiotensin converting enzyme inhibitor alone or in combination with an aldosterone blocker (e.g. spironolactone): mn=months, HRR=owner counted home resting respiration rate

[a] = Evaluation of a biochemistry panel prior to the initiation of any chronic oral cardiac medication is recommended, and in the case of an ACEI one should be rechecked 10-14 days after initiation and/or following any increase in dosage

[b] =Baseline thoracic radiographs should be recommended in dogs with a risk of developing congestive heart failure, particularly those at highest risk e.g. those with severe heart enlargement

[c] =an echocardiogram is the gold standard for confirmation and staging of dogs with degenerative valve disease

[d] =highest priority recommendation

include reduction in exercise capacity, collapse, fainting, reduction in appetite, unintended weight loss, increase in rate or effort of breathing, and new or worsening cough. Owners should be strongly encouraged to record their dog's home (resting or sleeping) breathing rate on a weekly basis, especially in stage B2 dogs. Several smartphone applications are available to facilitate this goal.

Recheck examinations

Typical scheduled recheck intervals for stage B1 dogs are every 12 months whereas stage B2 dogs should be seen every 6 to 8 months. Urgent or emergent reevaluation may be required if dogs develop clinical signs suggestive of disease progression. Rechecks should emphasize a thorough history with an emphasis on recorded home respiratory rates, physical examination, thoracic radiographs, and systemic BP measurement. Routine blood work is typically recommended annually in these patients, barring any obvious indications to perform it more frequently **Table 2 Box 3**

Diet and supplements

Owners should be encouraged to feed diets that fulfill the World Small Animal Veterinary Medical Association Global Nutrition Guidelines.[29] In general, the diets should be palatable with high-quality protein and fed with a goal of maintaining an optimum body and muscle condition score. Moderate sodium restriction is appropriate if well tolerated by the patient, particularly in stage B2. Severe sodium restriction should be avoided. Omega-3 fatty acid supplementation can be considered in stages B1 and B2.[30,31]

Exercise

Normal life stage appropriate exercise should be encouraged.

TREATMENT
Stage B1

No medical treatment is recommended in stage B1.[7]

Stage B2

Before publication of the EPIC study[8] and the 2019 consensus statement,[7] there were no strong evidence-based recommendations for treatment of stage B2 DVD, although treatment with an angiotensin-converting enzyme (ACE) inhibitor had been investigated and historically advocated for by some cardiologists to treat select stage B2 dogs.[6] Additionally, the potential benefit of pimobendan (Vetmedin; Boehringer Ingelheim, Ingelheim am Rhein, Germany) therapy in delaying or preventing the onset of clinical signs in dogs with stage B2 DVD had not been evaluated and information regarding its hemodynamic effects in dogs with stage B1 and B2 DVD was sparse.

Box 3
Pimobendan Recommended Dose for Stage B2 DVD:

- Same as registered dose for treatment of CHF secondary to DVD

- 0.4 to 0.6 mg/kg/day divided into 2 doses
  - Note: Doses do not need to be equal in am and pm

- Pimobendan does not need to be given on an empty stomach

Two small studies[32,33] evaluated the hemodynamic effects of pimobendan in dogs with stage B DVD. One did not find any evidence of benefit in dogs with stage B2 DVD over 6 months of follow-up,[33] and the other[32] reported adverse cardiac functional and morphologic effects in dogs with stage B1 DVD when compared with an ACE inhibitor.

The EPIC study was a prospective double-blind, randomized, multicenter/global, placebo-controlled clinical trial designed to evaluate the effectiveness of pimobendan to delay the onset of left-sided CHF (pulmonary edema) or cardiac-related death (if it occurred before CHF) in dogs with heart enlargement secondary to asymptomatic DVD (stage B2).[8] Experts in cardiology enrolled 360 dogs that were randomized to receive pimobendan or placebo (180 per treatment group) **Box 3**. The primary end point was a composite of the time to onset of left-sided CHF (pulmonary edema) or cardiac-related death (sudden or euthanasia) in the event that it happened before left-sided CHF. Additional secondary end point and safety analysis, including all-cause mortality, were also evaluated. The final analysis of the primary end point demonstrated a significant ($P = 0.0038$) and clinically relevant extension of symptom-free survival, with most of the benefits attributable to delaying the onset of left-sided CHF, and the magnitude and significance of the benefits attributable to pimobendan remained in subsequent analyses that evaluated the effect of baseline variables, including heart size, on the study outcome. On average, dogs receiving pimobendan met the primary end point in 1228 days (40.9 months) versus 766 days (25.5 months) in the placebo group, which translates into an average of 462 additional days (15.4 months). This represents a 60% extension in symptom-free survival. The results also can be expressed as the risk (hazard ratio) that a dog in the study would experience the primary end point. All dogs receiving pimobendan in the study experienced a 36% reduction in risk in comparison with the placebo group. It is important to note that all dogs in the study had a risk of experiencing the primary end point, although we know that the absolute risk is different for individual dogs. Whatever an individual dog's risk was, however, it was reduced by 36%. This is a good way in which to express the results of the study to an owner when discussing the recommendation to initiate lifelong pimobendan, as expressing benefit by citing median or average number of months of extension of symptom-free survival does not predict the fate of an individual dog, but understanding that your dog has a risk and that initiating pimobendan can reduce that risk by one-third are tangible. The results of the safety analyses supported the safety of pimobendan treatment in the study population, as number, type, and severity of adverse events were not different ($P = 0.82$) between the placebo and pimobendan group. The overall survival was also prolonged ($P = 0.012$).

In dogs with DVD, clinical signs related to pulmonary edema may not represent the first clinical signs a dog experiences that are attributable to DVD. Some dogs may develop clinical signs associated with poor perfusion, pulmonary hypertension (PH), ascites, or cough related to left mainstem bronchial compression (LMSBC) before the onset of left-sided CHF. The EPIC study included a prespecified secondary end point that attempted to address this aspect of preclinical DVD. This analysis showed that in asymptomatic dogs with cardiomegaly secondary to DVD, treatment with pimobendan extended the time to the "first event." The "first event" end point was a composite of many outcomes that a dog in the study could experience and resulted in treatment with a variety of precluded cardiovascular medications. In comparison with the primary end point analysis, this secondary end point was more inclusive and thus relevant to dogs and dog owners, as the need to start any medication for a cardiac indication, even if the indication is not pulmonary edema, represents morbidity for the dog and requires a visit to the veterinarian. The time to "first event" analysis was highly significant ($P < 0.0001$), demonstrating a clear statistical and clinically relevant difference between the two groups, with a median of 640 days (21.3 months) in the pimobendan group versus 406 days (13.5 months) in the placebo group. This translates into an average of 234 days (7.8 months) of symptom-free survival. These results can also be expressed as the risk (hazard ratio) that a dog in the study would experience a "first event." The 95% confidence interval for risk reduction in the time to "first event" analysis was 33.5% to 42.5% in favor of pimobendan. This suggests that the administration of pimobendan in dogs with stage B2 DVD may not only delay the onset of pulmonary edema, but it may also delay the onset of a myriad of other signs or symptoms attributable to DVD if they occur before pulmonary edema. The results of the EPIC study ushered in evidence-based recommendations for treatment of stage B2 DVD that are now incorporated into the updated 2019 DVD consensus statement.[7] It is important to note, however, that the EPIC study did not evaluate pimobendan treatment in dogs with stage B1 DVD, and thus, no conclusions regarding the safety or efficacy of treatment in this group can be drawn from the EPIC study.

Historical use of ACE inhibitors in stage B2 was based predominantly on the results of the VETPROOF (Veterinary Enalapril Trial to Prove Reduction in Onset of Heart Failure) study in combination with their well-known safety profile.[34–36] More recently, the DELAY (Delay of Appearance of Symptoms of Canine DVD Treated with Spironolactone and Benazepril) study[37] investigated the potential value of more comprehensive blockade of the renin–angiotensin–aldosterone system (RAAS) using a combination of an ACE inhibitor (benazepril) and an aldosterone blocker (spironolactone) in dogs with preclinical DVD characterized by heart enlargement. The dogs included in the DELAY study met the current criteria for diagnosis of stage B2 DVD.[7] This study was a large ($N = 184$), prospective, randomized (1:1), multicenter, single-blinded, placebo-controlled study. The DELAY study investigated whether comprehensive blockade of the RAAS (benazepril: 0.25–0.5 mg/kg q 24 h and spironolactone: 2–4 mg/kg q 24 h) could delay the onset of CHF or cardiac death (if cardiac death occurred before CHF). Enrolled dogs were not allowed to receive other cardiovascular medications including pimobendan. The primary end point was time to onset of CHF or cardiac death. Secondary end points included effects on disease progression including change in heart size and cardiac biomarker concentrations (NT-proBNP and cardiac troponin). The median time to CHF or cardiac death was not different between the treatment and placebo groups (902 days vs 1139 days, respectively). There were, however, beneficial effects on cardiac remodeling reported. This included decreases in some radiographic and echocardiographic measurements of heart size as well as lower NT-proBNP levels in the treatment group, which the authors interpreted to be of possible clinical relevance. These results do not resolve the controversy related to the role of RAAS inhibition in preclinical DVD.

The role of concurrent use of RAAS blockade in combination with pimobendan at later stages of B2 DVD is also controversial. **Box 4** The CEG and 2019 Consensus guidelines addressed this question before the publication of the DELAY Study. At that time, their recommendation was to continue ACE inhibitors in dogs already receiving them when the indication for pimobendan was met, but that initiation of an ACE inhibitor in stage B2 DVD should otherwise be reserved for stage C DVD. In addition, ACE inhibition can also be considered if reevaluation demonstrates an increase in VHS greater than 0.5 vertebral bodies in 6 months in dogs with stage B2 DVD already receiving pimobendan. Other medications can also be considered as appropriate when clinical signs of disease progression develop.

> **Box 4**
> **Current recommendation concerning the use of RAAS inhibbitors in Stage B2 DVD**
>
> - ACE inhibitors ± spironolactone can be continued in dogs already receiving them when they meet criteria to initiate pimobendan.
> - Initiation of RAAS inhibbition in Stage B2 dogs already receiving pimobendan is controversial and not evidence based but can be considered if reevaluation demonstrates progressive increase in heart size (e.g. VHS of $\geq$ 0.5 in 6 months).

Future therapies

Ideally, future therapies will be developed that focus on prevention or early termination of progressive valve degeneration in stage B1 dogs, rather than focusing exclusively on treatment options for dogs that have already progressed to more advanced stages of the disease. Frustratingly, despite the common nature of DVD in both humans and dogs, the pathophysiologic triggers that underlie the development of this disease remain largely unknown. One important structural transformation that has been associated with the development of DVD pathology involves the transformation of valvular interstitial cells, one of the two predominant cell types present in the mitral valve, from a typical quiescent cell to an activated myofibroblast phenotype.[38] Triggers for this transformation have been associated with both the serotonin and transforming growth factor ß1 pathways.[39] Research into these lines of investigation suggest that clinical trials studying serotonin antagonists or serotonin receptor antagonists may be one next step forward in DVD research in dogs.[40] Study in this area is ongoing. Another area of investigation, which holds promise for application in the near future, is related to the field of metabolomics. Metabolomics is defined by Wikipedia as "the scientific study of chemical processes involving metabolites, the small molecule substrates, intermediates and products of cell metabolism."[41] The outcome of this field of study has resulted in the identification of several abnormalities in dogs with DVD, and resultant dietary strategies to address these abnormalities are under investigation.[42] Recent publication of a small prospective randomized controlled dietary intervention study reported a reduction in left atrial size in dogs with early preclinical DVD.[43] The authors are optimistic that widespread application of these results to clinical practice is on the near horizon. Lastly, as open-heart surgery programs with high success rates[7,44–46] become more widely available, mitral valve repair will become an option for more stage B2 dogs. Repair interventions will also be expanded in stage B2, if and when minimally invasive options become available.

SPECIAL CONSIDERATIONS IN STAGE B DVD

Most clinical trials performed in dogs with asymptomatic DVD are designed to prove whether a given therapy can delay the onset of pulmonary edema (left-sided CHF),[8,34,35] but symptoms of pulmonary edema may not represent the first clinical signs a dog experiences that are attributable to DVD. In addition, the ACVIM staging scheme focuses on the development of clinical signs attributable to CHF secondary to DVD (stage C), in particular those attributable to pulmonary edema, but also includes those attributable to right heart failure, such as ascites. However, some dogs with stage B2 DVD develop clinical signs associated with poor perfusion, PH, or cough related to LMSBC (**Fig. 4**) before the onset of CHF and therefore remain classified as stage B2. The authors classify these dogs as stage B+: the "+" indicates the presence of clinical signs attributable to DVD that are not related to active CHF. In the updated consensus statement, cough attributed to LMSBC is designated as advanced stage B2.[7] Another way to include these dogs in the current staging scheme could be to broaden the definition of stage C to include dogs with any previous or current clinical signs attributable to DVD, rather than those attributed solely to CHF. Regardless of how these dogs are staged, they represent a subset of the DVD population with signs related to their heart disease but unrelated to CHF that can impair the quality of their life, and, by extension, their owners' quality of life. Thus, despite a lack of evidence-based recommendations, this group of dogs often requires therapy. Many therapeutic recommendations for stage B+ are therefore based on experience and professional opinion and often stem from treatment of these conditions when they occur as comorbidities in dogs with stage C and D DVD. The EPIC study[8] included a prespecified secondary end point that attempted to address this aspect of preclinical DVD. This analysis showed that the administration of pimobendan in asymptomatic dogs with cardiomegaly secondary to DVD may not only delay the onset of pulmonary edema, it may also significantly delay the onset of a myriad of other signs or symptoms attributable to DVD if they occur before pulmonary edema.

Pulmonary Hypertension in Stage B DVD

PH is a consequence of a variety of etiologies that are not mutually exclusive, one of which is DVD. This is more thoroughly discussed in the 2020 ACVIM consensus guidelines on canine PH.[47] Dogs with DVD develop evidence of concurrent PH as a complication of left-sided heart disease.[48–50] Development of PH has prognostic significance, as dogs with DVD and an echocardiographically estimated systolic pulmonary artery pressure of greater than 55 mm Hg (moderate PH) have a poorer long-term outcome.[50] Clinical signs associated with PH can mimic those characteristic of pulmonary edema, poor perfusion, and LMSBC and include exercise intolerance,

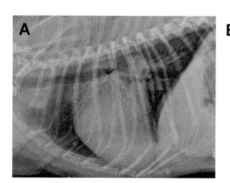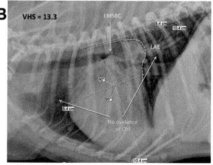

Fig. 4. A right lateral radiograph from a dog with DVD that presented for evaluation of a chronic, harsh cough. The dog had never been in congestive heart failure and was thus classified as stage B2. The VHS is 13.3. The left atrium is severely enlarged and appears to compress the airway directly dorsal to it consistent with left mainstem bronchial compression (LMSBC). There is no evidence of pulmonary edema. In some cases, direct visualization of LMSBC may not be possible, but it can be considered a possible rule-out or contributing cause for any dog with a cough and significant cardiomegaly, especially with moderate to severe left atrial enlargement. An echocardiogram should be recommended in this dog to confirm the diagnosis and directly assess left atrial and left ventricular size. If an echocardiogram is not available, initial treatment recommendations for this dog should include pimobendan (based on VHS $\geq$ 11.5). Other palliative treatments can be added as needed as outlined in the text.

syncope, cough, increased respiratory effort at rest or with exercise or dyspnea. In addition, dogs with PH can develop signs of right-sided CHF (ascites) or remain entirely asymptomatic.[48] The therapeutic approach to treating PH in dogs with DVD requires an understanding of the underlying disease pathophysiology. In these dogs, PH is typically a result of chronic elevation in left atrial pressure and pulmonary venous hypertension. In some dogs, secondary reactive pulmonary arterial vasoconstriction and remodeling also can develop as a result of chronic hypoxic change.[48] In both scenarios, PH secondary to DVD is almost always associated with left atrial enlargement, making its presence solely related to DVD very unlikely in stage B1 dogs and more likely as the disease progresses from stage B2 to stages C and D.[50,51] PH due solely to DVD is, however, typically mild to moderate and unlikely to be severe.[50] Other etiologies of PH should be considered, including heartworm disease, chronic pulmonary disease, or chronic pulmonary thromboembolic disease. If present, these comorbidities can contribute to the development of vascular remodeling and PH in dogs with DVD. Although PH associated with chronic elevations in left atrial pressure and pulmonary venous hypertension can improve with appropriate therapy, dogs with chronic pulmonary arterial remodeling likely have a more irreversible form of the disease.

Definitive diagnosis of PH in veterinary patients is typically dependent on Doppler echocardiography, which is specific, but not 100% sensitive.[49] That is, a definitive diagnosis is not always possible and often a presumptive diagnosis is made based on the presence of indirect evidence of PH that are identified during a complete echocardiogram. In some symptomatic cases, the diagnosis is based on the exclusion of other etiologies to explain the clinical signs and/or the response to therapy for PH, for example, in a dog with stage B2 DVD with active respiratory distress and no evidence of radiographic pulmonary infiltrates to support the presence of pulmonary edema (left-sided CHF) or with radiographic pulmonary infiltrates that do not resolve with diuretic therapy.[52]

Once PH is considered probable based on echocardiographic characteristics in a dog with DVD, optimization of treatment for their underlying left-sided heart disease should be the first course of action. Thoracic radiographs are recommended to screen for any evidence of active pulmonary edema and home monitoring of the resting respiratory rate should be emphasized (if not already on going) to gauge the likelihood of early CHF that was not radiographically obvious. If evidence of CHF is appreciated, standard therapy for stage C DVD should be instituted.[7] In asymptomatic stage B1 or B2 dogs, identification of mild PH (estimated systolic pulmonary artery pressure >30 to <50 mm Hg) would be monitored as recommended for all stage B dogs. In stage B2 dogs with mild PH that have already met the EPIC criteria to receive pimobendan[8] (see **Figs. 1–3**), the addition of an ACE inhibitor also can be considered if the dog is not already receiving one, particularly if and when clinical signs associated with PH are suspected. For stage B2 dogs that are receiving both an ACE inhibitor and pimobendan, documentation of moderate (>50 to <75 mm Hg) to severe (>75 mm Hg) PH in association with clinical signs, such as an increase in respiratory rate or effort (not attributable to pulmonary edema), exercise intolerance, or syncope, warrants treatment with a phosphodiesterase-5 (PDE-5) inhibitor, such as sildenafil, with or without the addition of L-arginine.[47,49] Documentation of moderate PH in a reportedly asymptomatic dog with stage B DVD is less clear-cut with regard to treatment recommendations. Dogs in this category that are stage B2 and meet the EPIC criteria for pimobendan should receive this drug. The addition of other medications, such as an ACE inhibitor and a PDE-5 inhibitor, with or without L-arginine, also can be considered, especially if the severity of PH worsens or clinical signs attributable to PH develop over time. Careful monitoring for disease progression and the development of clinical signs is warranted and emphasizes the need for follow-up evaluations in this population. Identification of severe PH in reportedly asymptomatic dogs with stage B DVD warrants evaluation for other potential causes of PH and likely therapy with a PDE-5 inhibitor, with or without L-arginine, regardless of a lack of reported clinical signs.

In all dogs with PH secondary solely to stage B DVD, severe PH is unlikely, particularly in stage B1. Additionally, noncardiac comorbidities causing PH of varying degrees can develop during any stage of DVD. This emphasizes the need to investigate for other possible concurrent etiologies of PH in many cases. Recommended diagnostics in these dogs include heartworm antigen test (if appropriate), complete blood count, biochemistry profile, and urinalysis to screen for other etiologies of PH, such as heartworm disease or prothrombotic conditions, including hyperadrenocorticism, protein-losing diseases, and neoplasia that could predispose to chronic pulmonary thromboembolic disease. Referral for advanced respiratory diagnostics, such as fluoroscopy, bronchoscopy, or airway cytology and culture via bronchoalveolar lavage, also may be indicated if uncontrolled chronic respiratory disease is suspected. If identified, definitive treatment for these conditions should be instituted as appropriate. See **Table 3** for a summary of these recommendations.

Left Mainstem Bronchial Compression in Stage B2 DVD

Cough attributable solely to LMSBC is not associated with concurrent tachypnea or dyspnea, is often chronic and exacerbated by excitement, and therefore mimics many primary airway diseases. This condition alone is rarely life threatening but coughing that is severe enough to impair a dog's or owner's quality of life represents a common complaint in older small-breed dogs with stage B2, C, and D DVD and frequently requires treatment. Cough in these dogs is often evidence of underlying respiratory disease, multifactorial, and generally not attributable to active pulmonary edema.[53] Some common etiologies for a severe cough in these dogs include collapsing trachea, bronchitis, and LMSBC. The first clinical step in these cases always includes the elimination of active pulmonary edema as a contributing cause to the cough and respiratory signs. In stage B dogs, this would represent first-onset CHF versus recurrence in stage C and D. Thoracic radiography will allow active pulmonary edema to be ruled out and assessment of VHS and VLAS (see **Fig. 4**). In some cases, there will be obvious evidence of bronchial collapse or compression dorsal to the enlarged left atrium; however, even if this is not clearly visualized, LMSBC should be considered a rule-out for cough in any small-breed dog with moderate to severe left atrial enlargement.[53] Fluoroscopy can be used to confirm the presence and severity of LMSBC and can be useful if cough can be induced with tracheal palpation but is not absolutely necessary. Treatment can be initiated based on a presumptive diagnosis when other etiologies are ruled out.

The interaction between cardiomegaly, in particular left atrial enlargement, and collapse of the left mainstem bronchus is not well defined. There is no single accepted hypothesis for cough in these dogs.[54] Breeds that are predisposed to DVD are also predisposed to the development of structural airway collapse and airway inflammation.[54] Regardless, the probable role of an underlying primary large airway disease in combination with left atrial enlargement and the relatively high chronic left atrial pressure in dogs with stage B2 DVD often leads to permanent or intermittent clinically relevant cough. LMSBC should not be considered a differential diagnosis in dogs with stage B1 DVD, as by definition these dogs do not have heart enlargement and

Table 3
Recommendations for chronic treatment of pulmonary hypertension in dogs with stage B DVD

Clinical signs/symptoms of PH	DVD Stage	Mild PH, 30–50 mm Hg	Moderate PH, 50–75 mm Hg	Severe PH, >75 mm Hg
Yes • Rule out active pulmonary edema with thoracic radiographs in dogs with DVD and active respiratory signs[a] • Monitor for PH and DVD progression[a]	B1	• Unlikely to cause clinical signs but severity of PH can be underestimated by echo. • Investigate other causes of PH for the clinical signs[a]	• Investigate other etiologies for PH.[a] • Treat underlying etiology of PH if possible.[a] • Intiate treatment with PDE-5 inhibitor ± L-arginine.[a] • Intiate treatment for right heart failure if ascites is documented.	
	B2	• As per stage B1 above. • If underestimation of severity of PH is possible, consider trail therapy with a PDE-5 inhibitor ± L-arginine and evaluate clinical response to treatment	• As per stage B1 above.[a] • Consider initiating an ACE inhibitor.	
	B2[a]	• Initiate pimobendan[a]	• Investigate other etiologies for PH.[a] • Treat underlying etiology of PH if possible.[a] • Initiate pimobendan[a] • Consider initiation of treatment with a PDE-5 inhibitor ± L-arginine, particularly if pimobendan alone fails to palliate clinical signs or if clinical signs are severe enough at the time of diagnoses of PH that they limit the ability to wait and determine if monotherapy with pimobenden is efficacious.[a] • Consider initiating an ACE inhibitor. • Add other medications as needed to treat right heart failure if ascites is present. • Monitor clinical response to treatment.[a]	

	No		
B1	• Monitor for PH and DVD progression[a]	• Investigate other etiologies for PH. • Treat underlying etiology of PH if possible.	• Investigate other etiologies for PH. • Treat underlying etiology of PH if possible. • Consider the initiation of a PDE-5 inhibitor ± L-arginine.[a]
B2[E]	• No specific recommendations.	• Investigate other etiologies for PH. • Treat underlying etiology of PH if possible. • Consider initiating an ACE inhibitor. • Monitor for PH and DVD progression[a]	• Investigate other etiologies for PH. • Treat underlying etiology of PH if possible. • Consider the initiation of a PDE-5 inhibitor ± L-arginine.[a]
B1[eterase]	• Initiate pimodendan.[a]	• Investigate other etiologies for PH. • Treat underlying etiology of PH if possible. • Consider initiating an ACE inhibitor. • Initiate treatment with pimodendan.[a] • Monitor for PH and DVD progression[a]	• Investigate other etiologies for PH. • Treat underlying etiology of PH if possible. • Initiate treatment with pimodendan.[a] • Consider the initiation of a PDE-5 inhibitor ± L-arginine.[a]

Abbreviations: ACE, angiotensin-converting enzyme; B2[E], stage B2 DVD that meets EPIC criteria for initiation of pimobendan; DVD, degenerative value disease; echo, Doppler echocardiography; PDE, phosphodiese; PH, pulmonary hypertension.

[a] Highest priority recommendation.

therefore other etiologies for cough should be investigated. The complex etiology for cough due to LMSBC is best approached conceptually as an airway disease that is exacerbated by an enlarged heart. Successful management, therefore, includes strategies that address both the heart disease and respiratory component and response to treatment through scheduled follow-up. Scheduled follow-up also should include surveillance for the development of CHF owner-recorded home breathing rates. Cough secondary to LMSBC is often not curable; thus, the goal for minimizing the cough to a clinically tolerable level should be clearly communicated to the owner. Nonspecific palliative treatment of dogs with stage B2 DVD and cough due to LMSBC includes cough suppressants, weight loss (if appropriate), and modification of any potential environmental contributing causes (smoking). Specific airway therapies include intermittent antibiotics (doxycycline), bronchodilators, and corticosteroids. Corticosteroids should be used with caution in these dogs but can be used in short courses at anti-inflammatory doses. Inhaled corticosteroids can be better tolerated if required chronically. Cardiac-specific therapies are aimed at reducing heart size and left atrial pressure and include pimobendan,[8] RAAS inhibition,[37] and in some cases low-dose furosemide. The optimum therapy must be tailored to an individual dog, and even therapies that are clinically successful can fail intermittently and need to be revisited. In general, the authors attempt to never initiate more than 2 to 3 therapies on a given day and then make changes based on clinical response. In some cases, changes to therapy may include changes in dose, and in other dogs, it may require discontinuation of one medication to initiate another one in the hope of a better clinical outcome. There is no recommended definitive therapy for this condition. Stenting for bronchial collapse is possible in select dogs without complicating concurrent bronchomalacia or chronic inflammatory airway disease and is considered palliative, not curative.[55] It has been associated with an increased risk of complications related to stent migration, infection, and clinical decompensation and is not routinely performed. Perhaps in the future, newer devices will make this possible. Reduction of heart size via valve repair or replacement could be considered if the patient was a good candidate for this procedure. Surgical repair of DVD can result in significant reductions in heart size and might be palliative for severe cough related to LMSBC, assuming the dog was considered a good candidate for repair.

CLINICS CARE POINTS

- Dogs diagnosed with Stage B2 DVD will benefit from receiving pimobendan.
- A Vertebral heart size >= 11.5 can be used to identify stage B2 dogs if a confirmation echocardiogram is not available.
- If an echocardiogram confirms a diagnosis of Stage B2, radiographs are not essential but are recommended. In this scenario a VHS > 10.5 is consistent Stage B2 DVD.
- Confirmation of normal blood pressure is recommended in all dogs with DVD.

DISCLOSURE

Drs S.G. Gordon and A.B. Saunders have received funding from Boehringer Ingelheim Animal Health GmbH within the last 5 years for some or all of the following activities: research, travel, speaking fees, consultancy fees, and preparation of educational materials. Drs S.G. Gordon and A.B. Saunders are authors of the EPIC Study, Dr S.G. Gordon is a member of the Cardiac Education Group.

REFERENCES

1. Buchanan JW. Chronic valvular disease (endocardiosis) in dogs. Adv Vet Sci Comp Med 1977;21:75–106.
2. Egenvall A, Bonnett BN, Hedhammar A, et al. Mortality in over 350,000 insured Swedish dogs from 1995-2000: II. Breed-specific age and survival patterns and relative risk for causes of death. Acta Vet Scand 2005;46(3):121–36.
3. Beardow AW, Buchanan JW. Chronic mitral valve disease in cavalier King Charles spaniels: 95 cases (1987-1991). J Am Vet Med Assoc 1993;203(7):1023–9.
4. Haggstrom J, Hansson K, Kvart C, et al. Chronic valvular disease in the cavalier King Charles spaniel in Sweden. Vet Rec 1992;131(24):549–53.
5. Borgarelli M, Zini E, D'Agnolo G, et al. Comparison of primary mitral valve disease in German Shepherd dogs and in small breeds. J Vet Cardiol 2004;6(2):27–34.
6. Atkins C, Bonagura J, Ettinger S, et al. Guidelines for the diagnosis and treatment of canine chronic valvular heart disease. J Vet Intern Med 2009;23(6):1142–50.
7. Keene BW, Atkins CE, Bonagura JD, et al. ACVIM consensus guidelines for the diagnosis and treatment of myxomatous mitral valve disease in dogs. J Vet Intern Med 2019;33(3):1127–40.
8. Boswood A, Haggstrom J, Gordon SG, et al. Effect of pimobendan in dogs with preclinical myxomatous mitral valve disease and cardiomegaly: the epic study-a randomized clinical trial. J Vet Intern Med 2016;30(6):1765–79.
9. Buchanan JW, Bucheler J. Vertebral scale system to measure canine heart size in radiographs. J Am Vet Med Assoc 1995;206(2):194–9.
10. Hansson K, Haggstrom J, Kvart C, et al. Left atrial to aortic root indices using two-dimensional and M-mode echocardiography in cavalier King Charles spaniels with and without left atrial enlargement. Vet Radiol Ultrasound 2002;43(6):568–75.
11. Cornell CC, Kittleson MD, Della Torre P, et al. Allometric scaling of M-mode cardiac measurements in normal adult dogs. J Vet Intern Med 2004;18(3):311–21.
12. Hansson K, Haggstrom J, Kvart C, et al. Interobserver variability of vertebral heart size measurements in dogs with normal and enlarged hearts. Vet Radiol Ultrasound 2005;46(2):122–30.
13. Jepsen-Grant K, Pollard RE, Johnson LR. Vertebral heart scores in eight dog breeds. Vet Radiol Ultrasound 2013;54(1):3–8.
14. Reynolds CA, Brown DC, Rush JE, et al. Prediction of first onset of congestive heart failure in dogs with degenerative mitral valve disease: the PREDICT cohort study. J Vet Cardiol 2012;14(1):193–202.
15. Lord P, Hansson K, Kvart C, et al. Rate of change of heart size before congestive heart failure in dogs with mitral regurgitation. J Small Anim Pract 2010;51(4):210–8.
16. Wesselowski S, Gordon SG, Meddaugh N, et al. Prediction of clinically important acquired cardiac disease without an echocardiogram in large breed dogs using a combination of clinical, radiographic and electrocardiographic variables. J Vet Cardiol 2021.
17. Duler L, Visser LC, Jackson KN, et al. Evaluation of radiographic predictors of left heart enlargement in dogs with known or suspected cardiovascular disease. Vet Radiol Ultrasound 2021;62(3):271–81.
18. Poad MH, Manzi TJ, Oyama MA, et al. Utility of radiographic measurements to predict echocardiographic left heart enlargement in dogs with preclinical myxomatous mitral valve disease. J Vet Intern Med 2020;34(5):1728–33.

19. Stepien RL, Rak MB, Blume LM. Use of radiographic measurements to diagnose stage B2 preclinical myxomatous mitral valve disease in dogs. J Am Vet Med Assoc 2020;256(10):1129–36.

20. The Cardiac Education Group (CEG). The EPIC trial: pimobendan in preclinical MVD. Cardiaceducationgroup.org. Avaialble at. http://cardiaceducationgroup.org/wp-content/uploads/2016/12/CEG_Recommendations_EPIC_121316.pdf. [Accessed 15 January 2017]. Accessed.

21. Malcolm EGS, Haggstrom J, Wesselowski S, et al. Reproducibility and repeatability of radiographic measurements of cardiac size in dogs [abstract]. J Vet Intern Med 2021;35:21.

22. Malcolm EL, Visser LC, Phillips KL, et al. Diagnostic value of vertebral left atrial size as determined from thoracic radiographs for assessment of left atrial size in dogs with myxomatous mitral valve disease. J Am Vet Med Assoc 2018; 253(8):1038–45.

23. Vezzosi T, Puccinelli C, Tognetti R, et al. Radiographic vertebral left atrial size: A reference interval study in healthy adult dogs. Vet Radiol Ultrasound 2020;61(5): 507–11.

24. Puccinelli C, Citi S, Vezzosi T, et al. A radiographic study of breed-specific vertebral heart score and vertebral left atrial size in Chihuahuas. Vet Radiol Ultrasound 2021;62(1):20–6.

25. Mikawa S, Nagakawa M, Ogi H, et al. Use of vertebral left atrial size for staging of dogs with myxomatous valve disease. J Vet Cardiol 2020;30:92–9.

26. Wilshaw J, Rosenthal SL, Wess G, et al. Accuracy of history, physical examination, cardiac biomarkers, and biochemical variables in identifying dogs with stage B2 degenerative mitral valve disease. J Vet Intern Med 2021;35(2):755–70.

27. Wesselowski SGS, Saunders A, Fries R, et al. Use of physical examination, electrocardiography, radiography and biomarkers to predict stage B2 myxomatous mitral valve disease in preclinical Cavalier King Charles Spaniels [abstract]. J Vet Intern Med 2021;35:17.

28. Acierno MJ, Brown S, Coleman AE, et al. ACVIM consensus statement: Guidelines for the identification, evaluation, and management of systemic hypertension in dogs and cats. J Vet Intern Med 2018;32(6):1803–22.

29. WSAVA global nutrition guidelines. Avaialble at. https://wsava.org/global-guidelines/global-nutrition-guidelines/. Accessed November 30, 2021.

30. Freeman LM. Part 1: Nutritional Management of Heart Disease. 2015. Avaialble at. http://cardiaceducationgroup.org/wp-content/uploads/2015/10/C_A_-NutritionalMgmt_Of_HD_LisaFreeman_FINAL.pdf. [Accessed 30 November 2021]. Accessed.

31. Freeman LM. Part 2: implementing an optimal nutrition plan for your cardiovascular patient 2015. Avaialble at. http://cardiaceducationgroup.org/wp-content/uploads/2015/10/C_A_ImplementingANutritionalProg_LisaFreeman_FINAL.pdf. [Accessed 30 November 2021]. Accessed.

32. Chetboul V, Lefebvre HP, Sampedrano CC, et al. Comparative adverse cardiac effects of pimobendan and benazepril monotherapy in dogs with mild degenerative mitral valve disease: a prospective, controlled, blinded, and randomized study. J Vet Intern Med 2007;21(4):742–53.

33. Ouellet M, Belanger MC, Difruscia R, et al. Effect of pimobendan on echocardiographic values in dogs with asymptomatic mitral valve disease. J Vet Intern Med 2009;23(2):258–63.

34. Atkins CE, Keene BW, Brown WA, et al. Results of the veterinary enalapril trial to prove reduction in onset of heart failure in dogs chronically treated with enalapril

alone for compensated, naturally occurring mitral valve insufficiency. J Am Vet Med Assoc 2007;231(7):1061–9.

35. Kvart C, Haggstrom J, Pedersen HD, et al. Efficacy of enalapril for prevention of congestive heart failure in dogs with myxomatous valve disease and asymptomatic mitral regurgitation. J Vet Intern Med 2002;16(1):80–8.

36. Atkins CE, Brown WA, Coats JR, et al. Effects of long-term administration of enalapril on clinical indicators of renal function in dogs with compensated mitral regurgitation. J Am Vet Med Assoc 2002;221(5):654–8.

37. Borgarelli M, Ferasin L, Lamb K, et al. DELay of Appearance of sYmptoms of Canine Degenerative Mitral Valve Disease Treated with Spironolactone and Benazepril: the DELAY Study. J Vet Cardiol 2020;27:34–53.

38. Black A, French AT, Dukes-McEwan J, et al. Ultrastructural morphologic evaluation of the phenotype of valvular interstitial cells in dogs with myxomatous degeneration of the mitral valve. Am J Vet Res 2005;66(8):1408–14.

39. Oyama MA, Levy RJ. Insights into serotonin signaling mechanisms associated with canine degenerative mitral valve disease. J Vet Intern Med 2010;24(1):27–36.

40. Oyama MA, Elliott C, Loughran KA, et al. Comparative pathology of human and canine myxomatous mitral valve degeneration: 5HT and TGF-beta mechanisms. Cardiovasc Pathol 2020;46:107196.

41. Metabolomics, From Wikipedia, the free encyclopedia. Avaialble at. https://en.wikipedia.org/wiki/Metabolomics. [Accessed 30 November 2021]. Accessed.

42. Li Q, Freeman LM, Rush JE, et al. Veterinary Medicine and Multi-Omics Research for Future Nutrition Targets: Metabolomics and Transcriptomics of the Common Degenerative Mitral Valve Disease in Dogs. OMICS 2015;19(8):461–70.

43. Li Q, Heaney A, Langenfeld-McCoy N, et al. Dietary intervention reduces left atrial enlargement in dogs with early preclinical myxomatous mitral valve disease: a blinded randomized controlled study in 36 dogs. BMC Vet Res 2019;15(1):425.

44. Uechi M. Mitral valve repair in dogs. J Vet Cardiol 2012;14(1):185–92.

45. Uechi M, Mizukoshi T, Mizuno T, et al. Mitral valve repair under cardiopulmonary bypass in small-breed dogs: 48 cases (2006-2009). J Am Vet Med Assoc 2012; 240(10):1194–201.

46. Mizuno T, Mizukoshi T, Uechi M. Long-term outcome in dogs undergoing mitral valve repair with suture annuloplasty and chordae tendinae replacement. J Small Anim Pract 2013;54(2):104–7.

47. Reinero C, Visser LC, Kellihan HB, et al. ACVIM consensus statement guidelines for the diagnosis, classification, treatment, and monitoring of pulmonary hypertension in dogs. J Vet Intern Med 2020;34(2):549–73.

48. Kellihan HB, Stepien RL. Pulmonary hypertension in canine degenerative mitral valve disease. J Vet Cardiol 2012;14(1):149–64.

49. Kellihan HB, Stepien RL. Pulmonary hypertension in dogs: diagnosis and therapy. Vet Clin North Am Small Anim Pract 2010;40(4):623–41.

50. Borgarelli M, Abbott J, Braz-Ruivo L, et al. Prevalence and prognostic importance of pulmonary hypertension in dogs with myxomatous mitral valve disease. J Vet Intern Med 2015;29(2):569–74.

51. Sudunagunta S, Green D, Christley R, et al. The prevalence of pulmonary hypertension in Cavalier King Charles spaniels compared with other breeds with myxomatous mitral valve disease. J Vet Cardiol 2019;23:21–31.

52. Kellihan HB, Waller KR, Pinkos A, et al. Acute resolution of pulmonary alveolar infiltrates in 10 dogs with pulmonary hypertension treated with sildenafil citrate: 2005-2014. J Vet Cardiol 2015;17(3):182–91.

53. Ferasin L, Crews L, Biller DS, et al. Risk factors for coughing in dogs with naturally acquired myxomatous mitral valve disease. J Vet Intern Med 2013;27(2):286–92.

54. Singh MK, Johnson LR, Kittleson MD, et al. Bronchomalacia in dogs with myxomatous mitral valve degeneration. J Vet Intern Med 2012;26(2):312–9.

55. Kramer G. Bronchial collapse and stenting. In: Weisse C, Berent A, editors. Veterinary image-guided interventions. Ames, IA: Blackwell; 2015. p. 83–90.

Moving?

Make sure your subscription moves with you!

To notify us of your new address, find your **Clinics Account Number** (located on your mailing label above your name), and contact customer service at:

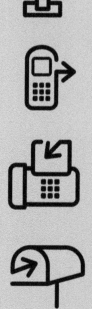

Email: journalscustomerservice-usa@elsevier.com

800-654-2452 (subscribers in the U.S. & Canada)
314-447-8871 (subscribers outside of the U.S. & Canada)

Fax number: 314-447-8029

Elsevier Health Sciences Division
Subscription Customer Service
3251 Riverport Lane
Maryland Heights, MO 63043

*To ensure uninterrupted delivery of your subscription, please notify us at least 4 weeks in advance of move.